Mechanisms of Adiponectin Action

Mechanisms of Adiponectin Action

Special Issue Editor

Tania Fiaschi

MDPI • Basel • Beijing • Wuhan • Barcelona • Belgrade

MDPI

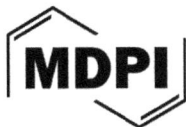

Special Issue Editor
Tania Fiaschi
Universita degli Studi di Firenze
Italy

Editorial Office
MDPI
St. Alban-Anlage 66
4052 Basel, Switzerland

This is a reprint of articles from the Special Issue published online in the open access journal *International Journal of Molecular Sciences* (ISSN 1422-0067) in 2019 (available at: https://www.mdpi.com/journal/ijms/special_issues/adiponectin_action)

For citation purposes, cite each article independently as indicated on the article page online and as indicated below:

LastName, A.A.; LastName, B.B.; LastName, C.C. Article Title. *Journal Name* **Year**, *Article Number, Page Range.*

ISBN 978-3-03921-245-3 (Pbk)
ISBN 978-3-03921-246-0 (PDF)

Contents

About the Special Issue Editor

Tania Fiaschi received her M.S. degree in Biological Sciences from the University of Florence, Italy. She then received her Ph.D. in Biochemistry and specialization in Biochemistry and Clinical Chemistry, also from the University of Florence. Since 2007, her research has focused on the regenerative effects of adiponectin in skeletal muscle. Her actual interest is in the study of adiponectin involvement in the amelioration of inherited myopathies such as Duchenne muscular dystrophy, Bethlem myopathy, and Ullrich congenital muscular dystrophy. She is currently serving as Associate Professor in Molecular Biology at the University of Florence.

International Journal of
Molecular Sciences

MDPI

Editorial

Mechanisms of Adiponectin Action

Tania Fiaschi

Dipartimento di Scienze Biomediche, Sperimentali e Cliniche "M. Serio", Università degli Studi di Firenze, Viale Morgagni 50, 50134 Firenze, Italy; tania.fiaschi@unifi.it; Tel.: +39-055-275-1233

Published: 13 June 2019

Adiponectin, the most abundant secreted adipokine, has received great attention from the scientific community since its discovery [1]. The huge number of studies is justified by the insulin-sensitizing role and the beneficial effects of adiponectin in diabetic conditions [2,3]. Over the years, a large body of evidence has supported a pleiotropic role of the hormone in different tissues in which it influences varied physiological aspects both in healthy and in diseased conditions.

This Special Issue, entitled "Mechanisms of Adiponectin Action", shows the pleiotropic role of adiponectin by presenting three research articles and seven reviews focused on recent findings about adiponectin in different target tissues. The Special Issue contains two reviews about adiponectin in skeletal muscle, a classical adiponectin target tissue, in which the hormone affects both metabolic [4] and regenerative properties [5]. Krause et al. report a close relationship between physical exercise and expression and circulating levels of adiponectin in both healthy and diseased population. Indeed, a higher adiponectin level is associated with greater physical activity, while some conditions, such as inactive obese, pre-diabetic, and diabetic patients, are characterized by decreased adiponectin levels. The restoration of proper adiponectin levels can be achieved with physical exercise, and this leads to increased insulin sensitivity [6]. Gamberi et al. discusses the current knowledge about adiponectin in myopathies (both non-inherited/acquired and inherited myopathies). The paper reports that some myopathies (as Duchenne muscular dystrophy and collagen VI-related myopathies) are characterized by a decreased circulating adiponectin level and that hormone replenishment induces beneficial effects in the diseased muscles [7]. Studies about the involvement of adiponectin in cancer have been growing in the last years. Parida et al. report how obesity and adiposity are closely related to cancer progression in several types of tumors (such as liver, pancreatic, prostate, and colorectal cancers). Obesity acts by dysregulating adipokine production, leading to the upregulation of oncogenic adipokines, such as leptin, and the downregulation of adiponectin, which plays a protective role in obesity-associated cancers [8]. About the relationship between obesity and cancer, Gelsomino et al. describe the role of adiponectin in the onset of obesity-associated female cancers (such as cervical, ovarian, endometrial, and breast cancers), reporting that adiponectin exerts anti-proliferative actions in some female cancers [9]. Barbe et al. report an overview of the expression levels and signaling pathways of adiponectin in male and female reproductive tract, from gametogenesis to embryo implantation and embryonal development. In addition, the authors describe some diseases associated with infertility, characterized by altered adiponectin levels (such as polycystic ovary syndrome, ovarian and endometrial cancers, endometriosis, gestational diseases, preeclampsia, and foetal growth restriction) [10]. Smolinska et al. report a research article describing a comparative transcriptomic study performed in control and adiponectin-treated endometrial tissues isolated from 15- to 16-day-pregnant pigs. The findings evidence that adiponectin affects processes important for reproductive success, such as cell proliferation, cell adhesion, and synthesis of steroids, prostaglandins, and cytokines [11]. The anti-atherogenic role of adiponectin has been widely recognized. Yanai et al. illustrate the mechanisms underlying the anti-atherogenic role of the hormone, describing methods (such as weight loss, exercise, administration of nutritional factors and anti-diabetic drugs) leading to the rise of circulating adiponectin, which have been proven to have protective effects against atherosclerotic progression [12]. A role of adiponectin in the mitigation of renal injury due to diabetes has been proposed. Kim et al. highlight recent advances about adiponectin and kidney diseases, describing adiponectin signaling pathways in healthy and disease conditions. In particular, the review discusses the possible strategies for upregulating adiponectin and adiponectin receptors and the possible use of the receptor agonist AdipoRon in the amelioration of overt diabetic kidney disease [13]. Furthermore, this Special Issue contains two research articles regarding adiponectin involvement in human follicular dermal papilla cells and the interaction of adiponectin with nerve growth factor β (NGFβ) and secreted protein acidic and rich in cysteine (SPARC). Park et al. report that kojyl cinnamate ester derivatives and Seletinoid G promote adiponectin secretion by human follicular dermal papilla cells. In addition, cell medium containing secreted adiponectin induces the expression of hair growth-related factors, thus suggesting an involvement of the hormone in the promotion of hair growth in humans [14]. Finally, Okura et al. investigate the interaction between adiponectin and NGFβ and SPARC. Surface plasmon resonance analysis demonstrated a physical interaction between adiponectin and NGFβ, and this interaction was confirmed in neuronal cultured PC12 cells [15].

Collectively, the papers reported in this Special Issue reinforce the idea that adiponectin plays an important role at the systemic level and that hypoadiponectinemia is associated with many diseases. The exogenous administration of adiponectin has often beneficial effects in diseased tissues, suggesting that the planning of new drugs able to activate adiponectin signaling could be a new tool for the amelioration of several pathologies.

Acknowledgments: This work was supported by the Italian Ministry of University and Research (MIUR).

Conflicts of Interest: The author declares no conflict of interest.

References

1. Scherer, P.E.; Williams, S.; Fogliano, M.; Baldini, G.; Lodish, H.F. A novel serum protein similar to C1q, produced exclusively in adipocytes. *J. Biol. Chem.* **1995**, *270*, 26746–26749. [CrossRef] [PubMed]
2. Yamauchi, T.; Hara, K.; Kubota, N.; Terauchi, Y.; Tobe, K.; Froguel, P.; Nagai, R.; Kadowaki, T. Dual roles of adiponectin/Acrp30 in vivo as an anti-diabetic and anti-atherogenic adipokine. *Curr. Drug Targets Immune Endocr. Metab. Disord.* **2003**, *3*, 243–253. [CrossRef]
3. Yamauchi, T.; Kamon, J.; Ito, Y.; Tsuchida, A.; Yokomizo, T.; Kita, S.; Sugiyama, T.; Miyagishi, M.; Hara, K.; Tsunoda, M.; et al. Cloning of adiponectin receptors that mediate antidiabetic metabolic effects. *Nature* **2003**, *423*, 762–769. [CrossRef] [PubMed]
4. Yamauchi, T.; Kamon, J.; Minokoshi, Y.; Ito, Y.; Waki, H.; Uchida, S.; Yamashita, S.; Noda, M.; Kita, S.; Ueki, K.; et al. Adiponectin stimulates glucose utilization and fatty-acid oxidation by activating AMP-activated protein kinase. *Nat. Med.* **2002**, *8*, 1288–1295. [CrossRef] [PubMed]
5. Fiaschi, T.; Magherini, F.; Gamberi, T.; Modesti, P.A.; Modesti, A. Adiponectin as a tissue regenerating hormone: More than a metabolic function. *Cell. Mol. Life Sci.* **2014**, *71*, 1917–1925. [CrossRef] [PubMed]
6. Krause, M.P.; Milne, K.J.; Hawke, T.J. Adiponectin—Consideration for its role in skeletal muscle health. *Int. J. Mol. Sci.* **2019**, *20*, 1528. [CrossRef] [PubMed]
7. Gamberi, T.; Magherini, F.; Fiaschi, T. Adiponectin in myopathies. *Int. J. Mol. Sci.* **2019**, *20*, 1544. [CrossRef] [PubMed]
8. Parida, S.; Siddharth, S.; Sharma, D. Adiponectin, obesity, and cancer: Clash of the bigwigs in health and disease. *Int. J. Mol. Sci.* **2019**, *20*, 2519. [CrossRef] [PubMed]
9. Gelsomino, L.; Naimo, G.D.; Catalano, S.; Mauro, L.; Andò, S. The emerging role of adiponectin in female malignancies. *Int. J. Mol. Sci.* **2019**, *20*, 2127. [CrossRef] [PubMed]
10. Barbe, A.; Bongrani, A.; Mellouk, N.; Estienne, A.; Kurowska, P.; Grandhaye, J.; Elfassy, Y.; Levy, R.; Rak, A.; Froment, P.; et al. Mechanisms of adiponectin action in fertility: An overview from gametogenesis to gestation in humans and animal models in normal and pathological conditions. *Int. J. Mol. Sci.* **2019**, *20*, 1526. [CrossRef] [PubMed]

11. Smolinska, N.; Szeszko, K.; Dobrzyn, K.; Kiezun, M.; Rytelewska, E.; Kisielewska, K.; Gudelska, M.; Bors, K.; Wyrebek, J.; Kopij, G.; et al. Transcriptomic analysis of porcine endometrium during implantation after in vitro stimulation by adiponectin. *Int. J. Mol. Sci.* **2019**, *20*, 1335. [CrossRef] [PubMed]
12. Yanai, H.; Yoshida, H. Beneficial effects of adiponectin on glucose and lipid metabolism and atherosclerotic progression: Mechanisms and perspectives. *Int. J. Mol. Sci.* **2019**, *20*, 1190. [CrossRef] [PubMed]
13. Kim, Y.; Park, C.W. Mechanisms of adiponectin action: Implication of adiponectin receptor agonism in diabetic Kidney disease. *Int. J. Mol. Sci.* **2019**, *20*, 1782. [CrossRef] [PubMed]
14. Park, P.J.; Cho, E.G. Kojyl cinnamate ester derivatives increase adiponectin expression and stimulate adiponectin-induced hair growth factors in human dermal papilla cells. *Int. J. Mol. Sci.* **2019**, *20*, 1859. [CrossRef] [PubMed]
15. Okura, Y.; Imao, T.; Murashima, S.; Shibata, H.; Kamikavwa, A.; Okamatsu-Ogura, Y.; Saito, M.; Kimura, K. Interaction of nerve growth factor β with adiponectin and SPARC oppositely modulates its biological activity. *Int. J. Mol. Sci.* **2019**, *20*, 1541. [CrossRef] [PubMed]

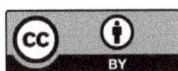

International Journal of
Molecular Sciences

MDPI

Review

Adiponectin—Consideration for its Role in Skeletal Muscle Health

Matthew P. Krause [1,*], Kevin J. Milne [1] and Thomas J. Hawke [2]

[1] Department of Kinesiology, Faculty of Human Kinetics, University of Windsor, 401 Sunset Avenue, Windsor, ON N9B 3P4, Canada; kjmilne@uwindsor.ca
[2] Department of Pathology and Molecular Medicine, Faculty of Health Sciences, McMaster University, 1280 Main Street, Hamilton, ON L8S 4L8, Canada; hawke@mcmaster.ca
*   Correspondence: mpkrause@uwindsor.ca; Tel.: 1-519-253-3000

Received: 8 March 2019; Accepted: 25 March 2019; Published: 27 March 2019

Abstract: Adiponectin regulates metabolism through blood glucose control and fatty acid oxidation, partly mediated by downstream effects of adiponectin signaling in skeletal muscle. More recently, skeletal muscle has been identified as a source of adiponectin expression, fueling interest in the role of adiponectin as both a circulating adipokine and a locally expressed paracrine/autocrine factor. In addition to being metabolically responsive, skeletal muscle functional capacity, calcium handling, growth and maintenance, regenerative capacity, and susceptibility to chronic inflammation are all strongly influenced by adiponectin stimulation. Furthermore, physical exercise has clear links to adiponectin expression and circulating concentrations in healthy and diseased populations. Greater physical activity is generally related to higher adiponectin expression while lower adiponectin levels are found in inactive obese, pre-diabetic, and diabetic populations. Exercise training typically restores plasma adiponectin and is associated with improved insulin sensitivity. Thus, the role of adiponectin signaling in skeletal muscle has expanded beyond that of a metabolic regulator to include several aspects of skeletal muscle function and maintenance critical to muscle health, many of which are responsive to, and mediated by, physical exercise.

Keywords: skeletal muscle; regeneration; adiponectin isoforms; exercise; training

1. Introduction

Since the discovery of adiponectin over 20 years ago [1], nearly 20,000 scientific articles have been published on this adipokine; reflecting an intense interest from the scientific community. Although originally identified as an adipose tissue secreted protein, adiponectin is now known to be expressed by multiple tissues including skeletal muscle. In conjunction with other canonical metabolic hormones (e.g., insulin, leptin, etc.), adiponectin helps to regulate metabolism through blood glucose control and fatty acid oxidation [2–5]. Despite being expressed and secreted by adipocytes, obesity-associated metabolic disorders such as insulin resistance and type 2 diabetes (T2D) are inversely related to adiponectin levels (i.e., circulating adiponectin decreases despite greater fat mass) [5,6]. Furthermore, low adiponectin levels are related to an increased rate of progression of diabetic complications such as nephropathy, retinopathy, and cardiomyopathy [7]. Thus, much of the research focus has been on elucidating the mechanistic roles played by adiponectin in regulating metabolism across multiple tissues, and how its expression is regulated under normal and pathophysiological circumstances. More recently, other physiological roles of adiponectin have emerged, including that skeletal muscle both expresses and is sensitive to adiponectin. Consequently, the purpose of this review is to highlight the physiological roles of adiponectin in skeletal muscle and the pathophysiology related to dysregulated adiponectin expression. Given the potency of regular physical exercise to improve metabolic control, this review will also examine how adiponectin expression is altered by exercise and whether benefits of exercise are mediated, at least in part, by the actions of adiponectin.

2. Expression and Post-Translational Modification of Adiponectin

Well over 200 proteins are reported to be expressed and secreted by human adipocytes, one of which is adiponectin (also referred to as adipocyte complement-related protein of 30 kDa [Acrp30], Adipocyte, C1q, and collagen domain-containing protein [ACDC], or Adipose most abundant gene transcript 1 protein [apM-1]) [8]. Originally, expression and release of adiponectin into the circulation was thought to be restricted to adipose tissue [1], however, it is now established that adiponectin is produced and secreted from a number of cell types, including skeletal and cardiac muscles [9–16]. Adiponectin is part of a large family of secreted protein hormones, the C1q TNFα Related Proteins (CTRP), many of which have overlapping biological functions [17]. At least eight isoforms of adiponectin exist following post-translational modifications of the initial gene product [18]. In the plasma, adiponectin exists as low molecular weight trimers (LMW) that can associate with one another to form middle molecular weight hexamers and high molecular weight (HMW) multimers of various sizes [19] (Figure 1), while the adiponectin monomer is not detected in the circulation. These post-translational modifications and associations impact the stability and biological activity of adiponectin in the circulation [18,19]. Indeed, HMW adiponectin has been shown to have a greater predictive power for insulin resistance than total plasma adiponectin [20]. Adiponectin is one of the most abundant adipokines in the plasma, circulating in the range of approximately 5 to 30 μg/mL with a half-life of 13 and 17.5 h for the HMW and low molecular weight isoforms, respectively [21]. This expression level is approximately 0.05% of total serum protein content. In comparison, other notable adipokines have been reported in the ng/mL scale. For example, leptin and plasminogen activator inhibitor (PAI)-1, range between 1 to 200 ng/mL [22,23] and 15 to 550 ng/mL [24], respectively.

Through proteolytic cleavage, adiponectin can also exist as globular adiponectin (gAd; Figure 1) and reports suggest that, although it is expressed at very low levels, gAd displays biological activities that are distinct from the properties of the full-length adiponectin protein [25–28]. Throughout the remainder of the review, the isoform of adiponectin (globular, trimeric, hexameric, or HMW) will be indicated where possible. However, a major limitation in how the findings of adiponectin studies are interpreted is that the adiponectin isoform is often not delineated, possibly due to the reliance on pan-adiponectin antibodies for detection.

The secretion, stability, and signaling function/potency of adiponectin is dependent not only on multimeric conformation, but how adiponectin is post-translationally modified. Adiponectin shares structural similarities with some collagen types and, similar to collagen, is glycosylated and hydroxylated as part of its post-translational modification [18,29,30]. Trimeric (LMW) adiponectin is stabilized by interactions of the collagenous domains, while the hexameric and HMW forms further require disulfide bond formation between cysteine residues [29,30]. Quenching of available cysteine residues (through excessive fumarate causing succination of cysteine) prevents the post-translational modifications necessary to produce competent hexamers and HMW adiponectin in type 2, but not type 1, diabetic rodents [31–33]. Succination is a post-translational modification for many proteins and appears to be upregulated in obese and diabetic rodents in multiple tissues including skeletal muscle [33]. Consequently, it is likely that adiponectin expressed by tissues other than adipose is similarly affected by excessive fumarate. The half-life of circulating adiponectin also appears to be dependent on post-translational modification. Consistent across species [34], adiponectin has been demonstrated to be modified by the addition of sialic acid to O-linked glycans (referred to as sialylation) and the desialylation of adiponectin results in accelerated clearance of adiponectin from the circulation [35].

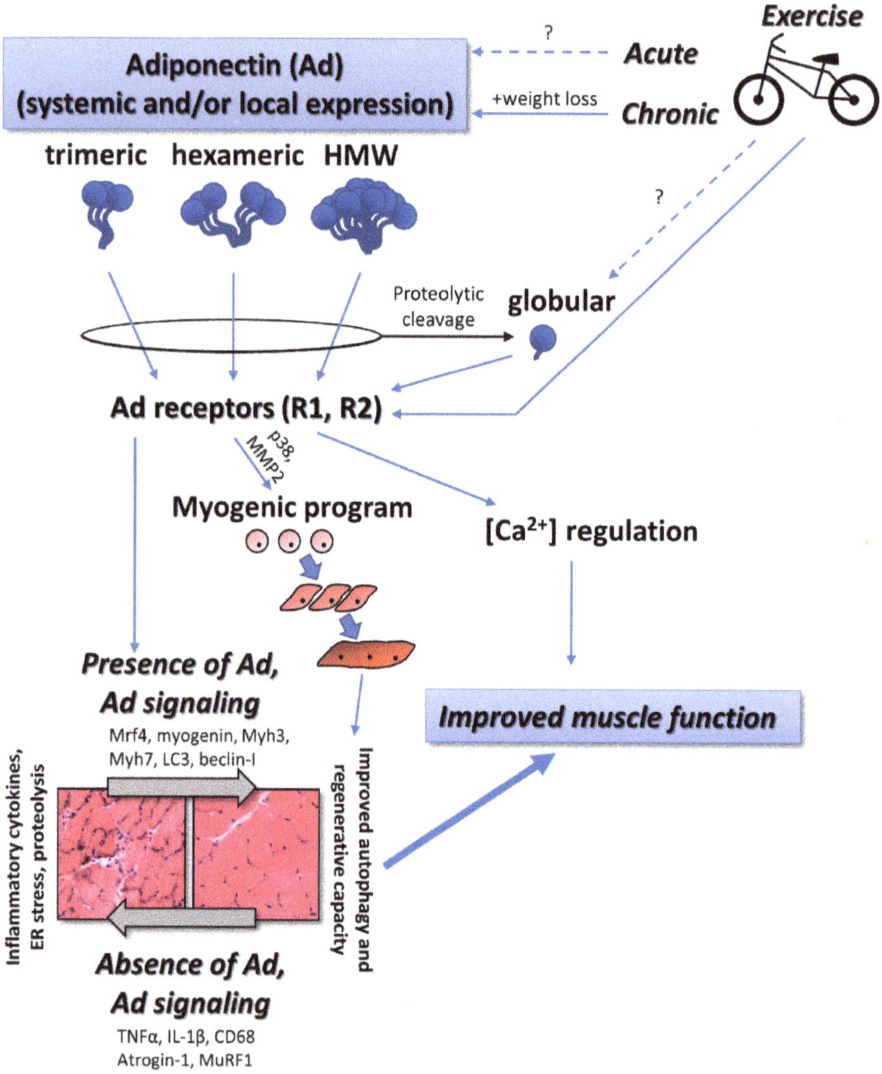

Figure 1. Proposed relationships between adiponectin, exercise, and skeletal muscle function. Multiple isoforms including the proteolytically cleaved globular isoform signal to tissue including skeletal muscle, satellite cells, myoblasts, and differentiated myotubes. Physical exercise generally stimulates increases in adiponectin expression and signaling. Skeletal muscle health is ultimately improved with sufficient adiponectin signaling via improved cellular functions such as autophagy and regeneration and suppression of inflammation, endoplasmic reticulum (ER) stress, and proteolysis. Solid arrows represent relationships, effects, or interactions that are clearly defined in the literature. Broken arrows with "?" represent relationships, effects, or interactions that are not clearly defined in the literature.

Adiponectin expression follows a circadian rhythm, with circulating concentrations peaking in the early afternoon [36,37], although the impact of this rhythm is not well understood. Obesity and the progression from insulin resistance to diabetes has been linked to disruptions in circadian rhythm stemming from a cycle of disrupted sleep and poor eating habits. A potential link between disrupted circadian rhythms and metabolic disease progression is the disruption of rhythmic adiponectin expression and signaling. For example, mice switched from a normal diet to a high fat diet (to induce obesity and insulin resistance) caused a phase delay and general decrease in adiponectin expression, as well as phase delays in adiponectin receptor mRNA peaks [38], similar to observations of obese, diabetic KK-A(y) mice [39]. Conversely, mice with disrupted expression of circadian rhythm regulators (Bmal1 and Clock) exhibited an increase in adiponectin expression [40,41]. Interestingly, mice that were subjected to repeated weight cycling demonstrated disrupted expression of several clock genes with no significant alteration to plasma adiponectin despite increased adiposity [42]. Clearly, this potential relationship between circadian rhythms, adiponectin expression, and metabolic diseases is of tremendous importance and requires further attention.

3. Adiponectin Effects in Skeletal Muscle

3.1. Muscle Function and Calcium Handling

There is little evidence of a direct relationship between adiponectin and skeletal muscle contractile capacity, and the studies inferring such a relationship are limited. While adiponectin KO mice displayed a reduction in peak force [13], adiponectin receptor 1 (AdipoR1) KO mice displayed poor capacity for endurance exercise and a decreased type I fiber percentage but were not tested for peak force [43]. In contrast, a study of young and elderly BMI- and physical activity habit-matched males and females reported no correlation between adiponectin levels and contractile force output [44].

Despite scattered evidence of an effect on contractile force, adiponectin does appear to regulate intramyocellular calcium concentration; important in dictating the contractile force output in muscle. For example, adding adiponectin to the culture media of differentiated C2C12 myotubes resulted in a rapid increase in intracellular calcium, an effect that is abolished by siRNA knockdown of AdipoR1 [43], while a similar effect is also observed in C2C12 myoblasts [45]. These studies offer evidence that the adiponectin-mediated calcium influx is mediated both by calcium from sarcoplasmic reticulum stores and the extracellular space [43,45]. Given that intramyocellular calcium modulates contractile force output, myosin light chain phosphorylation state, and a multitude of gene expression responses [46], adiponectin likely plays a role in calcium-mediated events in skeletal muscle, assuming that cellular observations translate *in vivo*. Indeed, an adiponectin-induced increase in myocellular calcium has been linked to activation of calmodulin-kinase activation and transcription of PGC-1α [43,45]. Further, adiponectin has recently been shown to influence calcium transients in cardiomyocytes through the regulation of sarcoplasmic reticulum calcium ATPase (SERCA) function [47], thereby presenting another method by which adiponectin may be linked to contractile function through calcium handling.

In both human and animal models of diabetes, reduced skeletal muscle contractile capacity is typically observed, however, a unified mechanism for this reduction remains elusive [13,48–50]. A recent study using a high-fat diet (HFD) rat model to induce diabetes (but also characterized by low adiponectin expression) found reduced peak twitch and tetanic force and a prolonged half-relaxation time, in addition to reduced SERCA gene expression in the gastrocnemius [51]. However, HFD rats treated with adiponectin transfection in one gastrocnemius saw partial restoration of force production, attributable to the restoration of SERCA expression. Further, exercise training had a similar effect on restoring SERCA expression and contractile parameters, although it is noteworthy that adiponectin transfection in combination with exercise training did not have a synergistic effect [51]. The observation of reduced muscle function is in agreement with previous studies on the effect of a HFD [49] or adiponectin-KO [13]. Consequently, we speculate that adiponectin has limited acute effects on muscle contraction, but that chronic muscle adiponectin signaling, or lack thereof, in diabetic or adiponectin KO models leads to changes in calcium handling, and thus influences contractile capacity via both calcium availability and changes in gene expression.

3.2. Muscle Development, Growth, Maintenance, and Aging

Adiponectin appears to play a role in regulating muscle mass, with recent mechanistic studies demonstrating it as a critical signal for muscle regeneration and suppression of proteolysis [25,52–58]. Epidemiological studies support the idea that adiponectin aids in the development and maintenance of muscle mass. For example, adiponectin was recently implicated in a study of adolescent idiopathic scoliosis (AIS), a common form of spinal deformity [59]. It is thought that unequal bilateral development of the paravertebral muscles leads to the development of lateral curvatures of the spine. Muscle samples of paravertebral muscles from the concave (more developed) and convex sides of AIS were analyzed via RNAseq. Interestingly, among other genes, adiponectin expression was found to be high on the concave side relative to the convex side [59], suggesting that this imbalance is related to unequal rates of paravertebral development.

Similarly, there is evidence that adiponectin provides a protective effect in muscle wasting conditions. Muscle wasting in sarcopenia is associated with aging and is driven by multiple factors including motor neuron degeneration and hormonal changes. Adiponectin was found to be significantly decreased in sarcopenic compared to non-sarcopenic adults [60]. However, in another study, young and elderly (non-sarcopenic) participants matched for physical activity habits demonstrated no difference in muscle mass or circulating adiponectin levels [44]. It is worth noting that in a study of young vs old mice, adiponectin expression was markedly higher in old EDL muscle compared to young, but AdipoR2 was not expressed as highly in old compared to young muscle [61], suggesting that disrupted adiponectin signaling, rather than adiponectin levels, may be problematic in some cases.

Together, these finding are surprisingly at odds with other studies suggesting that higher adiponectin levels drive muscle wasting. Adiponectin levels were found to be significantly elevated in sarcopenic males with cardiovascular disease (CVD) compared to non-sarcopenic, CVD controls [62]. Furthermore, adiponectin levels negatively correlated with functional measures such as grip strength and gait speed [62]. A similar negative relationship between adiponectin and muscle function has been demonstrated in other studies examining middle aged and elderly people with and without CVD [63–65]. As well, in a study of spinal and bulbar muscular atrophy patients, circulating adiponectin levels were found to be higher compared to age-matched healthy control participants, although circulating adiponectin levels did not significantly correlate with a composite muscle function score [66]. These epidemiological studies are supported by an *in vitro* study that manipulated adiponectin signaling with the use of AdipoRon [61], a small molecule agonist of AdipoR1 and R2 [67]. AdipoRon treatment reduced protein content and newly-formed myotube size in C2C12 cells, while reducing muscle fiber size in mouse plantaris muscle [61]. Given the well-defined role of adiponectin as an activator of adenosine monophosphate-activated protein kinase (AMPK) [4,68] and AMPK activity inhibits the mammalian target of rapamycin (mTOR) [69], perhaps it should not be surprising that elevated adiponectin signaling would negatively correlate with muscle mass/function. We speculate that there is a certain healthy range of adiponectin concentrations and/or signaling and significant deviations below or above that range is pathological. Further study is required to resolve these apparently opposing roles of adiponectin in the regulation of muscle mass in health and various disease states.

3.3. Skeletal Muscle Regeneration and Adaptive Capacity

Early studies by Fiaschi et al. provided evidence for the impact of adiponectin on skeletal muscle regeneration. This group first reported that proliferating skeletal muscle cells responded to the globular isoform of adiponectin by exiting the cell cycle, committing to the myogenic lineage, and driving differentiation [52]. This response appeared to be mediated through redox signaling since treatment with the ROS scavenger, N-acetyl cysteine (NAC), blunted the adiponectin-induced muscle differentiation [52]. A follow-up study demonstrated that satellite cells isolated from murine tibialis anterior muscles were sensitive to both full-length and globular adiponectin, though the latter induced a greater motility in satellite cells and encouraged expression of matrix metalloproteinase (MMP)-2, both key components of muscle regeneration [25]. In that study, it was also demonstrated that activated macrophages cleaved full-length adiponectin into the globular form, helping to stimulate satellite cells via p38 mitogen-activated protein kinase (MAPK) activation and serving as a chemoattractant for further macrophage numbers [25]. An earlier *in vitro* study had demonstrated that the monocyte cell line THP-1 cleaved full-length adiponectin into globular adiponectin whereas Fao hepatocytes, 3T3-L1 adipocytes, and L6 myocytes did not [28], consistent with the work of Fiaschi et al. [25].

Interestingly, recent work using the adiponectin knockout mouse model and adenovirally-mediated adiponectin overexpression was unable to significantly affect skeletal muscle regeneration when compared to wild-type mice [58]. However, (adenovirally-mediated) adiponectin overexpression was capable of improving muscle regeneration in both adiponectin knockout mice and in angiotensin II infused mice (to mimic chronic heart failure condition or aging conditions) [58], suggesting that while adiponectin may not be a primary mediator of skeletal muscle regeneration, its presence or absence can significantly affect the regenerative process. Consistent with this hypothesis, the ability of exercise training to restore regenerative capacity and contractile function in SAMP10 mouse skeletal muscle (a model of accelerated senescence) was nullified when the animals concurrently received adiponectin antibody treatment to lower available circulating adiponectin [56]. Interestingly, the spiny mouse Acomys cahirinus, notable for its exceptional skeletal muscle regenerative capacity, expresses ~2.5-fold greater adiponectin in regenerating muscle compared to that of a C57Bl6 mouse counterpart [70], again suggesting the importance of adiponectin to the regeneration process.

Beyond muscle regeneration, skeletal muscle is also highly adaptable to changes in load bearing (e.g., hypertrophy in response to chronic load bearing; atrophy in response to unloading). Exercise-trained SAMP10 mice demonstrated increased grip strength and muscle mass which as abrogated by anti-adiponectin antibody treatment [56], suggesting adiponectin plays a role in mediating the hypertrophic response to exercise, though it should be noted that endurance exercise was the mode of training in this study. To the best of our knowledge, no study has yet to test the necessity of adiponectin for the hypertrophic response to resistance exercise. Based on these data, it could be speculated that adiponectin is required for hypertrophy, although such speculation is at odds with its role of activating AMPK and therefore suppressing mTOR activity.

Skeletal muscle expression of adiponectin, its receptors AdipoR1 and R2, and the adaptor protein APPL1 are required to relay the adiponectin signal to the cell interior [71] and the state of load bearing in skeletal muscle dictates the level of expression of these proteins. When overloaded via synergist ablation, mouse soleus fibers increase expression of adiponectin, both adiponectin receptors (AdipoR1 and R2), and APPL1, similar to what occurs in myoblasts as they differentiate and become myotubes *in vitro* [55]. Conversely, after 2 weeks of hindlimb suspension, soleus AdipoR1 expression was reduced, but not adiponectin, AdipoR2, or APPL1. Upon resumption of normal ambulation patterns, soleus AdipoR1, adiponectin, and APPL1 significantly increased [55]. The importance of adiponectin in suppressing muscle atrophy has also been directly demonstrated. Using C2C12 cells, treatment with either globular adiponectin or with glucopyranosyl tetrahydroxydihydroflavonol (GTDF), a mimetic of globular adiponectin, stimulated cell differentiation [57]. Furthermore, GTDF or adiponectin protected against dexamethasone-induced expression of atrogin-1 and MuRF1 (the atrogenes), key genes of the proteolytic pathway which is highly active during muscle atrophy. This effect was consistent in rat gastrocnemius *in vivo* and prevented atrophy [57]. Low expression of adiponectin and elevated expression of the atrogenes was also noted in a study of cachexia in tumour-bearing mice [72]. Thus, muscle expression of adiponectin, its receptors, and associated adapter protein are sensitive to the state of loading and play a role in minimizing proteolysis. We speculate that adiponectin signaling is altered as a mechanism serving to carry out processes related to hypertrophy and atrophy (Figure 1).

3.4. Dystrophy and Inflammation

Adiponectin attenuates inflammatory signaling [73] and has recently been demonstrated to reduce degeneration of muscle in muscular dystrophy. Crossing adiponectin null mice with mdx mice (a murine model of muscular dystrophy), mdx/adiponectin-null mice were generated [74]. Without adiponectin, muscle contractile force was worsened compared to mdx mice, coinciding with higher levels of markers of muscle damage (e.g., plasma creatine kinase, pervading Evans Blue Dye). Restoring adiponectin levels via local gene electrotransfer resulted in reduced markers of inflammation (TNFα, IL-1β, CD68), greater expression of markers of regeneration (Mrf4, myogenin, Myh3, Myh7), and morphological improvements (larger muscle fibers, decreased inflammation and ECM in between fibers). Using adiponectin overexpression in mdx mice, similar improvements (i.e., reduced inflammation, greater expression of myogenic markers, morphological and functional improvements) were observed [75]. Furthermore, treating mdx mice with adiponectin reduced the expression of the Nlrp3 inflammasome, a caspase complex responsible for activating inflammatory cytokines IL-1β and IL-18 [76], providing a potential link between adiponectin and reduced inflammation in skeletal muscle. Importantly, adiponectin treatment of myoblasts isolated from Duchenne Muscular Dystrophy (DMD) patients and cultured into myotubes demonstrated similar results to rodent studies. Analysis of the secretome of DMD-myotubes treated with adiponectin revealed that expression of several inflammatory cytokines (TNFα, IL-17A, and CCL28) was repressed while expression of utrophin was increased [77]. Further, it was recently demonstrated that mesoangioblasts were capable of fusing with dystrophic muscle *in vivo* under the influence of exogenous adiponectin treatment [53]. This is important because treatment of dystrophic muscle with myogenic cells expressing competent dystrophin would ideally result in the replacement of the defective dystrophin gene. If adiponectin can help in these regards, support for adiponectin as an adjunct in novel treatments against muscular dystrophy and associated inflammation is warranted.

3.5. Regulation of Autophagy

Reductions in adiponectin and/or adiponectin signaling could be mediating deleterious effects on skeletal muscle through decreased stimulation of autophagy. Recently, it was demonstrated that insulin resistant L6 skeletal muscle cells have insulin sensitivity restored with adiponectin exposure [78]. Interestingly, this effect of adiponectin was mediated through restoration of autophagy and reduction of ER stress, an effect also captured by rapamycin treatment but lost in Atg5-dominant negative cells that are autophagy-deficient [78]. Activation of autophagy in response to adiponectin (in this case, globular adiponectin) has also been demonstrated in C2C12 cells, promoting myoblast survival and suppressing apoptosis [54]. Furthermore, skeletal muscle from adiponectin KO mice displayed reduced expression of LC3 and beclin-I, key markers of autophagy, as well as histological markers of myopathy (i.e., centrally located nuclei, accentuated fiber cross-sectional area heterogeneity, necrotic fibers) [54]. Interestingly, high fat diet-induced obesity stimulated autophagy, an effect lost in adiponectin-KO mice and restored with adiponectin treatment [79].

3.6. Adiponectin Mimetics and Related Proteins

Adiponectin mimetics and related proteins share effects on skeletal muscle similar to those of adiponectin itself. GTDF [57,80] and AdipoRon [67,81] are agonists of the AdipoR and have already been described earlier in this review. Evidence is accumulating that proteins closely related to adiponectin may also play similar roles in skeletal muscle. The C1q/TNF-related protein (CTRP) family has 16 identified family members including adiponectin, many of which form multimeric complexes and have biological functions similar to adiponectin [17]. CTRP3 in particular, is notable due to its positive effect on glucose homeostasis and anti-inflammatory functions [17]. Recently, CTRP3 was demonstrated to be expressed by embryonic skeletal muscle and by differentiating C2C12 myoblasts [82]. Despite being expressed during differentiation, CTRP3 signaling stimulates ERK1/2 activity, promotes proliferation, and delays differentiation of C2C12 myoblasts into myotubes [82]. Thus, it is possible that other members of the CTRP family also play key roles in developing and maintaining a healthy skeletal muscle but have yet to be examined.

4. Mechanisms of Benefits of Exercise Mediated by Adiponectin

Unlike most circulating adipokines, adiponectin is inversely associated with adiposity, visceral fat in particular [83]. In general, women express greater plasma adiponectin than men, independent of BMI and fat mass, and there has been suggestion that this relationship is partly influenced by sex hormones [83]. A number of investigations of the sex-related differences in circulating adiponectin throughout adolescence suggest that adiponectin is negatively associated with serum androgens given that there is a drop in adiponectin as young boys progress through puberty, a result not seen to the same extent in young girls and independent of body composition changes during this period [84,85].

4.1. Acute and Chronic Effects of Exercise on Adiponectin Expression

Circulating adiponectin is negatively associated with insulin resistance, poor glucose control, and diabetes [86,87], and has anti-inflammatory and anti-atherogenic properties [88]. Further, low levels of circulating adiponectin are observed in obese individuals [89,90], those with CVD [91], and some cancers [92]. Consequently, adiponectin has been a prime target for study and manipulation since its initial characterization. Not surprisingly, because physical activity is a potent countermeasure against metabolic and CVD [93,94], studies to determine the relationship between exercise and plasma adiponectin have been plentiful. In rodents, there is evidence to suggest that moderate physical activity (10 weeks voluntary wheel or treadmill running) can increase plasma adiponectin without changes in fat mass [56,95], but this is not clear given that neither 10 weeks of endurance running at 70% maximal running capacity nor 10 weeks of high intensity interval training (HIIT) were shown to significantly increase plasma LMW and HMW adiponectin (as measured by Western Blot) in mice [96]. Similarly, systematic summaries of the relationship between exercise and adiponectin in humans have shown equivocal findings [97,98]. Observations of plasma adiponectin after a single bout of aerobic or resistance exercise reveal small changes, if any, in either direction in acute timelines [90,98–101], while interventions of repeated bouts of exercise training over weeks or months may cause either an increase [90,98,102], decrease [98,103,104], or no change [98,104–106] in this adipokine. This is not unusual when attempting to summarize the results of exercise studies because, much like many of the benefits of an exercise training regime, outcomes are dependent on frequency, mode, intensity, and type of exercise in addition to a host of individual characteristics (e.g., age, health, fitness level, etc.). Similarly, there are challenges in interpreting adiponectin changes in response to exercise because of differences in the sex of study participants, initial body composition, separating fat loss from exercise related changes, and different methods of measuring adiponectin. For example, serum adiponectin was reduced in overweight and obese individuals, but not normal weight middle-age adults following 12 months of aerobic (supervised aquatic exercise for 60 min, twice a week) and resistance training exercise even though all groups improved cardiorespiratory fitness and no group exhibited changes in fat mass following training [104]. In another study, healthy adult men free of any known chronic diseases and grouped according to BMI (i.e., normal BMI versus overweight/obese) and activity level (i.e., sedentary versus active) partook in 2 months of cycle ergometer training (i.e., 3×60 min at 50% VO_2peak) [103]. The study authors measured LMW, MMW, and HMW adiponectin by several ELISA's and observed reduced total and HMW adiponectin concentrations only after training in the sedentary groups, but not the active groups, regardless of body composition [103]. The findings of these two studies suggest that adiponectin levels in normal weight and/or active adults do not respond to low intensity exercise, whereas overweight/obese individuals show reductions in circulating adiponectin to these exercise intensities, especially when body composition is unchanged.

In contrast, when exercise is associated with significant body fat loss, it appears that circulating adiponectin is increased. For example, sedentary and obese ($30\ kg/m^2 < BMI > 40\ kg/m^2$) but otherwise healthy adult (37 ± 7 y) men and women who participated in a supervised aerobic (60 to 75 min/session, three sessions/week at 500 to 600 kcal/session) exercise training regimen and/or reduced calorie diet for 12 weeks, only exhibited changes in adiponectin when the interventions were associated with weight loss [107]. Further, in relatively healthy older (71.2 ± 5.0 years) adult men and women who completed 12 weeks (3 d/wk) of combined moderate intensity endurance (20 min of walking at 60% to 70% of heart rate reserve) and resistance exercise, adiponectin increased over 50% following exercise training [102]. At a similar intensity (45 min at 70% of maximum heart rate, 3×/week) performed by middle-aged hypertensive men, plasma adiponectin was elevated at 8 and 12 weeks of the intervention [108]. Nonetheless, in both studies, increases in circulating adiponectin were either significantly correlated with body fat [102] or occurred in the presence of significant weight loss [108] (Figure 1). Future studies should consider the impact of progressive exercise training on the adipocyte secretome and related molecular signaling, perhaps best achieved with isolated adipocyte studies.

4.2. Physical Activity Behaviour and Adiponectin Expression

In contrast to training interventions, large cross-sectional studies of physical activity behaviour and adipokine/inflammatory biomarker expression tend to show a relationship between greater volumes of physical activity and/or moderate to vigorous physical activity (MVPA) and plasma adiponectin that is independent of body fat. For example, older (~60 y) adult women who exhibited greater accelerometer-measured total activity were found to have higher circulating adiponectin, and though this relationship was attenuated after adjusting for BMI, a significant correlation still existed [109]. Moreover, women in the highest quartiles of both total activity and MVPA had significantly higher serum adiponectin than the lowest quartiles (Alessa et al. 2017). This relationship was also observed in young boys and girls (~9 y), where plasma adiponectin was positively associated with VO_2peak, even though this correlation was weak [110]. In a recent study out of Japan, with one of the largest samples (>10,000) of middle-aged (40 to 69 y) adults, serum concentrations of total adiponectin and HMW adiponectin were greatest in those individuals who were in the highest quartiles of accelerometer-measured light-intensity physical activity (LPA) and MVPA [111]. Not surprisingly, the individuals in the highest quartiles of physical activity also had the lowest BMIs, however the authors used isotemporal substitution analysis to show that replacing 60 min of sedentary time with LPA could be linked to increased total and HMW adiponectin levels by 4% to 13%, respectively, even after adjusting for body fat [111]. In the latter two studies, both girls and women had higher adiponectin levels than boys and men, even though they had lower maximum aerobic capacity [110] or physical activity levels [111], respectively, indicating that the circulating expression of this adipokine is regulated by many factors. Indeed, in middle aged Japanese men and women followed over 3 years, lower plasma adiponectin was observed in individuals who developed type 2 diabetes independent of visceral fat mass even though self-reported physical activity was not different between those with and without diabetes [112].

4.3. The Link Between Exercise, Adiponectin, and Improved Metabolic Health

Understanding the metabolic signals linked to increased circulating adiponectin could help to explain some of the above observations. However, other than a general idea that adiponectin both regulates [68] and is regulated by plasma FFA [113], the specific trigger initiated by increased physical activity and exercise in humans is not clear [114,115]. It is likely that even this response is multifaceted and, much like many of the observations noted in this review, the data regarding differential processing of the LMW, MMW, and HMW adiponectin are scarce. Interestingly, in one exercise training study, middle-aged adult men and women separated by performance on an oral glucose tolerance test (normal glucose tolerance versus impaired glucose tolerance/non-diabetic) and by presentation with type 2 diabetes performed 20 min of supervised biking or running, 20 min of swimming, and 20 min of cool down sessions, 3 days/week for 4 weeks [116]. In older participants

(~50 y) and those with T2D or impaired glucose tolerance, circulating adiponectin was reduced, while following exercise, adiponectin was increased, a result associated with reduced fat mass. These authors also found, however, that muscle adiponectin receptor mRNA was increased following exercise training, and suggested that when translated to receptor protein expression, could be part of the insulin sensitizing effects of regular exercise [116]. Consequently, in addition to investigation into the different molecular weight forms of adiponectin, it would be prudent for exercise studies to examine muscle, liver, and/or other tissue expression of adiponectin receptor expression along with some measure of function. In this context, two recent reports out of the same lab showed that diet, exercise type, and tissue had different interactive effects of the expression of the different molecular weight forms of adiponectin in mice [96,117]. Chronic endurance and HIIT exercise were independently able to attenuate many of the metabolic impairments caused by a high fat diet. Yet, while the expression of LMW and HMW adiponectin in the plasma was relatively unchanged by both exercise types, exercise and high fat feeding interacted to markedly increase muscle HMW adiponectin and reduce adiponectin receptor mRNA versus untrained animals only in muscles suspected to be used during exercise (i.e., the gastrocnemius vs masseter) [96,117]. Further, the addition of a calorically-restricted diet to an endurance exercise program appears to be a potent stimulus to counter the inflammatory and metabolic deregulatory effects of prior high fat feeding, including elevating circulating adiponectin back to normal levels and increasing adiponectin receptor protein expression in responsive tissues, such as the liver [118]. Both the translational and functional implications of these observations remain to be determined, but in the aforementioned studies, the authors noted differential downstream signaling gene products that would indicate altered function of these muscles.

It is also important to note that although physical exercise benefits several of the processes also influenced by adiponectin, the mechanisms through which exercise mediates these benefits may occur independent of adiponectin expression. Indeed, many of the studies noted above showed some type of advantageous metabolic change regardless of whether circulating adiponectin was increased, decreased, or remained the same. Further, it has been shown that adiponectin KO mice, when exercise trained, demonstrate improvements in expression of mitochondrial markers and activation of intracellular signaling kinases similar to wild type animals, suggesting that adiponectin is not required to mediate exercise-induced benefits in skeletal muscle [119,120]. Nonetheless, it is likely that the physiological change linking exercise to adiponectin expression may or may not occur, but exercise and adiponectin can exert positive metabolic, muscular, and cardiovascular effects independent of each other.

5. Future Directions and Conclusions

The promise of adiponectin as a clinically relevant biomarker and potential therapeutic target continues to expand. Originally deemed an adipose tissue-specific hormone, the past decade has revealed adiponectin expression by numerous tissues including skeletal muscle and the potential for treating not just metabolic diseases but other skeletal muscle conditions such as muscular dystrophy. Its importance for normal physiologic function of skeletal muscle has been demonstrated in studies of muscle development, regeneration, protein turnover, and regulation of inflammatory signaling. The relationship between physical activity (quantity and quality/type) and circulating and local adiponectin isoforms (trimers, hexamers, HMW, and globular) is not yet clear, although a general relationship of high intensity exercise reducing body fat mass leading to greater adiponectin circulation has been established.

Author Contributions: Conceptualization, resources, writing—original draft preparation, writing—review and editing, visualization, M.P.K., K.J.M., and T.J.H.; supervision, T.J.H.; project administration, funding acquisition, M.P.K., T.J.H.

Funding: This research was funded by the Natural Sciences and Engineering Research Council of Canada (NSERC) Discovery Grants Program (M.P.K., T.J.H.).

Conflicts of Interest: The authors declare no conflict of interest.

Abbreviations

T2D	Type 2 Diabetes Mellitus
Acrp30	Adipocyte complement-related protein of 30 kDa
ACDC	Adipocyte, C1q, and collagen domain-containing protein
apM-1	Adipose most abundant gene transcript 1 protein
CTRP	C1q TNFα Related Proteins
LMW	Low molecular weight
HMW	High molecular weight
PAI-1	Plasminogen Activator Inhibitor-1
gAd	Globular adiponectin
AdipoR1,2	Adiponectin receptors 1,2
HFD	High-fat diet
AMPK	Adenosine monophosphate-activated protein kinase
mTOR	Mammalian target of rapamycin
SERCA	Sarcoplasmic reticulum calcium ATPase
CVD	Cardiovascular disease
AIS	adolescent idiopathic scoliosis
NAC	N-acetyl cysteine
MMP	Matrix metalloproteinase
MAPK	Mitogen-activated protein kinase
GTDF	glucopyranosyl tetrahydroxydihydroflavonol
DMD	Duchenne Muscular Dystrophy
HIIT	High intensity interval training
VO_2	Volume of oxygen consumption
BMI	Body mass index
LPA	Light-intensity physical activity
MVPA	Moderate to vigorous physical activity

References

1. Scherer, P.E.; Williams, S.; Fogliano, M.; Baldini, G.; Lodish, H.F. A novel serum protein similar to C1q, produced exclusively in adipocytes. *J. Biol. Chem.* **1995**, *270*, 26746–26749. [CrossRef] [PubMed]
2. Nicholson, T.; Church, C.; Baker, D.J.; Jones, S.W. The role of adipokines in skeletal muscle inflammation and insulin sensitivity. *J. Inflamm.* **2018**, *15*, 9. [CrossRef] [PubMed]
3. Wang, Z.V.; Scherer, P.E. Adiponectin, the past two decades. *J. Mol. Cell. Biol.* **2016**, *8*, 93–100. [CrossRef] [PubMed]
4. Yamauchi, T.; Kamon, J.; Minokoshi, Y.; Ito, Y.; Waki, H.; Uchida, S.; Yamashita, S.; Noda, M.; Kita, S.; Ueki, K.; et al. Adiponectin stimulates glucose utilization and fatty-acid oxidation by activating AMP-activated protein kinase. *Nat. Med.* **2002**, *8*, 1288–1295. [CrossRef] [PubMed]
5. Yamauchi, T.; Kamon, J.; Waki, H.; Terauchi, Y.; Kubota, N.; Hara, K.; Mori, Y.; Ide, T.; Murakami, K.; Tsuboyama-Kasaoka, N.; et al. The fat-derived hormone adiponectin reverses insulin resistance associated with both lipoatrophy and obesity. *Nat. Med.* **2001**, *7*, 941–946. [CrossRef] [PubMed]
6. Kikuko, H.; Tohru, F.; Yukio, A.; Masahiko, T.; Morihiro, M.; Yoshihisa, O.; Hiromi, I.; Hiroshi, K.; Noriyuki, O.; Kazuhisa, M.; et al. Plasma Concentrations of a Novel, Adipose-Specific Protein, Adiponectin, in Type 2 Diabetic Patients. *Arterioscler. Thromb. Vasc. Biol.* **2000**, *20*, 1595–1599.
7. Forbes, J.M.; Cooper, M.E. Mechanisms of diabetic complications. *Physiol. Rev.* **2013**, *93*, 137–188. [CrossRef] [PubMed]
8. Lehr, S.; Hartwig, S.; Lamers, D.; Famulla, S.; Müller, S.; Hanisch, F.-G.; Cuvelier, C.; Ruige, J.; Eckardt, K.; Ouwens, D.M.; et al. Identification and validation of novel adipokines released from primary human adipocytes. *Mol. Cell Proteom.* **2012**, *11*. [CrossRef] [PubMed]
9. Delaigle, A.M.; Senou, M.; Guiot, Y.; Many, M.-C.; Brichard, S.M. Induction of adiponectin in skeletal muscle of type 2 diabetic mice: In vivo and in vitro studies. *Diabetologia* **2006**, *49*, 1311–1323. [CrossRef] [PubMed]

10. Delaigle, A.M.; Jonas, J.-C.; Bauche, I.B.; Cornu, O.; Brichard, S.M. Induction of Adiponectin in Skeletal Muscle by Inflammatory Cytokines: In Vivo and in Vitro Studies. *Endocrinology* **2004**, *145*, 5589–5597. [CrossRef]

11. Ding, G.; Qin, Q.; He, N.; Francis-David, S.C.; Hou, J.; Liu, J.; Ricks, E.; Yang, Q. Adiponectin and its receptors are expressed in adult ventricular cardiomyocytes and upregulated by activation of peroxisome proliferator-activated receptor γ. *J. Mol. Cell. Cardiol.* **2007**, *43*, 73–84. [CrossRef]

12. Guo, Z.; Xia, Z.; Yuen, V.G.; McNeill, J.H. Cardiac expression of adiponectin and its receptors in streptozotocin-induced diabetic rats. *Metabolism* **2007**, *56*, 1363–1371. [CrossRef] [PubMed]

13. Krause, M.P.; Liu, Y.; Vu, V.; Chan, L.; Xu, A.; Riddell, M.C.; Sweeney, G.; Hawke, T.J. Adiponectin is expressed by skeletal muscle fibers and influences muscle phenotype and function. *Am. J. Physiol. Cell Physiol.* **2008**, *295*, C203–C212. [CrossRef] [PubMed]

14. Lan, H.; Rabaglia, M.E.; Stoehr, J.P.; Nadler, S.T.; Schueler, K.L.; Zou, F.; Yandell, B.S.; Attie, A.D. Gene expression profiles of nondiabetic and diabetic obese mice suggest a role of hepatic lipogenic capacity in diabetes susceptibility. *Diabetes* **2003**, *52*, 688–700. [CrossRef]

15. Piñeiro, R.; Iglesias, M.J.; Gallego, R.; Raghay, K.; Eiras, S.; Rubio, J.; Diéguez, C.; Gualillo, O.; González-Juanatey, J.R.; Lago, F. Adiponectin is synthesized and secreted by human and murine cardiomyocytes. *FEBS Lett.* **2005**, *579*, 5163–5169. [CrossRef] [PubMed]

16. Yang, B.; Chen, L.; Qian, Y.; Triantafillou, J.A.; McNulty, J.A.; Carrick, K.; Clifton, L.G.; Han, B.; Geske, R.; Strum, J.; et al. Changes of skeletal muscle adiponectin content in diet-induced insulin resistant rats. *Biochem. Biophys. Res. Commun.* **2006**, *341*, 209–217. [CrossRef] [PubMed]

17. Schäffler, A.; Buechler, C. CTRP family: Linking immunity to metabolism. *Trends Endocrinol. Metab.* **2012**, *23*, 194–204. [CrossRef] [PubMed]

18. Wang, Y.; Xu, A.; Knight, C.; Xu, L.Y.; Cooper, G.J.S. Hydroxylation and glycosylation of the four conserved lysine residues in the collagenous domain of adiponectin. Potential role in the modulation of its insulin-sensitizing activity. *J. Biol. Chem.* **2002**, *277*, 19521–19529. [CrossRef]

19. Schraw, T.; Wang, Z.V.; Halberg, N.; Hawkins, M.; Scherer, P.E. Plasma adiponectin complexes have distinct biochemical characteristics. *Endocrinology* **2008**, *149*, 2270–2282. [CrossRef] [PubMed]

20. Hara, K.; Horikoshi, M.; Yamauchi, T.; Yago, H.; Miyazaki, O.; Ebinuma, H.; Imai, Y.; Nagai, R.; Kadowaki, T. Measurement of the High-Molecular Weight Form of Adiponectin in Plasma Is Useful for the Prediction of Insulin. *Cardiovasc. Metab. Risk* **2006**, *29*, 1357–1362.

21. Peake, P.W.; Kriketos, A.D.; Campbell, L.V.; Shen, Y.; Charlesworth, J.A. The metabolism of isoforms of human adiponectin: Studies in human subjects and in experimental animals. *Eur. J. Endocrinol.* **2005**, *153*, 409–417. [CrossRef] [PubMed]

22. Ma, Z.; Gingerich, R.L.; Santiago, J.V.; Klein, S.; Smith, C.H.; Landt, M. Radioimmunoassay of leptin in human plasma. *Clin. Chem.* **1996**, *42*, 942–946. [PubMed]

23. Maffei, M.; Halaas, J.; Ravussin, E.; Pratley, R.E.; Lee, G.H.; Zhang, Y.; Fei, H.; Kim, S.; Lallone, R.; Ranganathan, S. Leptin levels in human and rodent: Measurement of plasma leptin and ob RNA in obese and weight-reduced subjects. *Nat. Med.* **1995**, *1*, 1155–1161. [CrossRef] [PubMed]

24. Gürlek, A.; Bayraktar, M.; Kirazli, S. Increased plasminogen activator inhibitor-1 activity in offspring of type 2 diabetic patients: Lack of association with plasma insulin levels. *Diabetes Care* **2000**, *23*, 88–92. [CrossRef]

25. Fiaschi, T.; Giannoni, E.; Taddei, M.L.; Chiarugi, P. Globular adiponectin activates motility and regenerative traits of muscle satellite cells. *PLoS ONE* **2012**, *7*, e34782. [CrossRef]

26. Fruebis, J.; Tsao, T.S.; Javorschi, S.; Ebbets-Reed, D.; Erickson, M.R.; Yen, F.T.; Bihain, B.E.; Lodish, H.F. Proteolytic cleavage product of 30-kDa adipocyte complement-related protein increases fatty acid oxidation in muscle and causes weight loss in mice. *Proc. Natl. Acad. Sci. USA* **2001**, *98*, 2005–2010. [CrossRef] [PubMed]

27. Vetvik, K.K.; Sonerud, T.; Lindeberg, M.; Lüders, T.; Størkson, R.H.; Jonsdottir, K.; Frengen, E.; Pietiläinen, K.H.; Bukholm, I. Globular adiponectin and its downstream target genes are up-regulated locally in human colorectal tumors: Ex vivo and in vitro studies. *Metab. Clin. Exp.* **2014**, *63*, 672–681. [CrossRef]

28. Waki, H.; Yamauchi, T.; Kamon, J.; Kita, S.; Ito, Y.; Hada, Y.; Uchida, S.; Tsuchida, A.; Takekawa, S.; Kadowaki, T. Generation of Globular Fragment of Adiponectin by Leukocyte Elastase Secreted by Monocytic Cell Line THP-1. *Endocrinology* **2005**, *146*, 790–796. [CrossRef] [PubMed]

29. Wang, Y.; Lam, K.S.L.; Yau, M.; Xu, A. Post-translational modifications of adiponectin: Mechanisms and functional implications. *Biochem. J.* **2008**, *409*, 623–633. [CrossRef]

30. Zhang, L.; Li, M.-M.; Corcoran, M.; Zhang, S.; Cooper, G.J.S. Essential roles of insulin, AMPK signaling and lysyl and prolyl hydroxylases in the biosynthesis and multimerization of adiponectin. *Mol. Cell. Endocrinol.* **2015**, *399*, 164–177. [CrossRef]

31. Frizzell, N.; Lima, M.; Baynes, J.W. Succination of proteins in diabetes. *Free Radic. Res.* **2011**, *45*, 101–109. [CrossRef] [PubMed]

32. Frizzell, N.; Rajesh, M.; Jepson, M.J.; Nagai, R.; Carson, J.A.; Thorpe, S.R.; Baynes, J.W. Succination of thiol groups in adipose tissue proteins in diabetes: Succination inhibits polymerization and secretion of adiponectin. *J. Biol. Chem.* **2009**, *284*, 25772–25781. [CrossRef] [PubMed]

33. Thomas, S.A.; Storey, K.B.; Baynes, J.W.; Frizzell, N. Tissue Distribution of S-(2-Succino)cysteine (2SC), a Biomarker of Mitochondrial Stress in Obesity and Diabetes. *Obesity* **2012**, *20*, 263–269. [CrossRef] [PubMed]

34. Richards, A.A.; Colgrave, M.L.; Zhang, J.; Webster, J.; Simpson, F.; Preston, E.; Wilks, D.; Hoehn, K.L.; Stephenson, M.; Macdonald, G.A.; et al. Sialic acid modification of adiponectin is not required for multimerization or secretion but determines half-life in circulation. *Mol. Endocrinol.* **2010**, *24*, 229–239. [CrossRef]

35. Simpson, F.; Whitehead, J.P. Adiponectin—It's all about the modifications. *Int. J. Biochem. Cell Biol.* **2010**, *42*, 785–788. [CrossRef]

36. Gamble, K.L.; Berry, R.; Frank, S.J.; Young, M.E. Circadian clock control of endocrine factors. *Nat. Rev. Endocrinol.* **2014**, *10*, 466–475. [CrossRef]

37. Garaulet, M.; Ordovás, J.M.; Gómez-Abellán, P.; Martínez, J.A.; Madrid, J.A. An approximation to the temporal order in endogenous circadian rhythms of genes implicated in human adipose tissue metabolism. *J. Cell. Physiol.* **2011**, *226*, 2075–2080. [CrossRef] [PubMed]

38. Barnea, M.; Madar, Z.; Froy, O. High-fat diet followed by fasting disrupts circadian expression of adiponectin signaling pathway in muscle and adipose tissue. *Obesity* **2010**, *18*, 230–238. [CrossRef] [PubMed]

39. Ando, H.; Yanagihara, H.; Hayashi, Y.; Obi, Y.; Tsuruoka, S.; Takamura, T.; Kaneko, S.; Fujimura, A. Rhythmic messenger ribonucleic acid expression of clock genes and adipocytokines in mouse visceral adipose tissue. *Endocrinology* **2005**, *146*, 5631–5636. [CrossRef]

40. Kennaway, D.J.; Owens, J.A.; Voultsios, A.; Wight, N. Adipokines and adipocyte function in Clock mutant mice that retain melatonin rhythmicity. *Obesity* **2012**, *20*, 295–305. [CrossRef]

41. Kennaway, D.J.; Varcoe, T.J.; Voultsios, A.; Boden, M.J. Global loss of bmal1 expression alters adipose tissue hormones, gene expression and glucose metabolism. *PLoS ONE* **2013**, *8*, e65255. [CrossRef] [PubMed]

42. Dankel, S.N.; Degerud, E.M.; Borkowski, K.; Fjære, E.; Midtbø, L.K.; Haugen, C.; Solsvik, M.H.; Lavigne, A.M.; Liaset, B.; Sagen, J.V.; et al. Weight cycling promotes fat gain and altered clock gene expression in adipose tissue in C57BL/6J mice. *Am. J. Physiol. Endocrinol. Metab.* **2014**, *306*, E210–E224. [CrossRef] [PubMed]

43. Iwabu, M.; Yamauchi, T.; Okada-Iwabu, M.; Sato, K.; Nakagawa, T.; Funata, M.; Yamaguchi, M.; Namiki, S.; Nakayama, R.; Tabata, M.; et al. Adiponectin and AdipoR1 regulate PGC-1alpha and mitochondria by Ca(2+) and AMPK/SIRT1. *Nature* **2010**, *464*, 1313–1319. [CrossRef] [PubMed]

44. Hioki, M.; Kanehira, N.; Koike, T.; Saito, A.; Takahashi, H.; Shimaoka, K.; Sakakibara, H.; Oshida, Y.; Akima, H. Associations of intramyocellular lipid in vastus lateralis and biceps femoris with blood free fatty acid and muscle strength differ between young and elderly adults. *Clin. Physiol. Funct. Imaging* **2016**, *36*, 457–463. [CrossRef] [PubMed]

45. Zhou, L.; Deepa, S.S.; Etzler, J.C.; Ryu, J.; Mao, X.; Fang, Q.; Liu, D.D.; Torres, J.M.; Jia, W.; Lechleiter, J.D.; et al. Adiponectin Activates AMP-activated Protein Kinase in Muscle Cells via APPL1/LKB1-dependent and Phospholipase C/Ca^{2+}/Ca^{2+}/Calmodulin-dependent Protein Kinase Kinase-dependent Pathways. *J. Biol. Chem.* **2009**, *284*, 22426–22435. [CrossRef]

46. Berchtold, M.W.; Brinkmeier, H.; Müntener, M. Calcium ion in skeletal muscle: Its crucial role for muscle function, plasticity, and disease. *Physiol. Rev.* **2000**, *80*, 1215–1265. [CrossRef]

47. Yan, W.; Zhang, F.; Zhang, R.; Zhang, X.; Wang, Y.; Zhou, F.; Xia, Y.; Liu, P.; Gao, C.; Wang, H.; et al. Adiponectin regulates SR Ca(2+) cycling following ischemia/reperfusion via sphingosine 1-phosphate-CaMKII signaling in mice. *J. Mol. Cell. Cardiol.* **2014**, *74*, 183–192. [CrossRef]

48. Krause, M.P.; Riddell, M.C.; Hawke, T.J. Effects of type 1 diabetes mellitus on skeletal muscle: Clinical observations and physiological mechanisms. *Pediatr. Diabetes* **2011**, *12*, 345–364. [CrossRef]

49. Shortreed, K.E.; Krause, M.P.; Huang, J.H.; Dhanani, D.; Moradi, J.; Ceddia, R.B.; Hawke, T.J. Muscle-specific adaptations, impaired oxidative capacity and maintenance of contractile function characterize diet-induced obese mouse skeletal muscle. *PLoS ONE* **2009**, *4*, e7293. [CrossRef]

50. Tallis, J.; James, R.S.; Seebacher, F. The effects of obesity on skeletal muscle contractile function. *J. Exp. Biol.* **2018**, *221*, jeb163840. [CrossRef]

51. Safwat, Y.; Yassin, N.; Gamal El Din, M.; Kassem, L. Modulation of skeletal muscle performance and SERCA by exercise and adiponectin gene therapy in insulin-resistant rat. *DNA Cell Biol.* **2013**, *32*, 378–385. [CrossRef]

52. Fiaschi, T.; Cirelli, D.; Comito, G.; Gelmini, S.; Ramponi, G.; Serio, M.; Chiarugi, P. Globular adiponectin induces differentiation and fusion of skeletal muscle cells. *Cell Res.* **2009**, *19*, 584–597. [CrossRef]

53. Fiaschi, T.; Tedesco, F.S.; Giannoni, E.; Diaz-Manera, J.; Parri, M.; Cossu, G.; Chiarugi, P. Globular adiponectin as a complete mesoangioblast regulator: Role in proliferation, survival, motility, and skeletal muscle differentiation. *Mol. Biol. Cell* **2010**, *21*, 848–859. [CrossRef]

54. Gamberi, T.; Modesti, A.; Magherini, F.; D'Souza, D.M.; Hawke, T.; Fiaschi, T. Activation of autophagy by globular adiponectin is required for muscle differentiation. *Biochim. Biophys. Acta* **2016**, *1863*, 694–702. [CrossRef] [PubMed]

55. Goto, A.; Ohno, Y.; Ikuta, A.; Suzuki, M.; Ohira, T.; Egawa, T.; Sugiura, T.; Yoshioka, T.; Ohira, Y.; Goto, K. Up-Regulation of Adiponectin Expression in Antigravitational Soleus Muscle in Response to Unloading Followed by Reloading, and Functional Overloading in Mice. *PLoS ONE* **2013**, *8*, e81929. [CrossRef] [PubMed]

56. Inoue, A.; Cheng, X.W.; Huang, Z.; Hu, L.; Kikuchi, R.; Jiang, H.; Piao, L.; Sasaki, T.; Itakura, K.; Wu, H.; et al. Exercise restores muscle stem cell mobilization, regenerative capacity and muscle metabolic alterations via adiponectin/AdipoR1 activation in SAMP10 mice. *J. Cachexia Sarcopenia Muscle* **2017**, *8*, 370–385. [CrossRef]

57. Singh, A.K.; Shree, S.; Chattopadhyay, S.; Kumar, S.; Gurjar, A.; Kushwaha, S.; Kumar, H.; Trivedi, A.K.; Chattopadhyay, N.; Maurya, R.; et al. Small molecule adiponectin receptor agonist GTDF protects against skeletal muscle atrophy. *Mol. Cell. Endocrinol.* **2017**, *439*, 273–285. [CrossRef] [PubMed]

58. Tanaka, Y.; Kita, S.; Nishizawa, H.; Fukuda, S.; Fujishima, Y.; Obata, Y.; Nagao, H.; Masuda, S.; Nakamura, Y.; Shimizu, Y.; et al. Adiponectin promotes muscle regeneration through binding to T-cadherin. *Sci. Rep.* **2019**, *9*, 16. [CrossRef] [PubMed]

59. Jiang, H.; Yang, F.; Lin, T.; Shao, W.; Meng, Y.; Ma, J.; Wang, C.; Gao, R.; Zhou, X. Asymmetric expression of H19 and ADIPOQ in concave/convex paravertebral muscles is associated with severe adolescent idiopathic scoliosis. *Mol. Med.* **2018**, *24*, 48. [CrossRef] [PubMed]

60. Can, B.; Kara, O.; Kizilarslanoglu, M.C.; Arik, G.; Aycicek, G.S.; Sumer, F.; Civelek, R.; Demirtas, C.; Ulger, Z. Serum markers of inflammation and oxidative stress in sarcopenia. *Aging Clin. Exp. Res.* **2017**, *29*, 745–752. [CrossRef] [PubMed]

61. Ito, R.; Higa, M.; Goto, A.; Aoshima, M.; Ikuta, A.; Ohashi, K.; Yokoyama, S.; Ohno, Y.; Egawa, T.; Miyata, H.; et al. Activation of adiponectin receptors has negative impact on muscle mass in C2C12 myotubes and fast-type mouse skeletal muscle. *PLoS ONE* **2018**, *13*, e0205645. [CrossRef]

62. Harada, H.; Kai, H.; Shibata, R.; Niiyama, H.; Nishiyama, Y.; Murohara, T.; Yoshida, N.; Katoh, A.; Ikeda, H. New diagnostic index for sarcopenia in patients with cardiovascular diseases. *PLoS ONE* **2017**, *12*, e0178123. [CrossRef]

63. Huang, C.; Tomata, Y.; Kakizaki, M.; Sugawara, Y.; Hozawa, A.; Momma, H.; Tsuji, I.; Nagatomi, R. High circulating adiponectin levels predict decreased muscle strength among older adults aged 70 years and over: A prospective cohort study. *Nutr. Metab. Cardiovasc. Dis.* **2015**, *25*, 594–601. [CrossRef] [PubMed]

64. Karvonen-Gutierrez, C.A.; Zheng, H.; Mancuso, P.; Harlow, S.D. Higher Leptin and Adiponectin Concentrations Predict Poorer Performance-based Physical Functioning in Midlife Women: The Michigan Study of Women's Health across the Nation. *J. Gerontol. A Biol. Sci. Med. Sci.* **2016**, *71*, 508–514. [CrossRef]

65. Loncar, G.; Bozic, B.; von Haehling, S.; Düngen, H.-D.; Prodanovic, N.; Lainscak, M.; Arandjelovic, A.; Dimkovic, S.; Radojicic, Z.; Popovic, V. Association of adiponectin with peripheral muscle status in elderly patients with heart failure. *Eur. J. Intern. Med.* **2013**, *24*, 818–823. [CrossRef] [PubMed]

66. Nakatsuji, H.; Araki, A.; Hashizume, A.; Hijikata, Y.; Yamada, S.; Inagaki, T.; Suzuki, K.; Banno, H.; Suga, N.; Okada, Y.; et al. Correlation of insulin resistance and motor function in spinal and bulbar muscular atrophy. *J. Neurol.* **2017**, *264*, 839–847. [CrossRef]

67. Okada-Iwabu, M.; Yamauchi, T.; Iwabu, M.; Honma, T.; Hamagami, K.; Matsuda, K.; Yamaguchi, M.; Tanabe, H.; Kimura-Someya, T.; Shirouzu, M.; et al. A small-molecule AdipoR agonist for type 2 diabetes and short life in obesity. *Nature* **2013**, *503*, 493–499. [CrossRef] [PubMed]
68. Yamauchi, T.; Iwabu, M.; Okada-Iwabu, M.; Kadowaki, T. Adiponectin receptors: A review of their structure, function and how they work. *Best Pract. Res. Clin. Endocrinol. Metab.* **2014**, *28*, 15–23. [CrossRef]
69. Rennie, M.J.; Wackerhage, H.; Spangenburg, E.E.; Booth, F.W. Control of the size of the human muscle mass. *Annu. Rev. Physiol.* **2004**, *66*, 799–828. [CrossRef] [PubMed]
70. Maden, M.; Brant, J.O.; Rubiano, A.; Sandoval, A.G.W.; Simmons, C.; Mitchell, R.; Collin-Hooper, H.; Jacobson, J.; Omairi, S.; Patel, K. Perfect chronic skeletal muscle regeneration in adult spiny mice, Acomys cahirinus. *Sci. Rep.* **2018**, *8*, 8920. [CrossRef] [PubMed]
71. Liu, Y.; Sweeney, G. Adiponectin action in skeletal muscle. *Best Pract. Res. Clin. Endocrinol. Metab.* **2014**, *28*, 33–41. [CrossRef] [PubMed]
72. Asp, M.L.; Tian, M.; Wendel, A.A.; Belury, M.A. Evidence for the contribution of insulin resistance to the development of cachexia in tumor-bearing mice. *Int. J. Cancer* **2010**, *126*, 756–763. [CrossRef] [PubMed]
73. Shibata, R.; Sato, K.; Pimentel, D.R.; Takemura, Y.; Kihara, S.; Ohashi, K.; Funahashi, T.; Ouchi, N.; Walsh, K. Adiponectin protects against myocardial ischemia-reperfusion injury through AMPK- and COX-2-dependent mechanisms. *Nat. Med.* **2005**, *11*, 1096–1103. [CrossRef] [PubMed]
74. Abou-Samra, M.; Boursereau, R.; Lecompte, S.; Noel, L.; Brichard, S.M. Potential Therapeutic Action of Adiponectin in Duchenne Muscular Dystrophy. *Am. J. Pathol.* **2017**, *187*, 1577–1585. [CrossRef]
75. Abou-Samra, M.; Lecompte, S.; Schakman, O.; Noel, L.; Many, M.C.; Gailly, P.; Brichard, S.M. Involvement of adiponectin in the pathogenesis of dystrophinopathy. *Skelet. Muscle* **2015**, *5*, 25. [CrossRef]
76. Boursereau, R.; Abou-Samra, M.; Lecompte, S.; Noel, L.; Brichard, S.M. Downregulation of the NLRP3 inflammasome by adiponectin rescues Duchenne muscular dystrophy. *BMC Biol.* **2018**, *16*, 33. [CrossRef]
77. Lecompte, S.; Abou-Samra, M.; Boursereau, R.; Noel, L.; Brichard, S.M. Skeletal muscle secretome in Duchenne muscular dystrophy: A pivotal anti-inflammatory role of adiponectin. *Cell. Mol. Life Sci.* **2017**, *74*, 2487–2501. [CrossRef] [PubMed]
78. Ahlstrom, P.; Rai, E.; Chakma, S.; Cho, H.H.; Rengasamy, P.; Sweeney, G. Adiponectin improves insulin sensitivity via activation of autophagic flux. *J. Mol. Endocrinol.* **2017**, *59*, 339–350. [CrossRef]
79. Liu, Y.; Palanivel, R.; Rai, E.; Park, M.; Gabor, T.V.; Scheid, M.P.; Xu, A.; Sweeney, G. Adiponectin stimulates autophagy and reduces oxidative stress to enhance insulin sensitivity during high-fat diet feeding in mice. *Diabetes* **2015**, *64*, 36–48. [CrossRef]
80. Singh, A.K.; Joharapurkar, A.A.; Khan, M.P.; Mishra, J.S.; Singh, N.; Yadav, M.; Hossain, Z.; Khan, K.; Kumar, S.; Dhanesha, N.A.; et al. Orally Active Osteoanabolic Agent GTDF Binds to Adiponectin Receptors, with a Preference for AdipoR1, Induces Adiponectin-Associated Signaling, and Improves Metabolic Health in a Rodent Model of Diabetes. *Diabetes* **2014**, *63*, 3530–3544. [CrossRef]
81. Holland, W.L.; Scherer, P.E. Ronning after the Adiponectin Receptors. *Science* **2013**, *342*, 1460–1461. [CrossRef]
82. Otani, M.; Furukawa, S.; Wakisaka, S.; Maeda, T. A novel adipokine C1q/TNF-related protein 3 is expressed in developing skeletal muscle and controls myoblast proliferation and differentiation. *Mol. Cell. Biochem.* **2015**, *409*, 271–282. [CrossRef]
83. Cnop, M.; Havel, P.J.; Utzschneider, K.M.; Carr, D.B.; Sinha, M.K.; Boyko, E.J.; Retzlaff, B.M. Relationship of adiponectin to body fat distribution, insulin sensitivity and plasma lipoproteins: Evidence for independent roles of age and sex. *Diabetologia* **2003**, *46*, 459–469. [CrossRef]
84. Böttner, A.; Kratzsch, J.; Müller, G.; Kapellen, T.M.; Blüher, S.; Keller, E.; Blüher, M.; Kiess, W.; Kratzsch, R.; Mu, G.; et al. Gender differences of adiponectin levels develop during the progression of puberty and are related to serum androgen levels. *J. Clin. Endocrinol. Metab.* **2004**, *89*, 4053–4061. [CrossRef]
85. Woo, J.G.; Dolan, L.M.; Daniels, S.R.; Goodman, E.; Martin, L.J. Adolescent sex differences in adiponectin are conditional on pubertal development and adiposity. *Obes. Res.* **2005**, *13*, 2095–2101. [CrossRef]
86. Spranger, J.; Kroke, A.; Möhlig, M.; Bergmann, M.M.; Ristow, M.; Boeing, H.; Pfeiffer, A.F. Adiponectin and Protection Against Type 2 Diabetes Mellitus. *Lancet* **2003**, *361*, 226–228. [CrossRef]
87. Li, S.; Shin, H.J.; Ding, E.L.; van Dam, R.M. Adiponectin Levels and Risk of Type 2 Diabetes. *JAMA* **2009**, *302*, 179–188. [CrossRef]

88. Ouchi, N.; Kihara, S.; Arita, Y.; Maeda, K.; Kuriyama, H.; Okamoto, Y.; Hotta, K.; Nishida, M.; Takahashi, M.; Nakamura, T.; et al. Novel modulator for endothelial adhesion molecules: Adipocyte-derived plasma protein adiponectin. *Circulation* **1999**, *100*, 2473–2476. [CrossRef] [PubMed]

89. Arita, Y.; Kihara, S.; Ouchi, N.; Takahashi, M.; Maeda, K.; Miyagawa, J.I.; Hotta, K.; Shimomura, I.; Nakamura, T.; Miyaoka, K.; et al. Paradoxical decrease of an adipose-specific protein, adiponectin, in obesity. *Biochem. Biophys. Res. Commun.* **1999**, *257*, 79–83. [CrossRef] [PubMed]

90. Saunders, T.J.; Palombella, A.; McGuire, K.A.; Janiszewski, P.M.; Després, J.-P.; Ross, R. Acute exercise increases adiponectin levels in abdominally obese men. *J. Nutr. Metab.* **2012**, *2012*, 148729. [CrossRef]

91. Pischon, T.; Girman, C.J.; Hotamisligil, G.S.; Rifai, N.; Hu, F.B.; Rimm, E.B. Plasma Adiponectin Levels and Risk of Myocardial Infarction in Men. *JAMA* **2004**, *291*, 1730–1737. [CrossRef] [PubMed]

92. Mantzoros, C.; Petridou, E.; Dessypris, N.; Chavelas, C.; Dalamaga, M.; Alexe, D.M.; Papadiamantis, Y.; Markopoulos, C.; Spanos, E.; Chrousos, G.; et al. Adiponectin and breast cancer risk. *J. Clin. Endocrinol. Metab.* **2004**, *89*, 1102–1107. [CrossRef] [PubMed]

93. Lakka, T.A.; Laaksonen, D.E.; Lakka, H.M.; Männikkö, N.; Niskanen, L.K.; Rauramaa, R.; Salonen, J.T. Sedentary lifestyle, poor cardiorespiratory fitness, and the metabolic syndrome. *Med. Sci. Sports Exerc.* **2003**, *35*, 1279–1286. [CrossRef] [PubMed]

94. Seyedmehdi, S.M.; Attarchi, M.; Cherati, A.S.; Hajsadeghi, S.; Tofighi, R.; Jamaati, H. Relationship of aerobic fitness with cardiovascular risk factors in firefighters. *Work* **2016**, *55*, 155–161. [CrossRef] [PubMed]

95. de Carvalho, F.P.; Moretto, T.L.; Benfato, I.D.; Barthichoto, M.; Ferreira, S.M.; Costa-Júnior, J.M.; de Oliveira, C.A.M. Central and peripheral effects of physical exercise without weight reduction in obese and lean mice. *Biosci. Rep.* **2018**, *38*, BSR20171033. [CrossRef]

96. Martinez-Huenchullan, S.F.; Maharjan, B.R.; Williams, P.F.; Tam, C.S.; Mclennan, S.V.; Twigg, S.M. Differential metabolic effects of constant moderate versus high intensity interval training in high-fat fed mice: Possible role of muscle adiponectin. *Physiol. Rep.* **2018**, *6*, e13599. [CrossRef]

97. Hayashino, Y.; Jackson, J.L.; Hirata, T.; Fukumori, N.; Nakamura, F.; Fukuhara, S.; Tsujii, S.; Ishii, H. Effects of exercise on C-reactive protein, inflammatory cytokine and adipokine in patients with type 2 diabetes: A meta-analysis of randomized controlled trials. *Metab. Clin. Exp.* **2014**, *63*, 431–440. [CrossRef]

98. Simpson, K.A.; Singh, M.A.F. Effects of exercise on adiponectin: A systematic review. *Obesity* **2008**, *16*, 241–256. [CrossRef]

99. Wiecek, M.; Szymura, J.; Maciejczyk, M.; Kantorowicz, M.; Szygula, Z. Acute Anaerobic Exercise Affects the Secretion of Asprosin, Irisin, and Other Cytokines—A Comparison Between Sexes. *Front. Physiol.* **2018**, *9*, 1782. [CrossRef] [PubMed]

100. Vardar, S.A.; Karaca, A.; Güldiken, S.; Palabıyık, O.; Süt, N.; Demir, A.M. High-intensity interval training acutely alters plasma adipokine levels in young overweight/obese women. *Arch. Physiol. Biochem.* **2018**, *124*, 149–155. [CrossRef] [PubMed]

101. Goto, K.; Shioda, K.; Uchida, S. Effect of 2 days of intensive resistance training on appetite-related hormone and anabolic hormone responses. *Clin. Physiol. Funct. Imaging* **2013**, *33*, 131–136. [CrossRef]

102. Markofski, M.M.; Carrillo, A.E.; Timmerman, K.L.; Jennings, K.; Coen, P.M.; Pence, B.D.; Flynn, M.G. Exercise training modifies ghrelin and adiponectin concentrations and is related to inflammation in older adults. *J. Gerontol. Ser. A Biol. Sci. Med. Sci.* **2014**, *69*, 675–681. [CrossRef] [PubMed]

103. Gastebois, C.; Villars, C.; Drai, J.; Canet-Soulas, E.; Blanc, S.; Bergouignan, A.; Lefai, E.; Simon, C. Effects of training and detraining on adiponectin plasma concentration and muscle sensitivity in lean and overweight men. *Eur. J. Appl. Physiol.* **2016**, *116*, 2135–2144. [CrossRef] [PubMed]

104. Gondim, O.S.; De Camargo, V.T.N.; Gutierrez, F.A.; De Oliveira Martins, P.F.; Passos, M.E.P.; Momesso, C.M.; Santos, V.C.; Gorjão, R.; Pithon-Curi, T.C.; Cury-Boaventura, M.F. Benefits of regular exercise on inflammatory and cardiovascular risk markers in normal weight, overweight and obese adults. *PLoS ONE* **2015**, *10*, e0140596. [CrossRef]

105. Balducci, S.; Zanuso, S.; Nicolucci, A.; Fernando, F.; Cavallo, S.; Cardelli, P.; Fallucca, S.; Alessi, E.; Letizia, C.; Jimenez, A.; et al. Anti-inflammatory effect of exercise training in subjects with type 2 diabetes and the metabolic syndrome is dependent on exercise modalities and independent of weight loss. *Nutr. Metab. Cardiovasc. Dis.* **2010**, *20*, 608–617. [CrossRef] [PubMed]

106. Beavers, K.M.; Ambrosius, W.T.; Nicklas, B.J.; Rejeski, W.J. Independent and combined effects of physical activity and weight loss on inflammatory biomarkers in overweight and obese older adults. *J. Am. Geriatr. Soc.* **2013**, *61*, 1089–1094. [CrossRef]

107. Christiansen, T.; Paulsen, S.K.; Bruun, J.M.; Pedersen, S.B.; Richelsen, B. Exercise training versus diet-induced weight-loss on metabolic risk factors and inflammatory markers in obese subjects: A 12-week randomized intervention study. *AJP Endocrinol. Metab.* **2010**, *298*, E824–E831. [CrossRef] [PubMed]

108. Baghaiee, B.; Karimi, P.; Ebrahimi, K.; Dabagh Nikoo kheslat, S.; Sadeghi Zali, M.H.; Daneshian Moghaddam, A.M.; Sadaghian, M. Effects of a 12-week aerobic exercise on markers of hypertension in men. *J. Cardiovasc. Thorac. Res.* **2018**, *10*, 162–168. [CrossRef] [PubMed]

109. Alessa, H.B.; Chomistek, A.K.; Hankinson, S.E.; Barnett, J.B.; Rood, J.; Matthews, C.E.; Rimm, E.B.; Willett, W.C.; Hu, F.B.; Tobias, D.K. Objective Measures of Physical Activity and Cardiometabolic and Endocrine Biomarkers. *Med. Sci. Sports Exerc.* **2017**, *49*, 1817–1825. [CrossRef] [PubMed]

110. Steene-Johannessen, J.; Kolle, E.; Andersen, L.B.; Anderssen, S.A. Adiposity, aerobic fitness, muscle fitness, and markers of inflammation in children. *Med. Sci. Sports Exerc.* **2013**, *45*, 714–721. [CrossRef] [PubMed]

111. Nishida, Y.; Higaki, Y.; Taguchi, N.; Hara, M.; Nakamura, K.; Nanri, H.; Imaizumi, T.; Sakamoto, T.; Shimanoe, C.; Horita, M.; et al. Intensity-Specific and Modified Effects of Physical Activity on Serum Adiponectin in a Middle-Aged Population. *J. Endocr. Soc.* **2019**, *3*, 13–26. [CrossRef]

112. Yamamoto, S.; Matsushita, Y.; Nakagawa, T.; Hayashi, T.; Noda, M.; Mizoue, T. Circulating adiponectin levels and risk of type 2 diabetes in the Japanese. *Nutr. Diabetes* **2014**, *4*, e130–e135. [CrossRef] [PubMed]

113. Bajaj, M.; Suraamornkul, S.; Piper, P.; Hardies, L.J.; Glass, L.; Cersosimo, E.; Pratipanawatr, T.; Miyazaki, Y.; Defronzo, R.A. Decreased Plasma Adiponectin Concentrations Are Closely Related to Hepatic Fat Content and Hepatic Insulin Resistance in Pioglitazone-Treated Type 2 Diabetic Patients. *J. Clin. Endocrinol. Metab.* **2004**, *89*, 200–206. [CrossRef] [PubMed]

114. Punyadeera, C.; Zorenc, A.H.G.; Koopman, R.; McAinch, A.J.; Smit, E.; Manders, R.; Keizer, H.A.; Cameron-Smith, D.; van Loon, L.J.C. The effects of exercise and adipose tissue lipolysis on plasma adiponectin concentration and adiponectin receptor expression in human skeletal muscle. *Eur. J. Endocrinol.* **2005**, *152*, 427–436. [CrossRef] [PubMed]

115. Bajaj, M.; Suraamornkul, S.; Kashyap, S.; Cusi, K.; Mandarino, L.; DeFronzo, R.A. Sustained reduction in plasma free fatty acid concentration improves insulin action without altering plasma adipocytokine levels in subjects with strong family history of type 2 diabetes. *J. Clin. Endocrinol. Metab.* **2004**, *89*, 4649–4655. [CrossRef]

116. Blüher, M.; Bullen, J.W.; Lee, J.H.; Kralisch, S.; Fasshauer, M.; Klöting, N.; Niebauer, J.; Schön, M.R.; Williams, C.J.; Mantzoros, C.S. Circulating adiponectin and expression of adiponectin receptors in human skeletal muscle: Associations with metabolic parameters and insulin resistance and regulation by physical training. *J. Clin. Endocrinol. Metab.* **2006**, *91*, 2310–2316. [CrossRef] [PubMed]

117. Martinez-Huenchullan, S.F.; Maharjan, B.R.; Williams, P.F.; Tam, C.S.; Mclennan, S.V.; Twigg, S.M. Skeletal muscle adiponectin induction depends on diet, muscle type/activity, and exercise modality in C57BL/6 mice. *Physiol. Rep.* **2018**, *6*, e13848. [CrossRef] [PubMed]

118. Cho, J.; Koh, Y.; Han, J.; Kim, D.; Kim, T.; Kang, H. Adiponectin mediates the additive effects of combining daily exercise with caloric restriction for treatment of non-alcoholic fatty liver. *Int. J. Obes.* **2016**, *40*, 1760–1767. [CrossRef]

119. Ritchie, I.R.W.; MacDonald, T.L.; Wright, D.C.; Dyck, D.J. Adiponectin is sufficient, but not required, for exercise-induced increases in the expression of skeletal muscle mitochondrial enzymes. *J. Physiol.* **2014**, *592*, 2653–2665. [CrossRef]

120. Ritchie, I.R.W.; Wright, D.C.; Dyck, D.J. Adiponectin is not required for exercise training-induced improvements in glucose and insulin tolerance in mice. *Physiol. Rep.* **2014**, *2*, e12146. [CrossRef]

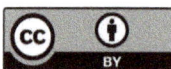

International Journal of
Molecular Sciences

MDPI

Review

Adiponectin in Myopathies

Tania Gamberi, Francesca Magherini and Tania Fiaschi *

Dipartimento di scienze Biomediche, Sperimentali e Cliniche "M. Serio", Università degli studi di Firenze, Viale Morgagni 50, 50134 Firenze, Italy; tania.gamberi@unifi.it (T.G.); francesca.magherini@unifi.it (F.M.)
* Correspondence: tania.fiaschi@unifi.it; Tel.: +39-055-275-1233

Received: 1 March 2019; Accepted: 26 March 2019; Published: 27 March 2019

Abstract: In skeletal muscle, adiponectin has varied and pleiotropic functions, ranging from metabolic, anti-inflammatory, insulin-sensitizing to regenerative roles. Despite the important functions exerted by adiponectin, the study of the hormone in myopathies is still marginal. Myopathies include inherited and non-inherited/acquired neuromuscular pathologies characterized by muscular degeneration and weakness. This review reports current knowledge about adiponectin in myopathies, regarding in particular the role of adiponectin in some hereditary myopathies (as Duchenne muscular dystrophy) and non-inherited/acquired myopathies (such as idiopathic inflammatory myopathies and fibromyalgia). These studies show that some myopathies are characterized by decreased concentration of plasma adiponectin and that hormone replenishment induces beneficial effects in the diseased muscles. Overall, these findings suggest that adiponectin could constitute a future new therapeutic approach for the improvement of the abnormalities caused by myopathies.

Keywords: adiponectin; muscle; myopathies

---

1. Introduction

1.1. Adiponectin in Skeletal Muscle

In skeletal muscle, adiponectin exerts several and pleiotropic biological effects, including the involvement in cellular metabolism that has been immediately evident since its discovery [1]. Adiponectin is mainly produced by adipose tissue as "full-length" (fAd) form, which can associate to form complexes circulating in the plasma. Circulating adiponectin oligomers comprise High Molecular Weight (HMW), Medium Molecular Weight (MMW), and Low Molecular Weight (LMW) forms [2]. fAd can be enzymatically cleaved to the smaller "globular form" (gAd) by the elastase produced by monocytes [3] or macrophages [4]. Skeletal muscle expresses two unusual, seven-transmembrane-spanning, and G-protein-independent adiponectin receptors, AdipoR1 and AdipoR2 [1]. The metabolic effects of adiponectin occur through the activation of intracellular signalling pathways initiated by the binding with the adiponectin receptors of the adaptor protein containing pleckstrin homology domain, phosphotyrosine binding domain, and leucine zipper domain (APPL1) [5]. APPL1 plays a crucial role in adiponectin-mediated effects, as the recruitment of glucose transporter GLUT4 to the plasma membrane [6] and the activation of AMP kinase (AMPK) [7]. Full AMPK activation occurs through both phosphorylation by liver kinase B1 (LKB1) and AMP binding [8]. In skeletal muscle, AMPK induces the inhibitory phosphorylation of Acetyl-CoA carboxylase (ACC), leading to decreased formation of malonyl CoA [9], activation of oxidation, and inhibition of fatty acid synthesis [9]. Moreover, adiponectin-dependent fatty acid oxidation in skeletal muscle occurs also through the activation of p38 MAPK and PPARα signalling pathways [10]. In addition, adiponectin regulates mitochondrial biogenesis through the binding with AdipoR1. This event leads to the activation and increased expression of peroxisome proliferator-activated receptor gamma coactivator 1-alpha (PGC-1α), which promotes mitochondrial biogenesis, the increase of oxidative metabolism, and formation of type I myofibers [11].

In skeletal muscle, adiponectin exerts an insulin-sensitizing role in which the decreased intracellular lipid content induced by the hormone is deeply involved [12]. Among the several types of lipids, elevated intracellular levels of ceramide have been reported to have cellular deleterious effects and greatly contribute to insulin resistance [13–15]. Adiponectin decreases intracellular ceramide content through the activation of ceramidase activity associated to AdipoR1/AdipoR2. Ceramide is then converted in sphingosine, which, in turn, became phosphorylated to sphingosine 1-phosphate (S1P) due to sphingosine kinase. Sphingosine and S1P are involved in PPARα and AMPK activation, respectively, thus leading to lipid oxidation, mitochondrial biogenesis, and glucose utilization [15–17]. This mechanism has been suggested to be involved in insulin sensitivity, since it decreases cellular availability of sphingolipid precursors and therefore enhances insulin signalling due to reduced ceramide content [17]. In addition, the sphingolipid-mediated pathway, involving probably ceramidase activity, has been reported to be involved in blocking apoptosis in cardiomyocytes [17].

1.2. Adiponectin Is a Myokine and a Myogenic Factor

Alongside adipose tissue, which secretes in the blood stream endocrine adiponectin through a largely elucidated molecular mechanism [18–20], a local secretion of the hormone has been reported by several tissues [21], including skeletal muscle. Several papers described skeletal muscle as secretory organ [22,23] able to locally secrete adiponectin [4,24–27]. In skeletal muscle, myotubes enhance the secretion of fAd in inflamed or pro-oxidant microenvironment [26,27] that is generated by a trauma. This condition could lead to the recruitment of macrophage which participate to the cleavage of fAd into gAd [4].

Besides the metabolic and insulin-sensitizing role, adiponectin acts as a myogenic factor through the participation in muscle differentiation and tissue regeneration, and influencing the behavior of muscle cells. Adiponectin acts on satellite cells, a population of stem cells involved in muscle regeneration in adult skeletal muscles, which undergo activation following trauma [28]. Adiponectin promotes satellite cell activation through the activation of the p38 MAPK signalling cascade [4]. In addition, adiponectin induces the expression of the transcription factors Snail and Twist, responsible for the activation of a motile program, thus permitting satellite cells to reach the site of damage. Cell motility induced by adiponectin involves the enhancement of metalloproteinase-2 secretion, thus facilitating the arrival of satellite cells to damaged site by degrading extracellular matrix [4]. In vitro, adiponectin acts as a myogenic factor both in myoblasts and in mesoangioblasts. In myoblasts, adiponectin induces the exit of cells from cell cycle and promotes myotubes formation [27]. We reported that adiponectin in myoblasts activates autophagy and that this autophagic process is strictly associated with the myogenic role of the hormone. Indeed, the inhibition of autophagy leads to the impairment of myotube formation due to adiponectin. These in vitro results were confirmed on adiponectin-KO mice, that showed decreased autophagy markers in skeletal muscle and a myopathic phenotype, thus demonstrating a close correlation between activation of autophagy and the differentiating role of adiponectin in skeletal muscle [29]. In addition to the role on resident muscle cells, as satellite cells and myoblasts, adiponectin also acts on the non-resident muscle precursors, mesoangioblasts [30]. These are multipotent cells capable of differentiation towards myogenic lineage and that gave promising results in gene therapy for the treatment of Duchenne muscular dystrophy [31,32]. Where mesoangioblasts are concerned, adiponectin affects in vitro several cellular features as the increased mesoangioblast migration towards myotubes, the enhancement of cell survival upon growth factor withdrawal or extracellular matrix detachment and promotes myogenesis [33]. The ex vivo treatment of mesoangioblasts with adiponectin and the following injection of treated cells into dystrophic muscles of sarcoglycan-null mice ameliorates in vivo mesoangioblast survival and improves their engraftment in the diseased muscles [33].

Decreased plasma adiponectin levels have been associated to different pathologies, including obesity and type 2 diabetes [34–36]. Obesity induced endoplasmic reticulum stress and impaired unfolded protein response in adipocytes, and both mechanisms seem to be responsible for the diminished adiponectin secretion in obese mice [37,38]. Hypoadiponectinemia alters several functions of skeletal muscle, such as glucose and lipid metabolism and muscle regeneration [39,40]. Indeed, obese mice display diminished regenerative capacity of skeletal muscle following injury, probably due to a reduced macrophage recruitment and angiogenesis [39], increased lipid accumulation and pro-inflammatory cytokines, and impaired satellite cell activity [40].

2. Adiponectin in Myopathies

Although the key role of adiponectin in healthy skeletal muscle has been well established, the study of the hormone in myopathies is just getting started. Myopathies refer to neuromuscular disorders of skeletal muscles characterized by muscular degeneration and weakness. Myopathies may be classified into two main categories: inherited and non-inherited/acquired myopathies. Inherited myopathies include muscular dystrophies, congenital myopathies, mitochondrial myopathies, and metabolic myopathies. Non inherited/acquired myopathies comprise inflammatory myopathies, toxic myopathies, and myopathies associated with systemic conditions [41].

Figure 1 summarizes the main results obtained on adiponectin in both inherited and non-inherited/acquired myopathies.

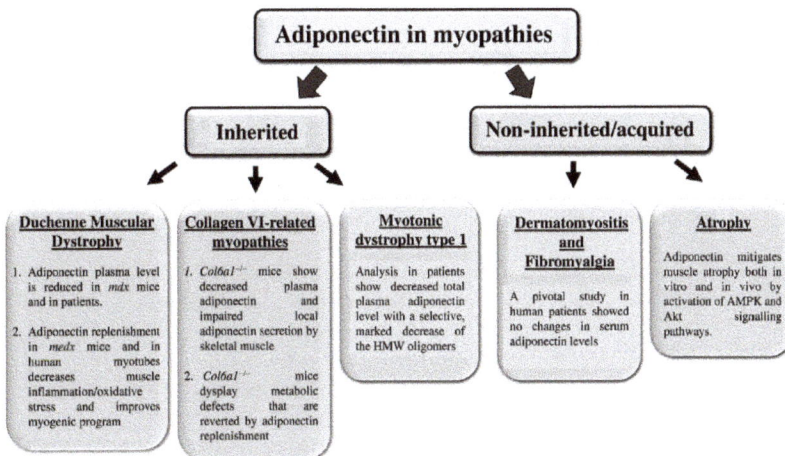

Figure 1. The state of the art about adiponectin in myopathies. Each panel reports the results obtained in the different myopathies (inherited and not inherited/acquired) about adiponectin. More details are explained in the text.

2.1. Adiponectin in Inherited Myopathies

Muscular dystrophies are inherited disorders, triggered by a genetic mutation that typically affects striated muscle tissue. Duchenne muscular dystrophy (DMD) is an X-linked recessive defect caused by dystrophin gene mutation. Dystrophin is a key scaffolding protein of the dystroglycan complex [42], which connects the myofibers to cytoskeleton and the extracellular matrix. Dystroglycan complex injuries lead to sarcolemma instability and vulnerability to mechanical stress, [43] thus permitting the infiltration of immune cells and generating inflammation, necrosis, and severe muscle degeneration. The chronic inflammation/oxidative stress plays a crucial role in DMD pathogenesis [44].

So far, most of the studies on adiponectin and dystrophies were mainly performed on mouse models. *mdx* mice, a widely used mouse model of DMD, show decreased plasma adiponectin level due to a reduced secretion of adiponectin by adipose tissue [45], probably as the result of the systemic inflamed and stressed environment present in *mdx* mice. Indeed, adiponectin secretion by adipose tissue is strictly dependent by stressed conditions. Decreased adiponectin level is associated with obesity [35], diabetes [34,36], and coronary artery disease [46], and is closely related with oxidative stress [38,47]. Impaired mitochondrial function in adipocytes induced endoplasmic reticulum stress, which leads to the activation of signalling pathways, involving c-Janus Kinase (JNK) and Cyclic AMP-dependent transcription factor (ATF)-3A, culminating in decreased adiponectin synthesis [20]. Replenishment of adiponectin, obtained by crossing *mdx* mice with transgenic mice moderately overexpressing adiponectin, counteracts muscle inflammation by reducing the expression of inflammation markers as Tumour Necrosis Factor (TNF) α and Interleukin (IL)-1β and upregulating the anti-inflammatory cytokine IL-10. Besides its anti-inflammatory properties, adiponectin also improves myogenic program as well as muscle function. Indeed, *mdx*–adiponectin mice displayed partial or complete restoration of the regulators of the early phase of differentiation MyoD, Myf5, as well as Mrf4 [45]. The importance of adiponectin in the physiology of the dystrophic muscle has been confirmed using adiponectin KO–*mdx* mice that displayed a worsened dystrophic phenotype. Conversely, reinsertion of adiponectin gene in the skeletal muscle of *mdx*–adiponectin KO mice lead to decreased expression levels of several oxidative stress/inflammatory markers as well as the activity of NF-κB, and the concomitant increased expression levels of the myogenic markers [48].

Studies performed on primary human cultures of myotubes from DMD patients confirmed the results obtained in *mdx* mice. In line with the studies on animal models, human dystrophic myotubes show a local decrease of adiponectin secretion [49]. Moreover, primary cultures of human myotubes isolated from DMD patients exposed to chronic inflammation, confirming the anti-inflammatory effects of adiponectin in skeletal muscle. This protective effect occurs through AdipoR1 binding and activation of AMPK-SIRT1-PGC-1α signalling pathway, thereby leading to NF-κB downregulation [45,49]. Analysis of the myokine secretion profile of DMD human myotubes treated with adiponectin following an inflammatory stimulus, pointed out the downregulation of several pro-inflammatory molecules (as TNFα, IL-17A, and CCL28) and the upregulation of anti-inflammatory IL6. Accordingly, adiponectin regulates the expression level of the NLRP3 inflammasome, which has been reported to be involved in the worsening of DMD [50]. DMD human myotubes expressed threefold increase of NLRP3 level in comparison to healthy myotubes, and their treatment with adiponectin or with miR-711—considered a strong candidate for the adiponectin anti-inflammatory action [51]—attenuates NLRP3 inflammasome expression level [50]. Concerning circulating adiponectin in DMD patients, a single study reports the increase with age of plasma adiponectin [52].

Inherited myopathies comprise the Collagen VI-related myopathies (COL6-RM). Collagen VI is one of the most abundant extracellular matrix proteins in adipose tissue [53–55] and its expression is positively regulated by glucose levels and negatively by PPAR-γ agonists and leptin [56,57]. COL6-RM refer to congenital muscular dystrophy caused by mutation in one of the human collagen VI genes (COL6A1, COL6A2, and COL6A3) and are characterized by a varied degree of muscle weakness and joint contractures. They include early severe forms (as Ullrich Congenital Muscular Dystrophy, UCMD), milder presentations (as Bethlem Myopathy, BM) and intermediate phenotypes [58].

Recently, we performed a study of adiponectin and collagen VI-related myopathies using collagen VI-null (*Col6a1$^{-/-}$*) mice that display myopathic phenotype close to human patients, thus representing a good animal model for the study of these genetic disorders [59]. Our findings show that *Col6a1$^{-/-}$* mice have decreased plasma adiponectin and impaired local adiponectin secretion by skeletal muscle. We found *Col6a1$^{-/-}$* myoblasts display several metabolic abnormalities, including impaired glucose uptake, altered mitochondria membrane potential, associated with a decreased oxygen consumption. These metabolic defects are reverted by adiponectin replenishment that restores *Col6a1$^{-/-}$* metabolic properties close to that of the healthy myoblasts [60].

Where human samples are concerned, transcriptome analysis performed using skeletal muscle biopsies of UCMD patients pointed out an increase of the mRNA levels of the main adipokines (as leptin and adiponectin). However, this transcriptomic data has not been confirmed at the intracellular protein level due to the small number of patients available [61].

Myotonic dystrophy type 1 (DM1) is a rare genetic disorder characterized by muscle wasting and metabolic comorbidity and increased risk of developing insulin resistance (IR) and type 2 diabetes [62]. An analysis carried out in 21 DM1 patients revealed a decrease of total plasma adiponectin with a selective, marked decrease of the HMW oligomers. Although not yet proven, it has been hypothesized that the decreased adiponectin level might contribute to the worsening of IR and metabolic complications observed in DM1 patients [63].

2.2. Adiponectin in Non-Inherited/Acquired Myopathies

Non-inherited myopathies include idiopathic inflammatory myopathies (IIM), which refers to a heterogeneous group of autoimmune muscle disorders classified in four phenotypes: dermatomyositis (DM), polymyositis (PM), necrotizing autoimmune myositis, and inclusion-body myositis.

A pivotal study in DM and PM patients focused on the analysis of serum adipokine levels useful as markers of disease, showed no changes in adiponectin amount [64]. However, it has been reported a close correlation between serum adipokine levels and the onset of the metabolic syndrome in DM young female patients. This study reported that serum adiponectin levels are positively correlated with the onset of metabolic syndrome, which is highly prevalent in DM patients in relation to age and disease progression [65].

Adiponectin has also been studied in other types of non-hereditary myopathies. These include fibromyalgia, which is a disorder characterized by widespread musculoskeletal pain accompanied by fatigue, sleep, memory, and mood issues [66]. This study, planned to evaluate leptin and adiponectin levels in patients with fibromyalgia with or without overweight or obesity, showed no difference of adiponectin amount in comparison to healthy subjects [67].

Recently, an involvement of adiponectin in blocking muscle atrophy has been reported [68]. Muscle atrophy is caused by excessive protein breakdown associated to a decreased protein synthesis as a consequence of several pathologies like AIDS, cancer, renal and cardiac failure [69]. Adiponectin is able to mitigate muscle atrophy both in vitro and in vivo, and this beneficial effect occurs through the activation of AMPK and Akt signalling pathways [68].

3. Future Perspectives

Although just beginning, the study of adiponectin in myopathies highlights a possible role of the hormone in the ameliorations of the abnormalities observed in these diseases. These preliminary studies reinforce the idea that the study of adiponectin in myopathies must proceed. As some inherited myopathies, such as DMD, are associated with a decreased content of plasma adiponectin, the hormone could potentially be used as a marker for the onset of the pathology. So far, several studies explored adiponectin as a biomarker in different diseases including hepatitis C, various types of cancers, inflammation, renal disease, and atherosclerosis [70]. More importantly, adiponectin treatment induces in some myopathies the amelioration of the defects induced by the pathology. This finding opens the possibility about the use of adiponectin as a new tool for the improvement of abnormalities caused by muscular pathologies. Several efforts were performed towards the planning of new pharmacological therapies able to induce adiponectin beneficial effects in pathologic conditions. In 2013, Kadowaki's group published a paper describing the discovery of an orally active synthetic small molecule (called AdipoRon) that binds to and activates both AdipoR1 and AdipoR2 receptors [71]. It has been reported that AdipoRon induces the same physiological effects of adiponectin in healthy tissues such as liver and skeletal muscle [71]. In addition, AdipoRon induces beneficial effects in some pathologic conditions as insulin resistance and type 2 diabetes in mice [71], cardiac disease induced by pressure overload [72], pancreatic cancer [73], liver injury by galactosamine [74], and diabetic nephropathy due to the decrease of ceramide content and lipotoxicity [75]. At the time, while gene therapy has not yet reached the desired results for the cure of congenital muscular myopathies, the treatment of myopathic patients with adiponectin or its agonists could be considered.

Author Contributions: Original Draft Preparation, T.F.; Writing: T.F., T.G.; Review & Editing: T.F., T.G.; F.M.; Supervision: T.F.

Funding: This work was supported by the Italian Ministry of University and Research (MIUR).

Conflicts of Interest: The authors declare no conflict of interest.

References

1. Yamauchi, T.; Kamon, J.; Ito, Y.; Tsuchida, A.; Yokomizo, T.; Kita, S.; Sugiyama, T.; Miyagishi, M.; Hara, K.; Tsunoda, M.; et al. Cloning of adiponectin receptors that mediate antidiabetic metabolic effects. *Nature* **2003**, *423*, 762–769. [CrossRef] [PubMed]

2. Waki, H.; Yamauchi, T.; Kamon, J.; Ito, Y.; Uchida, S.; Kita, S.; Hara, K.; Hada, Y.; Vasseur, F.; Froguel, P.; et al. Impaired multimerization of human adiponectin mutants associated with diabetes. Molecular structure and multimer formation of adiponectin. *J. Biol. Chem.* **2003**, *278*, 40352–40363. [CrossRef] [PubMed]

3. Waki, H.; Yamauchi, T.; Kamon, J.; Kita, S.; Ito, Y.; Hada, Y.; Uchida, S.; Tsuchida, A.; Takekawa, S.; Kadowaki, T. Generation of globular fragment of adiponectin by leukocyte elastase secreted by monocytic cell line THP-1. *Endocrinology* **2005**, *146*, 790–796. [CrossRef] [PubMed]

4. Fiaschi, T.; Giannoni, E.; Taddei, M.L.; Chiarugi, P. Globular adiponectin activates motility and regenerative traits of muscle satellite cells. *PLoS ONE* **2012**, *7*, e34782. [CrossRef] [PubMed]

5. Mao, X.; Kikani, C.K.; Riojas, R.A.; Langlais, P.; Wang, L.; Ramos, F.J.; Fang, Q.; Christ-Roberts, C.Y.; Hong, J.Y.; Kim, R.Y.; et al. APPL1 binds to adiponectin receptors and mediates adiponectin signalling and function. *Nat. Cell Biol.* **2006**, *8*, 516–523. [CrossRef]

6. Ceddia, R.B.; Somwar, R.; Maida, A.; Fang, X.; Bikopoulos, G.; Sweeney, G. Globular adiponectin increases GLUT4 translocation and glucose uptake but reduces glycogen synthesis in rat skeletal muscle cells. *Diabetologia* **2005**, *48*, 132–139. [CrossRef] [PubMed]

7. Zhou, L.; Deepa, S.S.; Etzler, J.C.; Ryu, J.; Mao, X.; Fang, Q.; Liu, D.D.; Torres, J.M.; Jia, W.; Lechleiter, J.D.; et al. Adiponectin activates AMP-activated protein kinase in muscle cells via APPL1/LKB1-dependent and phospholipase C/Ca^{2+}/Ca^{2+}/calmodulin-dependent protein kinase kinase-dependent pathways. *J. Biol. Chem.* **2009**, *284*, 22426–22435. [CrossRef]

8. Thomson, D.M. The Role of AMPK in the Regulation of Skeletal Muscle Size, Hypertrophy, and Regeneration. *Int. J. Mol. Sci.* **2018**, *19*, 3125. [CrossRef]

9. Yamauchi, T.; Kamon, J.; Minokoshi, Y.; Ito, Y.; Waki, H.; Uchida, S.; Yamashita, S.; Noda, M.; Kita, S.; Ueki, K.; et al. Adiponectin stimulates glucose utilization and fatty-acid oxidation by activating AMP-activated protein kinase. *Nat. Med.* **2002**, *8*, 1288–1295. [CrossRef]

10. Yoon, M.J.; Lee, G.Y.; Chung, J.J.; Ahn, Y.H.; Hong, S.H.; Kim, J.B. Adiponectin increases fatty acid oxidation in skeletal muscle cells by sequential activation of AMP-activated protein kinase, p38 mitogen-activated protein kinase, and peroxisome proliferator-activated receptor alpha. *Diabetes* **2006**, *55*, 2562–2570. [CrossRef]

11. Iwabu, M.; Yamauchi, T.; Okada-Iwabu, M.; Sato, K.; Nakagawa, T.; Funata, M.; Yamaguchi, M.; Namiki, S.; Nakayama, R.; Tabata, M.; et al. Adiponectin and AdipoR1 regulate PGC-1alpha and mitochondria by Ca(2+) and AMPK/SIRT1. *Nature* **2010**, *464*, 1313–1319. [CrossRef] [PubMed]

12. Yamauchi, T.; Iwabu, M.; Okada-Iwabu, M.; Kadowaki, T. Adiponectin receptors: A review of their structure, function and how they work. *Best Pract. Res. Clin. Endocrinol. Metab.* **2014**, *28*, 15–23. [CrossRef] [PubMed]

13. Holland, W.L.; Brozinick, J.T.; Wang, L.P.; Hawkins, E.D.; Sargent, K.M.; Liu, Y.; Narra, K.; Hoehn, K.L.; Knotts, T.A.; Siesky, A.; et al. Inhibition of ceramide synthesis ameliorates glucocorticoid-, saturated-fat-, and obesity-induced insulin resistance. *Cell Metab.* **2007**, *5*, 167–179. [CrossRef] [PubMed]

14. Xia, J.Y.; Holland, W.L.; Kusminski, C.M.; Sun, K.; Sharma, A.X.; Pearson, M.J.; Sifuentes, A.J.; McDonald, J.G.; Gordillo, R.; Scherer, P.E. Targeted Induction of Ceramide Degradation Leads to Improved Systemic Metabolism and Reduced Hepatic Steatosis. *Cell Metab.* **2015**, *22*, 266–278. [CrossRef]

15. Sharma, A.X.; Holland, W.L. Adiponectin and its Hydrolase-Activated Receptors. *J. Nat. Sci.* **2017**, *3*, e396. [PubMed]

16. Holland, W.L.; Xia, J.Y.; Johnson, J.A.; Sun, K.; Pearson, M.J.; Sharma, A.X.; Quittner-Strom, E.; Tippetts, T.S.; Gordillo, R.; Scherer, P.E. Inducible overexpression of adiponectin receptors highlight the roles of adiponectin-induced ceramidase signaling in lipid and glucose homeostasis. *Mol. Metab.* **2017**, *6*, 267–275. [CrossRef]

17. Holland, W.L.; Miller, R.A.; Wang, Z.V.; Sun, K.; Barth, B.M.; Bui, H.H.; Davis, K.E.; Bikman, B.T.; Halberg, N.; Rutkowski, J.M.; et al. Receptor-mediated activation of ceramidase activity initiates the pleiotropic actions of adiponectin. *Nat. Med.* **2011**, *17*, 55–63. [CrossRef]
18. Wang, Z.V.; Schraw, T.D.; Kim, J.Y.; Khan, T.; Rajala, M.W.; Follenzi, A.; Scherer, P.E. Secretion of the adipocyte-specific secretory protein adiponectin critically depends on thiol-mediated protein retention. *Mol. Cell. Biol.* **2007**, *27*, 3716–3731. [CrossRef]
19. Qiang, L.; Wang, H.; Farmer, S.R. Adiponectin secretion is regulated by SIRT1 and the endoplasmic reticulum oxidoreductase Ero1-L alpha. *Mol. Cell. Biol.* **2007**, *27*, 4698–4707. [CrossRef]
20. Koh, E.H.; Park, J.Y.; Park, H.S.; Jeon, M.J.; Ryu, J.W.; Kim, M.; Kim, S.Y.; Kim, M.S.; Kim, S.W.; Park, I.S.; et al. Essential role of mitochondrial function in adiponectin synthesis in adipocytes. *Diabetes* **2007**, *56*, 2973–2981. [CrossRef]
21. Fiaschi, T.; Magherini, F.; Gamberi, T.; Modesti, P.A.; Modesti, A. Adiponectin as a tissue regenerating hormone: More than a metabolic function. *Cell. Mol. Life Sci.* **2014**, *71*, 1917–1925. [CrossRef]
22. Pedersen, B.K.; Febbraio, M.A. Muscles, exercise and obesity: Skeletal muscle as a secretory organ. *Nat. Rev. Endocrinol.* **2012**, *8*, 457–465. [CrossRef]
23. Trayhurn, P.; Drevon, C.A.; Eckel, J. Secreted proteins from adipose tissue and skeletal muscle—Adipokines, myokines and adipose/muscle cross-talk. *Arch. Physiol. Biochem.* **2011**, *117*, 47–56. [CrossRef]
24. Amin, R.H.; Mathews, S.T.; Camp, H.S.; Ding, L.; Leff, T. Selective activation of PPARgamma in skeletal muscle induces endogenous production of adiponectin and protects mice from diet-induced insulin resistance. *Am. J. Physiol. Endocrinol. Metab.* **2010**, *298*, E28–E37. [CrossRef]
25. Delaigle, A.M.; Senou, M.; Guiot, Y.; Many, M.C.; Brichard, S.M. Induction of adiponectin in skeletal muscle of type 2 diabetic mice: In vivo and in vitro studies. *Diabetologia* **2006**, *49*, 1311–1323. [CrossRef]
26. Delaigle, A.M.; Jonas, J.C.; Bauche, I.B.; Cornu, O.; Brichard, S.M. Induction of adiponectin in skeletal muscle by inflammatory cytokines: In vivo and in vitro studies. *Endocrinology* **2004**, *145*, 5589–5597. [CrossRef]
27. Fiaschi, T.; Cirelli, D.; Comito, G.; Gelmini, S.; Ramponi, G.; Serio, M.; Chiarugi, P. Globular adiponectin induces differentiation and fusion of skeletal muscle cells. *Cell Res.* **2009**, *19*, 584–597. [CrossRef]
28. Giordani, L.; Parisi, A.; Le Grand, F. Satellite Cell Self-Renewal. *Curr. Top. Dev. Biol.* **2018**, *126*, 177–203.
29. Gamberi, T.; Modesti, A.; Magherini, F.; D'Souza, D.M.; Hawke, T.; Fiaschi, T. Activation of autophagy by globular adiponectin is required for muscle differentiation. *Biochim. Biophys. Acta* **2016**, *1863*, 694–702. [CrossRef]
30. Sampaolesi, M.; Torrente, Y.; Innocenzi, A.; Tonlorenzi, R.; D'Antona, G.; Pellegrino, M.A.; Barresi, R.; Bresolin, N.; De Angelis, M.G.; Campbell, K.P.; et al. Cell therapy of alpha-sarcoglycan null dystrophic mice through intra-arterial delivery of mesoangioblasts. *Science* **2003**, *301*, 487–492. [CrossRef]
31. Sampaolesi, M.; Blot, S.; D'Antona, G.; Granger, N.; Tonlorenzi, R.; Innocenzi, A.; Mognol, P.; Thibaud, J.L.; Galvez, B.G.; Barthélémy, I.; et al. Mesoangioblast stem cells ameliorate muscle function in dystrophic dogs. *Nature* **2006**, *444*, 574–579. [CrossRef]
32. Galvez, B.G.; Sampaolesi, M.; Brunelli, S.; Covarello, D.; Gavina, M.; Rossi, B.; Constantin, G.; Costantin, G.; Torrente, Y.; Cossu, G. Complete repair of dystrophic skeletal muscle by mesoangioblasts with enhanced migration ability. *J. Cell Biol.* **2006**, *174*, 231–243. [CrossRef]
33. Fiaschi, T.; Tedesco, F.S.; Giannoni, E.; Diaz-Manera, J.; Parri, M.; Cossu, G.; Chiarugi, P. Globular adiponectin as a complete mesoangioblast regulator: Role in proliferation, survival, motility, and skeletal muscle differentiation. *Mol. Biol. Cell* **2010**, *21*, 848–859. [CrossRef]
34. Hotta, K.; Funahashi, T.; Arita, Y.; Takahashi, M.; Matsuda, M.; Okamoto, Y.; Iwahashi, H.; Kuriyama, H.; Ouchi, N.; Maeda, K.; et al. Plasma concentrations of a novel, adipose-specific protein, adiponectin, in type 2 diabetic patients. *Arterioscler. Thromb. Vasc. Biol.* **2000**, *20*, 1595–1599. [CrossRef]
35. Arita, Y.; Kihara, S.; Ouchi, N.; Takahashi, M.; Maeda, K.; Miyagawa, J.; Hotta, K.; Shimomura, I.; Nakamura, T.; Miyaoka, K.; et al. Paradoxical decrease of an adipose-specific protein, adiponectin, in obesity. *Biochem. Biophys. Res. Commun.* **1999**, *257*, 79–83. [CrossRef]
36. Weyer, C.; Funahashi, T.; Tanaka, S.; Hotta, K.; Matsuzawa, Y.; Pratley, R.E.; Tataranni, P.A. Hypoadiponectinemia in obesity and type 2 diabetes: Close association with insulin resistance and hyperinsulinemia. *J. Clin. Endocrinol. Metab.* **2001**, *86*, 1930–1935. [CrossRef]

37. Torre-Villalvazo, I.; Bunt, A.E.; Alemán, G.; Marquez-Mota, C.C.; Diaz-Villaseñor, A.; Noriega, L.G.; Estrada, I.; Figueroa-Juárez, E.; Tovar-Palacio, C.; Rodriguez-López, L.A.; et al. Adiponectin synthesis and secretion by subcutaneous adipose tissue is impaired during obesity by endoplasmic reticulum stress. *J. Cell. Biochem.* **2018**, *119*, 5970–5984. [CrossRef]

38. Furukawa, S.; Fujita, T.; Shimabukuro, M.; Iwaki, M.; Yamada, Y.; Nakajima, Y.; Nakayama, O.; Makishima, M.; Matsuda, M.; Shimomura, I. Increased oxidative stress in obesity and its impact on metabolic syndrome. *J. Clin. Investig.* **2004**, *114*, 1752–1761. [CrossRef]

39. Nguyen, M.H.; Cheng, M.; Koh, T.J. Impaired muscle regeneration in ob/ob and db/db mice. *Sci. World J.* **2011**, *11*, 1525–1535. [CrossRef]

40. Akhmedov, D.; Berdeaux, R. The effects of obesity on skeletal muscle regeneration. *Front. Physiol.* **2013**, *4*, 371. [CrossRef]

41. Chawla, J. Stepwise approach to myopathy in systemic disease. *Front. Neurol.* **2011**, *2*, 49. [CrossRef]

42. Blake, D.J.; Weir, A.; Newey, S.E.; Davies, K.E. Function and genetics of dystrophin and dystrophin-related proteins in muscle. *Physiol. Rev.* **2002**, *82*, 291–329. [CrossRef]

43. Deconinck, N.; Dan, B. Pathophysiology of duchenne muscular dystrophy: Current hypotheses. *Pediatr. Neurol.* **2007**, *36*, 1–7. [CrossRef] [PubMed]

44. De Paepe, B.; De Bleecker, J.L. Cytokines and chemokines as regulators of skeletal muscle inflammation: Presenting the case of Duchenne muscular dystrophy. *Mediat. Inflamm.* **2013**, *2013*, 540370. [CrossRef]

45. Abou-Samra, M.; Lecompte, S.; Schakman, O.; Noel, L.; Many, M.C.; Gailly, P.; Brichard, S.M. Involvement of adiponectin in the pathogenesis of dystrophinopathy. *Skelet Muscle* **2015**, *5*, 25. [CrossRef] [PubMed]

46. Kumada, M.; Kihara, S.; Sumitsuji, S.; Kawamoto, T.; Matsumoto, S.; Ouchi, N.; Arita, Y.; Okamoto, Y.; Shimomura, I.; Hiraoka, H.; et al. Association of hypoadiponectinemia with coronary artery disease in men. *Arterioscler. Thromb. Vasc. Biol.* **2003**, *23*, 85–89. [CrossRef]

47. Hattori, S.; Hattori, Y.; Kasai, K. Hypoadiponectinemia is caused by chronic blockade of nitric oxide synthesis in rats. *Metabolism* **2005**, *54*, 482–487. [CrossRef]

48. Abou-Samra, M.; Boursereau, R.; Lecompte, S.; Noel, L.; Brichard, S.M. Potential Therapeutic Action of Adiponectin in Duchenne Muscular Dystrophy. *Am. J. Pathol.* **2017**, *187*, 1577–1585. [CrossRef] [PubMed]

49. Lecompte, S.; Abou-Samra, M.; Boursereau, R.; Noel, L.; Brichard, S.M. Skeletal muscle secretome in Duchenne muscular dystrophy: A pivotal anti-inflammatory role of adiponectin. *Cell. Mol. Life Sci.* **2017**, *74*, 2487–2501. [CrossRef]

50. Boursereau, R.; Abou-Samra, M.; Lecompte, S.; Noel, L.; Brichard, S.M. Downregulation of the NLRP3 inflammasome by adiponectin rescues Duchenne muscular dystrophy. *BMC Biol.* **2018**, *16*, 33. [CrossRef]

51. Ge, Q.; Gérard, J.; Noël, L.; Scroyen, I.; Brichard, S.M. MicroRNAs regulated by adiponectin as novel targets for controlling adipose tissue inflammation. *Endocrinology* **2012**, *153*, 5285–5296. [CrossRef]

52. Hathout, Y.; Marathi, R.L.; Rayavarapu, S.; Zhang, A.; Brown, K.J.; Seol, H.; Gordish-Dressman, H.; Cirak, S.; Bello, L.; Nagaraju, K.; et al. Discovery of serum protein biomarkers in the *mdx* mouse model and cross-species comparison to Duchenne muscular dystrophy patients. *Hum. Mol. Genet.* **2014**, *23*, 6458–6469. [CrossRef]

53. Nakajima, I.; Muroya, S.; Tanabe, R.; Chikuni, K. Extracellular matrix development during differentiation into adipocytes with a unique increase in type V and VI collagen. *Biol. Cell* **2002**, *94*, 197–203. [CrossRef]

54. Khan, T.; Muise, E.S.; Iyengar, P.; Wang, Z.V.; Chandalia, M.; Abate, N.; Zhang, B.B.; Bonaldo, P.; Chua, S.; Scherer, P.E. Metabolic dysregulation and adipose tissue fibrosis: Role of collagen VI. *Mol. Cell. Biol.* **2009**, *29*, 1575–1591. [CrossRef]

55. Pasarica, M.; Gowronska-Kozak, B.; Burk, D.; Remedios, I.; Hymel, D.; Gimble, J.; Ravussin, E.; Bray, G.A.; Smith, S.R. Adipose tissue collagen VI in obesity. *J. Clin. Endocrinol. Metab.* **2009**, *94*, 5155–5162. [CrossRef] [PubMed]

56. Dankel, S.N.; Svärd, J.; Matthä, S.; Claussnitzer, M.; Klöting, N.; Glunk, V.; Fandalyuk, Z.; Grytten, E.; Solsvik, M.H.; Nielsen, H.J.; et al. COL6A3 expression in adipocytes associates with insulin resistance and depends on PPARγ and adipocyte size. *Obesity (Silver Spring)* **2014**, *22*, 1807–1813. [CrossRef]

57. McCulloch, L.J.; Rawling, T.J.; Sjöholm, K.; Franck, N.; Dankel, S.N.; Price, E.J.; Knight, B.; Liversedge, N.H.; Mellgren, G.; Nystrom, F.; et al. COL6A3 is regulated by leptin in human adipose tissue and reduced in obesity. *Endocrinology* **2015**, *156*, 134–146. [CrossRef]

58. Cruz, S.; Figueroa-Bonaparte, S.; Gallardo, E.; de Becdelièvre, A.; Gartioux, C.; Allamand, V.; Piñol, P.; Garcia, M.A.; Jiménez-Mallebrera, C.; Llauger, J.; et al. Bethlem Myopathy Phenotypes and Follow Up: Description of 8 Patients at the Mildest End of the Spectrum. *J. Neuromuscul. Dis.* **2016**, *3*, 267–274. [CrossRef] [PubMed]

59. Irwin, W.A.; Bergamin, N.; Sabatelli, P.; Reggiani, C.; Megighian, A.; Merlini, L.; Braghetta, P.; Columbaro, M.; Volpin, D.; Bressan, G.M.; et al. Mitochondrial dysfunction and apoptosis in myopathic mice with collagen VI deficiency. *Nat. Genet.* **2003**, *35*, 367–371. [CrossRef]

60. Gamberi, T.; Magherini, F.; Mannelli, M.; Chrisam, M.; Cescon, M.; Castagnaro, S.; Modesti, A.; Braghetta, P.; Fiaschi, T. Role of adiponectin in the metabolism of skeletal muscles in collagen VI-related myopathies. *J. Mol. Med.* **2019**, in press. [CrossRef]

61. Paco, S.; Kalko, S.G.; Jou, C.; Rodríguez, M.A.; Corbera, J.; Muntoni, F.; Feng, L.; Rivas, E.; Torner, F.; Gualandi, F.; et al. Gene expression profiling identifies molecular pathways associated with collagen VI deficiency and provides novel therapeutic targets. *PLoS ONE* **2013**, *8*, e77430. [CrossRef]

62. Meola, G.; Cardani, R. Myotonic dystrophies: An update on clinical aspects, genetic, pathology, and molecular pathomechanisms. *Biochim. Biophys. Acta* **2015**, *1852*, 594–606. [CrossRef]

63. Daniele, A.; De Rosa, A.; De Cristofaro, M.; Monaco, M.L.; Masullo, M.; Porcile, C.; Capasso, M.; Tedeschi, G.; Oriani, G.; Di Costanzo, A. Decreased concentration of adiponectin together with a selective reduction of its high molecular weight oligomers is involved in metabolic complications of myotonic dystrophy type 1. *Eur. J. Endocrinol.* **2011**, *165*, 969–975. [CrossRef]

64. Loaiza-Félix, J.; Moreno-Ramírez, M.; Pérez-García, F.L.; Jiménez-Rojas, V.; Sánchez-Muñoz, F.; Amezcua-Guerra, M.L. Serum levels of adipokines in patients with idiopathic inflammatory myopathies: A pilot study. *Rheumatol. Int.* **2017**, *37*, 1341–1345. [CrossRef]

65. Silva, M.G.; Borba, E.F.; Mello, S.B.; Shinjo, S.K. Serum adipocytokine profile and metabolic syndrome in young adult female dermatomyositis patients. *Clinics (Sao Paulo)* **2016**, *71*, 709–714. [CrossRef]

66. Chinn, S.; Caldwell, W.; Gritsenko, K. Fibromyalgia Pathogenesis and Treatment Options Update. *Curr. Pain Headache Rep.* **2016**, *20*, 25. [CrossRef] [PubMed]

67. Paiva, E.S.; Andretta, A.; Batista, E.D.; Lobo, M.M.M.T.; Miranda, R.C.; Nisihara, R.; Schieferdecker, M.E.M.; Boguszewski, C.L. Serum levels of leptin and adiponectin and clinical parameters in women with fibromyalgia and overweight/obesity. *Arch. Endocrinol. Metab.* **2017**, *61*, 249–256. [CrossRef] [PubMed]

68. Singh, A.K.; Shree, S.; Chattopadhyay, S.; Kumar, S.; Gurjar, A.; Kushwaha, S.; Kumar, H.; Trivedi, A.K.; Chattopadhyay, N.; Maurya, R.; et al. Small molecule adiponectin receptor agonist GTDF protects against skeletal muscle atrophy. *Mol. Cell. Endocrinol.* **2017**, *439*, 273–285. [CrossRef] [PubMed]

69. Sacheck, J.M.; Hyatt, J.P.; Raffaello, A.; Jagoe, R.T.; Roy, R.R.; Edgerton, V.R.; Lecker, S.H.; Goldberg, A.L. Rapid disuse and denervation atrophy involve transcriptional changes similar to those of muscle wasting during systemic diseases. *FASEB J.* **2007**, *21*, 140–155. [CrossRef]

70. Cardoso, A.L.; Fernandes, A.; Aguilar-Pimentel, J.A.; de Angelis, M.H.; Guedes, J.R.; Brito, M.A.; Ortolano, S.; Pani, G.; Athanasopoulou, S.; Gonos, E.S.; et al. Towards frailty biomarkers: Candidates from genes and pathways regulated in aging and age-related diseases. *Ageing Res. Rev.* **2018**, *47*, 214–277. [CrossRef]

71. Okada-Iwabu, M.; Yamauchi, T.; Iwabu, M.; Honma, T.; Hamagami, K.; Matsuda, K.; Yamaguchi, M.; Tanabe, H.; Kimura-Someya, T.; Shirouzu, M.; et al. A small-molecule AdipoR agonist for type 2 diabetes and short life in obesity. *Nature* **2013**, *503*, 493–499. [CrossRef] [PubMed]

72. Zhang, N.; Wei, W.Y.; Liao, H.H.; Yang, Z.; Hu, C.; Wang, S.S.; Deng, W.; Tang, Q.Z. AdipoRon, an adiponectin receptor agonist, attenuates cardiac remodeling induced by pressure overload. *J. Mol. Med. (Berl.)* **2018**, *96*, 1345–1357. [CrossRef] [PubMed]

73. Akimoto, M.; Maruyama, R.; Kawabata, Y.; Tajima, Y.; Takenaga, K. Antidiabetic adiponectin receptor agonist AdipoRon suppresses tumour growth of pancreatic cancer by inducing RIPK1/ERK-dependent necroptosis. *Cell Death Dis.* **2018**, *9*, 804. [CrossRef] [PubMed]

74. Wang, Y.; Wan, Y.; Ye, G.; Wang, P.; Xue, X.; Wu, G.; Ye, B. Hepatoprotective effects of AdipoRon against d-galactosamine-induced liver injury in mice. *Eur. J. Pharm. Sci.* **2016**, *93*, 123–131. [CrossRef]
75. Kim, Y.; Lim, J.H.; Kim, M.Y.; Kim, E.N.; Yoon, H.E.; Shin, S.J.; Choi, B.S.; Kim, Y.S.; Chang, Y.S.; Park, C.W. The Adiponectin Receptor Agonist AdipoRon Ameliorates Diabetic Nephropathy in a Model of Type 2 Diabetes. *J. Am. Soc. Nephrol.* **2018**, *29*, 1108–1127. [CrossRef] [PubMed]

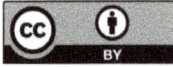

International Journal of
Molecular Sciences

MDPI

Review

Adipose Tissue, Obesity and Adiponectin: Role in Endocrine Cancer Risk

Andrea Tumminia, Federica Vinciguerra, Miriam Parisi, Marco Graziano, Laura Sciacca, Roberto Baratta and Lucia Frittitta *

Endocrinology, Department of Clinical and Experimental Medicine, University of Catania, Garibaldi Hospital, Via Palermo 636, 95122 Catania, Italy; andreatumminia@libero.it (A.T.); vinciguerrafederica@gmail.com (F.V.); mrmparisi@gmail.com (M.P.); graziano.marco91@gmail.com (M.G.); lsciacca@unict.it (L.S.); rob.baratta@gmail.com (R.B.)
* Correspondence: lfritti@unict.it; Tel.: +39-095-7598702

Received: 24 April 2019; Accepted: 10 June 2019; Published: 12 June 2019

Abstract: Adipose tissue has been recognized as a complex organ with endocrine and metabolic roles. The excess of fat mass, as occurs during overweight and obesity states, alters the regulation of adipose tissue, contributing to the development of obesity-related disorders. In this regard, many epidemiological studies shown an association between obesity and numerous types of malignancies, comprising those linked to the endocrine system (e.g., breast, endometrial, ovarian, thyroid and prostate cancers). Multiple factors may contribute to this phenomenon, such as hyperinsulinemia, dyslipidemia, oxidative stress, inflammation, abnormal adipokines secretion and metabolism. Among adipokines, growing interest has been placed in recent years on adiponectin (APN) and on its role in carcinogenesis. APN is secreted by adipose tissue and exerts both anti-inflammatory and anti-proliferative actions. It has been demonstrated that APN is drastically decreased in obese individuals and that it can play a crucial role in tumor growth. Although literature data on the impact of APN on carcinogenesis are sometimes conflicting, the most accredited hypothesis is that it has a protective action, preventing cancer development and progression. The aim of the present review is to summarize the currently available evidence on the involvement of APN and its signaling in the etiology of cancer, focusing on endocrine malignancies.

Keywords: adiponectin; adipose tissue; obesity; endocrine cancer

---

1. Introduction

Obesity represents a condition of chronic excess fat mass. Several epidemiological studies have revealed an alarming increase in the number of obese individuals worldwide [1]. It is important to emphasize that obesity represents a risk factor for the onset of different metabolic disorders, such as type 2 diabetes, as well as for the development of cardiovascular diseases [2]. Moreover, it has been well established that the risk of many types of malignancies is increased in obese individuals [3]. Recent evidence indicates, indeed, that excess adiposity is associated with about 20% of all cancers [4]. For these reasons, obesity is a substantial public health challenge, representing one of the major causes of avoidable mortality and morbidity [5].

Molecular mechanisms linking excessive adiposity with the development of cancer are complex and still not completely known. Multiple factors potentially contribute to this relationship. Obesity is, in fact, often related to metabolic defects that may favor not only cancer initiation, but also its progression [6]. These abnormalities include: adipose tissue low-grade inflammation, which implies the production of specific inflammatory adipocytokines, oxidative stress, peripheral insulin resistance with hyperinsulinemia and dyslipidemia [7,8]. In particular, growing interest has been recently placed on the role of adipose tissue-secreted molecules in the development of cancer [9]. Adipose tissue, initially thought as a mere fat mass depot, is now widely recognized as an active endocrine organ [10]. It secretes different types of molecules called adipokines, which are implicated in the pathogenesis of numerous types of malignancies [9,11]. Among others, adiponectin (APN) has been demonstrated to have several functions in human physiology balancing glucose and lipid metabolism and revealing insulin-sensitizing, anti-apoptotic and immune regulatory effects [10,12,13]. Hypoadiponectinemia has been, in fact, consistently associated with obesity-related insulin resistance and type 2 diabetes, as well as with a higher risk of various cancer types [9,14], and thus this molecule has generally been considered a beneficial adipokine. Indeed, several studies have demonstrated that increasing plasma APN levels and, therefore, the activation of its intracellular signaling, are able to mitigate the deleterious effects of metabolic dysfunctions on tumor development and progression [15]. Thus, the possibility of mimicking some of the cancer-protective properties of APN has attracted significant interest within the scientific community for the potential therapeutic applications of this approach. However, research on the role of APN on tumor growth has provided evidence for both positive and negative influences, raising doubts on the previously thought protective role of APN on cancer risk and progression [16]. Even more unexpected were data on the role of APN on the risk of all-cause mortality. In fact, a positive, rather than negative, relationship has been reported between APN and death rates across various clinical conditions, including different types of malignancy [17]. Therefore, understanding the complexity of APN's metabolism, and linking its signaling pathway to cancer development and prognosis, represent a challenging task.

In this review we will summarize the currently available data on this topic, mainly focusing on endocrine malignancies (e.g., breast, endometrial, ovarian, thyroid and prostate cancers), which seem to be deeply linked to dysfunctional APN secretion and action.

2. APN Structure and Receptors

APN is encoded by AdipoQ, a gene that makes a monomeric molecule made up of 244 amino acids and consists of a signal region at the NH2-terminus, a variable region, a collagenous domain and a globular domain at the COOH-terminus (Figure 1) [18].

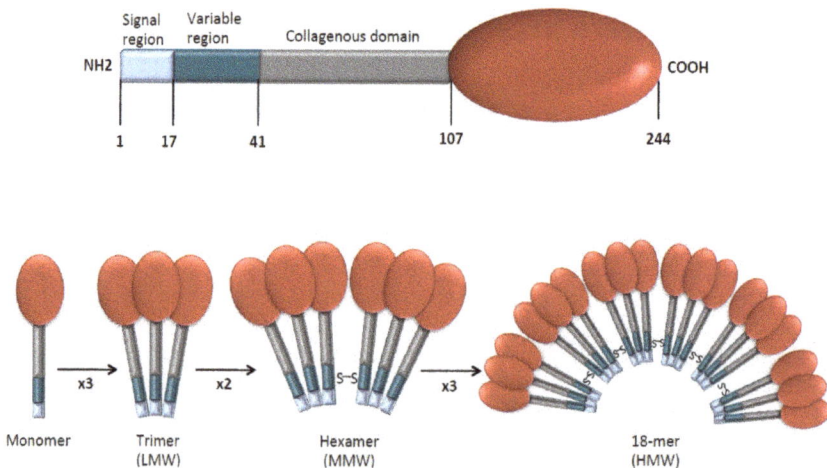

Figure 1. APN's molecular structure and isoforms. Monomeric APN is able to trimerize to form low molecular weight (LMW) APN. Two trimers can then combine to form middle molecular weight (MMW) hexamers. The trimers are able to form 12- or 18-mers with high molecular weight (HMW).

After post-translational modifications, APN circulates in trimeric, hexameric, and multimeric high-molecular weight (HMW) isoforms. Each isoform is able to activate distinct signal transduction pathways, regulating various biological functions [10]. Moreover, a globular version of APN, resulting from proteolytic cleavage of the COOH-terminal domain, circulates in small concentrations in plasma.

The different APN isoforms mediate distinct effects in various tissues and organs. For example, the HMW isoform, which is the most biologically active, is believed to mediate the pro-inflammatory effects of APN, whereas the trimeric isoform has been suggested as responsible for its anti-inflammatory activity [19].

APN acts through its classical receptors, AdipoR1 and AdipoR2, which have been demonstrated to have different binding affinity for the different APN isoforms [20]. There are seven trans-membrane domain receptors that activate a signaling cascade, leading to numerous metabolic and immune-related effects. AdipoR1 is expressed almost ubiquitously, whereas AdipoR2 is mostly expressed in hepatocytes and white adipose tissue [20]. In addition, a non-classical APN receptor, the T-Cadherin (which acts through calcium dependent mechanisms) has been found to bind the hexameric and HMW species of APN, but not the trimeric or globular species [21].

3. Adiponectin Signaling and Mechanisms of Carcinogenesis

The role of APN in endocrine cancer risk is deeply linked to many complex dysfunctions, including an altered adipose tissue homeostasis and the activation of multiple epigenetic pathways within tumor cells and neoplastic microenvironment [22]. A correlation between hypoadiponectinemia, obesity and hormonally influenced cancers has been found in several clinical studies [23,24]. While the majority of evidence shows an inverse correlation between APN and endocrine malignancies, another group of studies associates increased circulating APN levels with tumor progression [25]. Indeed, it has been proposed that low APN concentrations could be associated with cancers linked to an excess of fat mass and to sex steroid hormones, while higher plasma APN levels might indicate high levels of inflammation and advanced stages of malignancy [25,26].

A robust amount of studies in the past two decades have suggested that APN exerts its antineoplastic effects on endocrine cancers via two main mechanisms. First, it can affect endocrine tumor growth by acting directly on cancer cells through receptor-mediated pathways. Secondly, it may indirectly influence cancer biology by modulating insulin sensitivity, inflammation and tumor angiogenesis [23]. In the following section we will briefly discuss the in vitro and in vivo observations of these different mechanisms.

3.1. Direct Mechanisms: Receptor-Mediated and Paracrine

The main direct mechanism determining APN's protective role on endocrine cancer cells is the activation of adenosine monophosphate-activated protein kinase (AMPK). This protein represents a crucial regulator of energy balance, as it is responsible for cellular adaptation to metabolically challenging states such as inflammation and oxidative stress. In such conditions, AMPK turns off anabolic and proliferative pathways, while increasing the production of adenosine triphosphate (ATP) [27]. APN stimulates AMPK through an increase of AMP levels, and by means of various cellular mediators comprising the adaptor protein APPL-1, calcium-dependent kinases and the liver kinase B1 (LKB1) [28]. Specifically, it has been demonstrated that LKB1 plays a fundamental role in necessitating breast cancer cells for AMPK activation, and for the consequent inhibition of tumor cell adhesion, migration and invasiveness [29]. AMPK activation negatively influences cancer development by affecting some of the key mechanisms that regulate cell growth [30]. In fact, it is able to induce the expression of important molecules involved in cell cycle arrest and apoptosis, such as p53 and p21 [31]. This mechanism of action has been proven in many types of malignancies, especially endocrine cancers. APN treatment was in fact shown to stimulate AMPK in breast [32,33], prostate [34,35] and endometrial cancers [36], mediating tumor growth inhibition. Down-regulation of the mammalian target of rapamycin (mTOR) signaling pathway was implicated in many of these studies [29,34]. Moreover, in MDA-MB-231 breast cancer cells, APN-related AMPK pathway activation has been demonstrated to induce protein phosphatase 2A (PP2A), a tumor suppressor protein involved in Akt dephosphorylation [37,38]. Additionally, some studies have shown a direct negative influence of APN on the PI3K/Akt signaling pathway, which determines a series of events leading to cell death and, therefore, to tumor growth inhibition (Figure 2) [11].

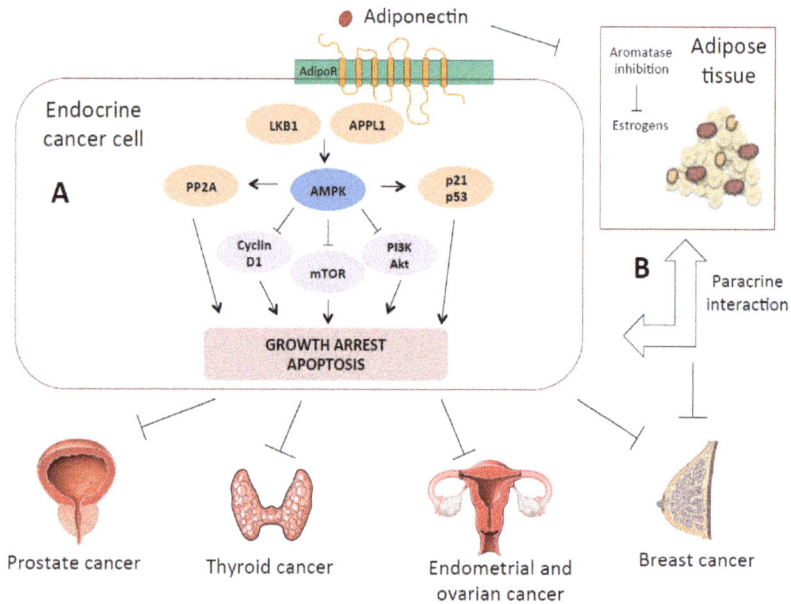

Figure 2. APN's receptor-mediated and paracrine actions on endocrine cancer cells. (**A**) APN activates adenosine monophosphate-activated protein kinase (AMPK) via an increased expression of the adaptor protein APPL-1 as well as the Ser/Thr kinase LKB1. AMPK activation affects cell growth by inducing p53, p21 and phosphatase 2A (PP2A) expression. Down-regulation of the mammalian target of rapamycin (mTOR), PI3K/Akt and Cyclin D1 signaling is also implicated in the APN-mediated growth arrest and apoptosis; (**B**) In adipocytes, APN inhibits aromatase activity, lowering estrogen production and reducing ERα-stimulation in adjacent breast cancer cells. It negatively affects pro-survival pathways.

APN also modulates signal transducer and activator of transcription 3 (STAT3) signaling. STAT3 is activated by adipokine-induced JAK phosphorylation and regulates various processes related to cancer development and progression [39]. For example, it has been demonstrated that APN treatment is able to down-regulate leptin-induced STAT3 phosphorylation, reducing tumor cell growth [39]. Furthermore, APN has been shown to regulate the cAMP/PKA pathway, modulating anti-proliferative actions leading to cell apoptosis in MCF7 breast cancer cells [32].

Of note, APN influence in endocrine cancer cells may also depend on paracrine interactions between adipocytes and tumor cells, being that these cell types are in close proximity to each other [40]. A typical example of this mechanism can be seen in the case of breast cancer [40]. In that situation, APN determines an inhibition of aromatase activity in adipocytes, lowering estrogen production and reducing estrogen receptor alpha (ERα) stimulation in adjacent breast cancer cells. This phenomenon negatively affects pro-survival pathways [40,41]. However, it is important to emphasize that the molecular links between adipose tissue and endocrine cancer cells are far more complex and not yet fully characterized. They involve, in fact, other adipocyte-secreted molecules (e.g., leptin and resistin), numerous inflammatory cytokines (e.g., TNFα, IL-6), extracellular matrix elements, pro-angiogenic factors (e.g., vascular endothelial growth factor (VEGF)), as well as metabolic regulators like insulin and insulin-like growth factor I (IGF-I) [40,42].

3.2. Indirect Mechanisms: Insulin-Sensitizing, Immune-Related, Anti-Angiogenic Effects

Through different mechanisms, APN can exert indirect antineoplastic actions, including insulin-sensitizing, immune-related and angiogenesis-related effects, although conflicting evidence has been published [23]. An indirect link between the insulin pathway, AP, and endocrine carcinogenesis has been shown in many studies. It is well documented that insulin supports tumor cell proliferation [43,44]. Serum APN levels appear to be inversely related to fasting insulin concentrations, and are reduced in conditions of insulin resistance [45]. Since these metabolic conditions represent risk factors for endocrine cancer development, APN might act as an anticancer agent due to its significant effect on insulin post-receptor signaling [46]. Specifically, APN is a strong inhibitor of the PI3K/Akt/mTOR pathway, being able to reduce tumor cell growth induced by insulin and by other growth factors [47].

Immune system deregulation represents a crucial pathophysiological factor in determining increased cancer risk [48,49]. Abnormal immune response is an important constituent of obesity, and contributes to the development of obesity-related disorders such as cancer. Adipose tissue overgrowth accompanies the infiltration of various types of immune cells from both innate and adaptive immunity [50]. Immune cells infiltrating tumor microenvironments and adipocytes secrete pro-inflammatory adipocytokines, providing a condition of low-grade inflammation which favors cancer initiation and progression [51]. Specifically, macrophage infiltration and its phenotypic switching toward an M1 phenotype, constitute critical mechanisms related to increased tumor growth in settings of excess adiposity [52]. In pathological conditions characterized by a chronic inflammatory response such as an infection, but also metabolic diseases such as obesity, type 2 diabetes and atherosclerosis, a lowering of serum APN concentrations has been observed [53]. Obesity, in particular, is associated with increased pro-inflammatory markers such as IL-6, TNF-α and c-reactive protein (CRP). APN has been shown to exert immune regulatory and anti-inflammatory actions and may thus mitigate the increased risk of cancer development related to states of obesity-induced inflammation [54]. Particularly, APN influences the function of myelomonocytic cells that are important regulators of innate immunity. Moreover, APN negatively affects macrophage phagocytic activity [55].

One of the main mechanisms of cancer development is the recruitment of blood vessels to provide nutrients and oxygen to cancer cells [56]. Inhibition of angiogenesis has been demonstrated to suppress tumor growth and may therefore represent a promising therapeutic option [57,58]. Regarding the role of APN in angiogenesis and cellular proliferation, the literature appears to be contradictory. Several studies suggest, in fact, that APN has an anti-angiogenic effect both in vitro and in vivo. In particular, Brakenhielm et al. characterized the strong inhibition of angiogenesis exerted by APN [57], which involves specific signaling pathways such as the mitogen-activated protein kinase (MAPK) and cAMP-PKA pathways [59]. Conversely, convincing molecular data suggest that APN might have a powerful pro-angiogenic effect that could promote cancer development particularly in murine mammary tumor models [60]. Further studies are needed to better define the role of APN on tumor angiogenesis.

4. Breast Cancer

Breast cancer represents the most common malignancy in the female sex and the second most frequent tumor worldwide [61]. In both premenopausal and postmenopausal patients, obesity is considered an important risk factor for the development and progression of breast cancer, lowering a patient's chances of survival [62].

Several studies have investigated the role of adipocytokines in breast cancer, suggesting a pivotal role of APN in its development and recurrence [63,64]. Within the mammary gland, epithelial cells included in peri-glandular adipose tissue are exposed to both circulating and locally secreted adipokines from adjacent adipocytes. As mentioned above, this paracrine interaction, in addition to the circulating effect of the hormone, may influence breast cancer development [65,66].

APN demonstrated in vitro anti-proliferative and pro-apoptotic effects on breast cancer cells, suppressing cell growth and proliferation, and inhibiting the migration and invasion capabilities of cancer cells [33,67–69]. Moreover, epidemiological studies reported a significant inverse association between APN and breast cancer risk (Table 1) [70–72]. This association appears to be stronger for postmenopausal women, although contrasting data have been sometimes published [73]. Significantly lower APN levels have been shown in women with breast cancer compared to healthy controls, especially during the postmenopausal period, suggesting that APN might influence proliferation of breast cancer cells in a low estrogen environment [70,74–76]. Conversely, other studies have indicated a stronger association in women of childbearing age [33,77]. A randomized trial conducted on premenopausal women with intraepithelial neoplasia or micro-invasive breast cancer demonstrated that baseline APN levels predict new breast events. After a median of 7.2 years, a 12% reduction in the risk of developing breast cancer was reported per unit increase of APN [78]. Recently, a large meta-analysis of 31 studies concluded that low serum APN concentrations might be linked to an increased risk of breast cancer in female patients regardless of age [79]. An inverse association between plasma APN levels and increased tumor aggressiveness has also been shown: low APN concentrations were associated with larger tumors, higher histological grade and increased metastasis rate [70,74,80]. Moreover, it has been reported that lower plasma APN concentrations represent a risk factor for progression from intraepithelial to invasive cancer, regardless of age or body mass index (BMI) [78]. Another recent meta-analysis including 27 case–control studies confirmed that serum APN might be inversely associated with breast cancer, but suggested differences in ethnicity, showing higher associations in Asian than Caucasian women [81]. These differences across ethnicity have not been reported in other previously published meta-analyses [73,82]. Authors speculate that several factors influencing serum APN concentrations, like different lifestyle and dietary habits or fat distribution, may explain these results [81,83].

The mechanisms through which APN determines its protective role against breast cancer are yet unclear, but various molecular mechanisms have been proposed [79]. Specifically, it is known that low serum APN levels are associated with hyperinsulinemia, which has been demonstrated to promote the proliferation of tumor cells acting as a growth factor through insulin and IGF-I receptors [84,85]. Furthermore, Brakenhielm et al. demonstrated that APN acts as a negative modulator of angiogenesis by suppressing endothelial cell proliferation [57]. It also induces a signaling cascade that results in apoptosis through the activation of caspases 3, 8 and 9 [57]. APN may also affect breast cancer risk by altering serum estrogen levels; it has, in fact, been demonstrated that APN levels are negatively associated with estrogen concentrations [86]. While these data contribute to understanding the crucial role of APN on breast cancer pathophysiology, several studies have not confirmed these findings [75–77,87]. According to some authors [88], this discrepancy could be partially due to the presence of various APN isoforms with different molecular weights. In particular, an increased breast cancer risk has been specifically related to low levels of the HMW isoform, rather than to total APN [88].

It has been also suggested that APN's effect on breast cancer growth may differ in relation to ERα expression. Most studies show that in ERα-negative breast cancer cells, APN has an anti-proliferative and pro-apoptotic effect [89–91]. Instead, ERα positivity seems to negatively interfere with the anti-proliferative effect of APN on breast cancer cell growth [92,93]. In ERα-positive cells, low APN levels favor the interaction of APPL1 (a mediator of signaling pathways of cell proliferation, apoptosis and cell survival) with AdipoR1, ERα, IGF-IR and c-Src, determining MAPK phosphorylation. This interaction promotes ERα activation at genomic levels, inducing breast cancer cell proliferation [92]. In contrast, APN-induced AMPK/LKB1 pathway activation results in mTOR inhibition in ERα-negative cells, limiting breast cancer progression [94]. Different genes appear to be involved in the anti-proliferative action of APN in ERα-negative breast cancer cells. They include p53, Bax, Bcl-2, c-myc and cyclin D1 [67,90,95]. Therefore, APN is able to inhibit ERα-negative cell growth and progression both in vitro and in vivo.

Table 1. Epidemiological associations between APN and endocrine cancers according to available metanalyses or major case–control studies.

Endocrine Cancer	APN Association to Cancer	Year	# of Studies	Ref.
Breast cancer	Inverse association. Low serum APN levels are associated with breast cancer in pre- and postmenopausal Asian women.	2019	27	[81]
	Inverse association. APN is a biomarker of breast cancer risk in pre- and postmenopausal women, especially among Asians.	2018	31	[79]
	Inverse association. Low APN concentrations are associated with an increased risk of breast cancer.	2014	15	[71]
	Inverse association. Lower APN levels correlate with a higher risk of breast cancer in postmenopausal women.	2014	8	[73]
	Inverse association. High APN level might decrease the risk of postmenopausal breast cancer.	2013	17	[82]
Endometrial cancer	Inverse association. Low APN level increases the risk of endometrial cancer.	2016	18	[96]
	Inverse association. Higher APN levels might have a protective effect against endometrial cancer in postmenopausal women.	2015	12	[97]
	Inverse association. Higher serum APN concentrations are associated with a reduced risk of endometrial cancer, especially in postmenopausal women.	2015	12	[98]
	Inverse association. Each 1 μg/mL increase of APN level is associated with a 3% reduction in endometrial cancer risk.	2015	12	[99]
	Inverse association. Increased circulating APN and adiponectin/leptin ratio are associated with a decreased risk of endometrial cancer.	2015	13	[100]
Ovarian cancer	Inverse association. The mean APN concentrations in patients with ovarian cancer are lower than those of the control group.	2016	1	[101]
Thyroid cancer	Inverse association. APN is inversely associated with thyroid cancer risk among women, but not among men.	2018	1	[102]
	No association. No direct association between decreased levels of APN and papillary thyroid carcinoma size or stage was found.	2018	1	[103]
	No association. Serum APN levels are not significantly different between patients with or without medullary thyroid carcinomas.	2016	1	[104]
	Inverse association. Circulating APN is inversely associated with thyroid cancer risk.	2011	1	[105]
Prostate cancer	Inverse association. Decreased concentration of APN is associated with a greater risk of prostate cancer.	2015	11	[106]
	Direct association. The incidence of prostate cancer is increased in overweight men with high APN concentrations.	2015	1	[107]
	Inverse association. Higher APN levels reduce both the risk of developing high-grade prostate cancer and a risk of dying from the cancer.	2010	1	[108]
	Direct association. Serum APN levels are higher in advanced outside (relative to organ-confined) prostate cancers.	2008	1	[25]
	No association. APN was not of significantly associated with prostate cancer risk or high-grade disease.	2006	1	[109]
	Inverse association. APN levels are decreased in patients with prostate cancer and are also inversely associated with the histologic grade of the tumor.	2005	1	[110]

Despite the complexity of the association between APN and breast cancer, the preponderance of evidence suggests a correlation between low serum PN concentrations and breast cancer risk (Table 1). Further large case–control studies are necessary to better explain the role of APN on the different breast cancer phenotypes and among different ethnicities.

5. Endometrial Cancer

Endometrial cancer is the most frequent gynecologic malignancy and the fourth most common type of cancer among women. It has a worldwide incidence of about 280,000 new cases annually [111].

Obesity represents one of the most important risk factors for the onset of endometrial cancer [112]. An excess of fat mass leads to reduced serum levels of sex hormone binding globulin (SHBG) and progesterone, which results in an increased amount of bioavailable testosterone and estrogen. These hormonal alterations constitute a stimulus for the proliferation of the endometrium and, therefore, for the development of endometrial cancer. It has been estimated that patients with first-degree obesity (BMI 30–35 kg/m^2) or severe obesity (BMI > 35 Kg/m^2) have respectively a 2.5 times and 5 times higher risk of developing endometrial cancer than average-weight patients [113]. This correlation appears to be even more critical because it has been recently reported that pre-pubertal obesity (7–13 years) is associated with the onset of this type of cancer in adult age [114]. Moreover, several studies correlate a patient's weight loss with a reduction of endometrial cancer risk [16].

The excess of adipose tissue may exacerbate endometrial cancer risk through several other mechanisms, including insulin resistance, excessive aromatization of adrenal androgens in the adipocytes (resulting in higher levels of endogenous estrogens), chronic inflammation and the production of several adipokines (including APN) [115]. In a recent meta-analysis, low APN levels, typical of obese women, were associated with a 53% greater risk of developing endometrial cancer [99]. This inverse correlation between plasma APN concentration and endometrial cancer risk is supported by most of the data published on this topic [96,100,116,117]. In particular, a strong inverse association was demonstrated in peri- or post-menopausal patients, while the association for women of fertile age was not univocal [97,98,118]. Furthermore, some authors have shown an inverse correlation between the circulating levels of APN and endometrial cancer staging, and women with lower APN levels, in fact, showed a more advanced endometrial cancer stage with a greater frequency [119].

The mechanisms by which APN inhibits the growth of endometrial cancer cells are not yet well known. However, several hypotheses have been formulated which imply the previously mentioned activation of AMPK (resulting in cell growth suppression and apoptosis), the extracellular signal-regulated protein kinase (ERK) and Akt pathway inhibition and the reduction of Cyclin D1 expression [120]. Furthermore, some authors have suggested that APN may reduce the Bcl2/Bax ratio, which causes an increase in the permeability of the mitochondrial membrane, resulting in the release of Cytochrome-C in the cell cytoplasm and, ultimately, in the activation of caspases-induced apoptosis [117]. Finally, the pro-apoptotic effect mediated by the APN seems to also occur in the endothelial cells of blood vessels, which makes it act as a strong anti-angiogenic factor [121].

Not only a lack of APN, but also a defect in its action seems to represent a negative prognostic factor that underlines the importance of this molecule in the prevention of the endometrial cancer [121]. Several authors have in fact shown that a lower expression of AdipoR1 in endometrial cancer cells is associated with more advanced tumor stages, a higher percentage of myometrial invasion and lymph node diffusion [117,120,121].

Summarizing, low circulating APN levels appear to be associated with an increased risk and worse prognosis of endometrial cancer (Table 1). APN might, therefore, represent a promising tool for the prevention and early diagnosis of this type of malignancy.

6. Ovarian Cancer

Ovarian cancer is the neoplasm burdened by the highest rate of lethality among female genital tract malignancies, and affects mainly peri- and postmenopausal women [122]. The main reason for this very high mortality rate is due to the fact that the majority of the cases of ovarian cancer are detected in advanced stages. About 80–90% of ovarian malignancies originate in cells of the ovarian epithelium, located on the surface of the gland. Other, less frequent histopathological phenotypes are stromal and germinal tumors, which develop from stromal tissue and germ cells, respectively [122].

The causes of ovarian cancer are not fully understood. The most important risk factors that have been identified are: genetic predisposition and history of ovarian neoplasia, Caucasian ethnicity, nulliparity, infertility, a high-fat diet and obesity [123].

Little evidence is available on the role of APN in ovarian cancer risk and progression. Some authors analyzed serum levels of APN and leptin in 52 patients with ovarian cancer, showing that both APN and leptin concentrations were significantly lower in women with ovarian cancer than in healthy individuals [101]. Other authors showed that women affected by ovarian cancer with a low leptin/adiponectin ratio had statistically longer progression-free survival times (using Kaplan–Meier survival estimates) than those with a higher leptin/adiponectin ratio [124]. The same trend was found in relation to the tumor responsiveness to chemotherapy, and women with a lower ratio in fact showed a better clinical response [125].

Furthermore, Li et al. showed that AdipoR1 expression levels in cancerous ovarian tissues represents an independent prognostic factor of the disease, being positively associated with overall survival in patients [126]. Finally, some authors showed that APN is able to repress human ovarian cancer cell growth and reverse the stimulatory effects of 17β-estradiol and IGF-1 on cell proliferation through the downregulation of their receptors [127]. In conclusion, although little available evidence has suggested a protective role of APN on ovarian carcinogenesis, additional studies are necessary to elucidate its function in ovarian tumor onset and progression.

7. Thyroid Cancer

Thyroid cancer is the most common endocrine malignancy [61]. The majority of lesions are represented by well-differentiated carcinomas, mainly papillary thyroid carcinoma and follicular carcinoma (85% and 12% of cases, respectively), while only a small part of thyroid neoplasms is represented by anaplastic carcinoma and medullary carcinoma [128]. The association between increased adiposity and the risk of thyroid cancer has not been univocally established. In a large meta-analysis, increase of weight, BMI, waist or hip circumference and waist-to-hip ratio were associated with a greater risk of papillary, follicular and anaplastic thyroid cancers [129]. Several hypotheses have been formulated to suggest potential mechanisms for this link, implicating factors such as inflammation, oxidative stress, hyperinsulinemia and a deregulated secretion of adipokines (mainly leptin and adiponectin) [130].

In 2011, Mitsiades et al. showed that patients with any form of thyroid cancer had significantly lower levels of circulating APN compared to healthy subjects [105]. These data were partially confirmed by a large, multicenter prospective study, which showed a relationship between low serum APN concentrations and the presence of thyroid cancer in female patients (but not male, probably due to the low percentage of males recruited for the study). The negative relationship with APN was, however, absent, even among women, when the time interval between blood collection and thyroid cancer diagnosis was less than six years [102]. Finally, in a recent paper, no direct association between decreased levels of APN and tumor size or stages was found [103].

Several in vitro studies have shown that even if thyroid cancer cells express both AdipoR1 and AdipoR2, papillary thyroid carcinoma cell lines express a significantly lower number of receptors than normal thyrocytes [105,131]. Finally, when APN levels were measured in patients with medullary carcinoma, no significantly different blood concentrations were found compared to controls [104]. Further studies are needed to elucidate the role of APN in thyroid cancer risk.

8. Prostate Cancer

Prostate cancer is the most common malignancy in males and represents the fifth leading cause of cancer death in men [61]. A sedentary lifestyle, together with a high-calorie and high-fat diet, are risk factors for the development of prostate cancer. Extensive evidence has shown that the excess adipose tissue is deeply involved in the onset and progression of prostate cancer [132,133]. Recent studies have highlighted the central role of APN and its receptors in prostate cancer, even if some evidence appears to be contradictory [134]. Immunohistochemistry analyses have shown a decreased expression of both AdipoR1 and AdipoR2 receptor isoforms in prostate neoplastic tissues in comparison to healthy prostate tissue [135]. Results of a meta-analysis indicated that concentrations of APN in prostate cancer patients were significantly lower than in controls [106]. Specifically, some authors showed that reduced concentrations of APN were related to prostate cancer development and progression [110]. Other authors showed that knockdown of APN leads to increased tumor proliferation and invasion, decreasing tumor suppressing genes [136]. A large prospective study on plasma APN levels and prostate cancer risk and survival showed that men with higher circulating APN concentrations had a decreased risk of developing poorly differentiated cancer or metastases [108]. Moreover, APN treatment has been demonstrated to increase cellular anti-oxidative protection and decrease oxidative stress in a dose-dependent manner in human prostate cancer cell lines [137]. Growing evidences indicate that APN performs an anti-proliferative action in prostate cancer cells, inhibiting dihydrotestosterone-activated cell proliferation [138]. The over-expression of APN in prostate cancer cell lines has been demonstrated to inhibit mTOR-mediated neoplastic cells proliferation [139]. Finally, Gao et al. showed that microRNA 323 is able to stimulate VEGF-A-mediated neo-angiogenesis in prostate cancer tissues through the downregulation of APN's receptors [140].

In contrast with these results, several authors have indicated that there is no significant association between APN expression and prostate malignancy [109], or that there is even a significant positive correlation between APN concentrations and incidence of low or intermediate-risk prostate cancer [107]. Plasma APN levels were reported detectable at higher concentrations in subjects with T3 (advanced outside) than in subjects with T2 (confined within the prostate) stage cancer. Authors have notably suggested that cachexia during the final stages of prostate cancer could be a reason for this phenomenon [25]. Furthermore, some evidence has indicated that AdipoR2 expression is directly associated with prostate cancer progression and metastatization [141,142].

Several genetic polymorphisms can result in a predisposition to increased prostate cancer risk. In a metanalysis of 133 published studies, AdipoQ rs2241766 and AdipoR1 rs10920531 variants were related to a higher risk of prostate neoplasia. Conversely, AdipoR1 rs2232853 variant was associated with a lower risk of developing this type of malignancy [134]. Finally, three common AdipoQ polymorphisms were evaluated in a large cohort of patients with localized prostate cancer who underwent radical prostatectomy: AdipoQ rs182052 allele was associated with both a higher risk of biochemical recurrence and decreased APN levels. Stratified analyses showed that this correlation was more evident in patients with abdominal fat distribution [143].

In conclusion, according to the predominance of literature showing an inverse correlation between APN and the risk of prostate neoplasia, APN deficiency might be a potential biomarker for the early detection of prostate cancer. Elevating APN levels in prostate cancer patients could be, therefore, a useful therapeutic target. Nevertheless, considering that literature data appear to be sometimes conflicting, further studies, both epidemiological and experimental, are warranted to clarify the association between APN and the development of prostate neoplasia.

9. Adiponectin Role in Endocrine Cancer Metastasis

Metastasis is an extremely complex process that represents a major issue in the management of cancer. Besides its role in cancer promotion, aberrant APN secretion has also been associated with tumor spread and metastasis [144]. Regarding endocrine malignancies, APN has been demonstrated to be able to suppress many important processes related to metastatization such as adhesion, invasion and migration of breast cancer cells [29]. This may occur in an LKB1-mediated manner: APN increases the expression of LKB1, determining an increased phosphorylation of AMPK. This phenomenon is of crucial importance for the modulation of two tumor suppressors, TSC2 and TSC1, and leads to a decreased phosphorylation of p70S6 kinase (S6K) and, ultimately, to reduced cancer cell migration and invasion [144]. APN's protective role on endocrine cancer metastasis is also partially regulated through the AMPK/Akt pathway. It has been in fact shown that APN-activated AMPK decreases the invasiveness of MDA-MB-231 cells by inducing PP2A-mediated Akt dephosphorylation [38].

APN was also demonstrated to have a suppressive effect on metastatic endometrial cancer cells [145]. APN was, in fact, able to inhibit leptin-induced cancer invasion, which requires the inactivation of the JAK/STAT3 pathway and the stimulation of AMPK signaling.

Future studies on the role of APN and other adipose tissue-secreting molecules on cancer invasion and metastatization should, therefore, focus also on LKB1-mediated effects, on the signaling pathways APN uses and on the potential interactions with other adipose tissue-secreting molecules that might contribute to the spreading of tumors.

10. Future Perspectives and Therapeutic Implications

Since many studies associate endocrine cancer protection with APN-mediated signaling, drugs intended to bypass APN by directly activating its molecular pathways have been investigated in order to find potential strategies (both prophylactic and therapeutic) and counteract tumor development [146]. However, efforts to engineer APN protein have often been challenging, partly due to a lack of knowledge on the peculiar actions of different APN isoforms [147]. Two suggestions have been proposed to possibly take advantage of the anti-cancer properties of APN: the identification/development of APN receptor agonists, and the increase of endogenous APN concentrations [16]. The first APN receptor agonist that was produced, ADP355, included several amino acids in its structure, which were able to stabilize the molecule protecting it from proteolytic enzymes. In vivo, intraperitoneal administration of 1 mg/kg/day ADP355 for 28 days in immunocompromised mice was demonstrated to suppress the development of human breast cancer xenografts by 31%, with a good safety profile [147]. It was also able to modulate different signaling pathways such as AMPK, STAT3, PIK3/Akt and ERK1/2 [147,148]. Using a high throughput assay, several naturally occurring APN receptor agonists were recently identified [149]. These compounds, acting preferably on AdipoR1 (e.g., matairesinol, arctiin, arctigenin, gramine) or AdipoR2 (e.g., syringin, parthenolide, taxifoliol, deoxyschizandrin) were demonstrated to share important anti-cancer properties with APN, including anti-proliferative and anti-inflammatory effects [149].

Furthermore, it is also conceivable to increase endogenous levels of APN. Peroxisome proliferator-activated receptor-gamma (PPARγ) ligands have been proposed as a promising tool to reach this therapeutic target. It has been demonstrated that thiazolidinediones (synthetic PPARγ ligands) are able to increase APN concentrations in a dose- and time-dependent manner [150]. Even if promising data have been initially produced on the anti-cancer role of several thiazolidinediones (such as troglitazone and efatutazone), their effects on tumors remain to be clarified, given that phase 2 trials failed to show sufficient efficacy [151,152]. Moreover, we must consider that modifying these receptor interactions could also result in unfavorable effects. In this regard, several possible side effects derived from chronic APN treatment (such as infertility, cardiac damage and reduced bone density) have been proposed by some authors [153,154]. For these reasons, further studies are needed to elucidate the clinical relevance of such therapeutic approaches. Finally, it must be remembered that APN may also be regulated by dietary or lifestyle habits. Daily consumption of fish, omega-3 and fiber supplements [83], together with aerobic exercise of moderate intensity, have in fact been demonstrated to significantly increase circulating APN concentrations [155].

11. Conclusions

Obesity represents a major health and social problem strongly increasing the risk for various severe complications comprising endocrine cancer development. Our understanding on obesity-associated malignancies has been rapidly improving during recent years. Among other mechanisms, growing interest has been placed on the regulation of adipocyte-secreted molecules as a critical factor influencing cancer pathophysiology.

APN has been recognized as a key mediator linking obesity and endocrine-related malignancies. The multifaceted role of APN includes a series of complex biological actions on different cancer metabolic pathways and tumor microenvironments. The majority of epidemiological evidence clearly demonstrates that hypoadiponectinemia is related to an increased risk of obesity-related malignancies and poor cancer prognosis. Nevertheless, APN has sometimes shown potentially contradicting actions in endocrine-related tumorigenesis. We believe that this topic represents a promising research field, but there remain several challenges before uniquely considering APN as a treatment strategy in cancer. A more profound understanding of the pathophysiological links between the different APN isoforms and endocrine-related malignancies is therefore required in order to develop effective and safe therapies. Moreover, molecular and environmental settings under which APN acts as an anti-inflammatory or pro-inflammatory adipokine need to be further examined. Finally, the specific roles of each APN receptor and signaling pathway on the different types of endocrine cancers also remain largely unknown. Further studies are therefore needed to clarify these aspects.

Author Contributions: Conceptualization, A.T. and L.F.; Resources, A.T., F.V., M.P., M.G., L.S., R.B. and L.F.; Original Draft Preparation, A.T., F.V., M.P., M.G., L.S., R.B. and L.F.; Review and Editing, A.T. and L.F.; Supervision, A.T. and L.F.

Funding: This research received no external funding.

Acknowledgments: M.P is a recipient of a post-doctoral fellowship founded by the Department of Clinical and Experimental Medicine, University of Catania, Catania (Italy).

Conflicts of Interest: The authors declare no conflict of interest.

Abbreviations

APN	Adiponectin
AdipoR1/2	Adiponectin receptor 1/2
BMI	Body mass index
TNF	Tumor necrosis factor
LMW	Low molecular weight
MMW	Middle molecular weight
HMW	High molecular weight
AMPK	Adenosine monophosphate-activated protein kinase
LKB1	Liver kinase B1
ATP	Adenosine triphosphate
mTOR	Mammalian target of rapamycin
JAK	Janus kinase
IL-6	Interleukin-6
STAT3	Signal transducer and activator of transcription 3
ERK1/2	Extracellular signal-regulated protein kinases 1 and 2
PP2A	Protein phosphatase 2A
ERα	Estrogen receptor alpha
VEGF	Vascular endothelial growth factor
CRP	C-reactive protein

MAPK   Mitogen-activated protein kinase
IGF-I   Insulin-like growth factor I
SHBG   Sex hormones binding globulin
PPARγ   Proliferator-activated receptor-gamma
S6K   p70S6 kinase

References

1. NCD Risk Factor Collaboration (NCD-RisC). Trends in adult body-mass index in 200 countries from 1975 to 2014: A pooled analysis of 1698 population-based measurement studies with 19.2 million participants. *Lancet* **2016**, *387*, 1377–1396. [CrossRef]
2. Global Burden of Metabolic Risk Factors for Chronic Diseases Collaboration (BMI Mediated Effects); Lu, Y.; Hajifathalian, K.; Ezzati, M.; Woodward, M.; Rimm, E.B.; Danaei, G. Metabolic mediators of the effects of body-mass index, overweight, and obesity on coronary heart disease and stroke: A pooled analysis of 97 prospective cohorts with 1.8 million participants. *Lancet* **2014**, *383*, 970–983. [CrossRef]
3. Renehan, A.G.; Tyson, M.; Egger, M.; Heller, R.F.; Zwahlen, M. Body-mass index and incidence of cancer: A systematic review and meta-analysis of prospective observational studies. *Lancet* **2008**, *371*, 569–578. [CrossRef]
4. Khandekar, M.J.; Cohen, P.; Spiegelman, B.M. Molecular mechanisms of cancer development in obesity. *Nat. Rev. Cancer* **2011**, *11*, 886–895. [CrossRef] [PubMed]
5. Global BMI Mortality Collaboration; Di Angelantonio, E.; Bhupathiraju Sh, N.; Wormser, D.; Gao, P.; Kaptoge, S.; Berrington de Gonzalez, A.; Cairns, B.J.; Huxley, R.; Jackson Ch, L.; et al. Body-mass index and all-cause mortality: Individual-participant-data meta-analysis of 239 prospective studies in four continents. *Lancet* **2016**, *388*, 776–786. [CrossRef]
6. Sciacca, L.; Vigneri, R.; Tumminia, A.; Frasca, F.; Squatrito, S.; Frittitta, L.; Vigneri, P. Clinical and molecular mechanisms favoring cancer initiation and progression in diabetic patients. *Nutr. Metab. Cardiov. Dis.* **2013**, *23*, 808–815. [CrossRef]
7. Vigneri, R.; Goldfine, I.D.; Frittitta, L. Insulin, insulin receptors, and cancer. *J. Endocrinol. Invest.* **2016**, *39*, 1365–1376. [CrossRef] [PubMed]
8. Vigneri, P.; Frasca, F.; Sciacca, L.; Frittitta, L.; Vigneri, R. Obesity and cancer. *Nutr. Metab. Cardiov. Dis.* **2006**, *16*, 1–7. [CrossRef] [PubMed]
9. Booth, A.; Magnuson, A.; Fouts, J.; Foster, M. Adipose tissue, obesity and adipokines: Role in cancer promotion. *Hormone Mol. Biol. Clin. Invest.* **2015**, *21*, 57–74. [CrossRef]
10. Scherer, P.E. The Multifaceted Roles of Adipose Tissue-Therapeutic Targets for Diabetes and Beyond: The 2015 Banting Lecture. *Diabetes* **2016**, *65*, 1452–1461. [CrossRef] [PubMed]
11. Di Zazzo, E.; Polito, R.; Bartollino, S.; Nigro, E.; Porcile, C.; Bianco, A.; Daniele, A.; Moncharmont, B. Adiponectin as Link Factor between Adipose Tissue and Cancer. *Int. J. Mol. Sci.* **2019**, *20*, 839. [CrossRef] [PubMed]
12. Baratta, R.; Amato, S.; Degano, C.; Farina, M.G.; Patane, G.; Vigneri, R.; Frittitta, L. Adiponectin relationship with lipid metabolism is independent of body fat mass: Evidence from both cross-sectional and intervention studies. *J. Clin. Endocrinol. Metab.* **2004**, *89*, 2665–2671. [CrossRef] [PubMed]
13. Patane, G.; Caporarello, N.; Marchetti, P.; Parrino, C.; Sudano, D.; Marselli, L.; Vigneri, R.; Frittitta, L. Adiponectin increases glucose-induced insulin secretion through the activation of lipid oxidation. *Acta Diabetol.* **2013**, *50*, 851–857. [CrossRef] [PubMed]
14. Yamauchi, T.; Kamon, J.; Ito, Y.; Tsuchida, A.; Yokomizo, T.; Kita, S.; Sugiyama, T.; Miyagishi, M.; Hara, K.; Tsunoda, M.; et al. Cloning of adiponectin receptors that mediate antidiabetic metabolic effects. *Nature* **2003**, *423*, 762–769. [CrossRef] [PubMed]
15. Vansaun, M.N. Molecular pathways: Adiponectin and leptin signaling in cancer. *Clin. Cancer Res.* **2013**, *19*, 1926–1932. [CrossRef] [PubMed]
16. Katira, A.; Tan, P.H. Evolving role of adiponectin in cancer-controversies and update. *Cancer Biol. Med.* **2016**, *13*, 101–119. [CrossRef] [PubMed]
17. Menzaghi, C.; Trischitta, V. The Adiponectin Paradox for All-Cause and Cardiovascular Mortality. *Diabetes* **2018**, *67*, 12–22. [CrossRef] [PubMed]

18. Wong, G.W.; Wang, J.; Hug, C.; Tsao, T.S.; Lodish, H.F. A family of Acrp30/adiponectin structural and functional paralogs. *Proc. Natl. Acad. Sci. USA* **2004**, *101*, 10302–10307. [CrossRef]

19. Takemura, Y.; Ouchi, N.; Shibata, R.; Aprahamian, T.; Kirber, M.T.; Summer, R.S.; Kihara, S.; Walsh, K. Adiponectin modulates inflammatory reactions via calreticulin receptor-dependent clearance of early apoptotic bodies. *J. Clin. Invest.* **2007**, *117*, 375–386. [CrossRef]

20. Yamauchi, T.; Iwabu, M.; Okada-Iwabu, M.; Kadowaki, T. Adiponectin receptors: A review of their structure, function and how they work. *Best Pract. Res. Clin. Endocrinol. Metab.* **2014**, *28*, 15–23. [CrossRef]

21. Hug, C.; Wang, J.; Ahmad, N.S.; Bogan, J.S.; Tsao, T.S.; Lodish, H.F. T-cadherin is a receptor for hexameric and high-molecular-weight forms of Acrp30/adiponectin. *Proc. Natl. Acad. Sci. USA* **2004**, *101*, 10308–10313. [CrossRef] [PubMed]

22. Hebbard, L.; Ranscht, B. Multifaceted roles of adiponectin in cancer. *Best Pract. Res. Clin. Endocrinol. Metab.* **2014**, *28*, 59–69. [CrossRef] [PubMed]

23. Dalamaga, M.; Diakopoulos, K.N.; Mantzoros, C.S. The role of adiponectin in cancer: A review of current evidence. *Endocr. Rev.* **2012**, *33*, 547–594. [CrossRef] [PubMed]

24. Hefetz-Sela, S.; Scherer, P.E. Adipocytes: Impact on tumor growth and potential sites for therapeutic intervention. *Pharmacol. Ther.* **2013**, *138*, 197–210. [CrossRef] [PubMed]

25. Housa, D.; Vernerova, Z.; Heracek, J.; Prochazka, B.; Cechak, P.; Kuncova, J.; Haluzik, M. Adiponectin as a potential marker of prostate cancer progression: Studies in organ-confined and locally advanced prostate cancer. *Physiol. Res.* **2008**, *57*, 451–458. [PubMed]

26. Izadi, V.; Farabad, E.; Azadbakht, L. Serum adiponectin level and different kinds of cancer: A review of recent evidence. *ISRN Oncol.* **2012**, *2012*, 982769. [CrossRef] [PubMed]

27. Steinberg, G.R.; Kemp, B.E. AMPK in Health and Disease. *Physiol. Rev.* **2009**, *89*, 1025–1078. [CrossRef] [PubMed]

28. Shackelford, D.B.; Shaw, R.J. The LKB1-AMPK pathway: Metabolism and growth control in tumour suppression. *Nat. Rev. Cancer* **2009**, *9*, 563–575. [CrossRef] [PubMed]

29. Taliaferro-Smith, L.; Nagalingam, A.; Zhong, D.; Zhou, W.; Saxena, N.K.; Sharma, D. LKB1 is required for adiponectin-mediated modulation of AMPK-S6K axis and inhibition of migration and invasion of breast cancer cells. *Oncogene* **2009**, *28*, 2621–2633. [CrossRef] [PubMed]

30. Manieri, E.; Herrera-Melle, L.; Mora, A.; Tomas-Loba, A.; Leiva-Vega, L.; Fernandez, D.I.; Rodriguez, E.; Moran, L.; Hernandez-Cosido, L.; Torres, J.L.; et al. Adiponectin accounts for gender differences in hepatocellular carcinoma incidence. *J. Exp. Med.* **2019**, *216*, 1108–1119. [CrossRef] [PubMed]

31. Luo, Z.; Saha, A.K.; Xiang, X.; Ruderman, N.B. AMPK, the metabolic syndrome and cancer. *Trends Pharmacol. Sci.* **2005**, *26*, 69–76. [CrossRef] [PubMed]

32. Li, G.; Cong, L.; Gasser, J.; Zhao, J.; Chen, K.; Li, F. Mechanisms underlying the anti-proliferative actions of adiponectin in human breast cancer cells, MCF7-dependency on the cAMP/protein kinase-A pathway. *Nutr. Cancer* **2011**, *63*, 80–88. [CrossRef] [PubMed]

33. Korner, A.; Pazaitou-Panayiotou, K.; Kelesidis, T.; Kelesidis, I.; Williams, C.J.; Kaprara, A.; Bullen, J.; Neuwirth, A.; Tseleni, S.; Mitsiades, N.; et al. Total and high-molecular-weight adiponectin in breast cancer: In vitro and in vivo studies. *J. Clin. Endocrinol. Metab.* **2007**, *92*, 1041–1048. [CrossRef] [PubMed]

34. Zakikhani, M.; Dowling, R.J.; Sonenberg, N.; Pollak, M.N. The effects of adiponectin and metformin on prostate and colon neoplasia involve activation of AMP-activated protein kinase. *Cancer Prev. Res.* **2008**, *1*, 369–375. [CrossRef] [PubMed]

35. Barb, D.; Neuwirth, A.; Mantzoros, C.S.; Balk, S.P. Adiponectin signals in prostate cancer cells through Akt to activate the mammalian target of rapamycin pathway. *Endocr. Relat. Cancer* **2007**, *14*, 995–1005. [CrossRef] [PubMed]

36. Cong, L.; Gasser, J.; Zhao, J.; Yang, B.; Li, F.; Zhao, A.Z. Human adiponectin inhibits cell growth and induces apoptosis in human endometrial carcinoma cells, HEC-1-A and RL95 2. *Endocr. Relat. Cancer* **2007**, *14*, 713–720. [CrossRef]

37. Sablina, A.A.; Hahn, W.C. The role of PP2A A subunits in tumor suppression. *Cell Adhes. Migr.* **2007**, *1*, 140–141. [CrossRef]

38. Kim, K.Y.; Baek, A.; Hwang, J.E.; Choi, Y.A.; Jeong, J.; Lee, M.S.; Cho, D.H.; Lim, J.S.; Kim, K.I.; Yang, Y. Adiponectin-activated AMPK stimulates dephosphorylation of AKT through protein phosphatase 2A activation. *Cancer Res.* **2009**, *69*, 4018–4026. [CrossRef]

39. Bowman, T.; Garcia, R.; Turkson, J.; Jove, R. STATs in oncogenesis. *Oncogene* **2000**, *19*, 2474–2488. [CrossRef]
40. Park, J.; Euhus, D.M.; Scherer, P.E. Paracrine and endocrine effects of adipose tissue on cancer development and progression. *Endocr. Rev.* **2011**, *32*, 550–570. [CrossRef]
41. Brown, K.A.; Simpson, E.R. Obesity and breast cancer: Progress to understanding the relationship. *Cancer Res.* **2010**, *70*, 4–7. [CrossRef] [PubMed]
42. Stephens, J.M.; Elks, C.M. Oncostatin M: Potential Implications for Malignancy and Metabolism. *Curr. Pharm. Des.* **2017**, *23*, 3645–3657. [CrossRef] [PubMed]
43. Pollak, M. Insulin and insulin-like growth factor signalling in neoplasia. *Nat. Rev. Cancer* **2008**, *8*, 915–928. [CrossRef] [PubMed]
44. Sciacca, L.; Vella, V.; Frittitta, L.; Tumminia, A.; Manzella, L.; Squatrito, S.; Belfiore, A.; Vigneri, R. Long-acting insulin analogs and cancer. *Nutr. Metab. Cardiov. Dis.* **2018**, *28*, 436–443. [CrossRef] [PubMed]
45. Weyer, C.; Funahashi, T.; Tanaka, S.; Hotta, K.; Matsuzawa, Y.; Pratley, R.E.; Tataranni, P.A. Hypoadiponectinemia in obesity and type 2 diabetes: Close association with insulin resistance and hyperinsulinemia. *J. Clin. Endocrinol. Metab.* **2001**, *86*, 1930–1935. [CrossRef]
46. Kelesidis, I.; Kelesidis, T.; Mantzoros, C.S. Adiponectin and cancer: A systematic review. *Br. J. Cancer* **2006**, *94*, 1221–1225. [CrossRef]
47. Sengupta, S.; Peterson, T.R.; Sabatini, D.M. Regulation of the mTOR complex 1 pathway by nutrients, growth factors, and stress. *Mol. Cell* **2010**, *40*, 310–322. [CrossRef]
48. Mantovani, A.; Marchesi, F.; Malesci, A.; Laghi, L.; Allavena, P. Tumour-associated macrophages as treatment targets in oncology. *Nat. Rev. Clin. Oncol.* **2017**, *14*, 399–416. [CrossRef]
49. Stacker, S.A.; Williams, S.P.; Karnezis, T.; Shayan, R.; Fox, S.B.; Achen, M.G. Lymphangiogenesis and lymphatic vessel remodelling in cancer. *Nat. Rev. Cancer* **2014**, *14*, 159–172. [CrossRef]
50. Catalan, V.; Gomez-Ambrosi, J.; Rodriguez, A.; Fruhbeck, G. Adipose tissue immunity and cancer. *Front. Physiol.* **2013**, *4*, 275. [CrossRef]
51. Mraz, M.; Haluzik, M. The role of adipose tissue immune cells in obesity and low-grade inflammation. *J. Endocrinol.* **2014**, *222*, R113–R127. [CrossRef] [PubMed]
52. Castoldi, A.; Naffah de Souza, C.; Camara, N.O.; Moraes-Vieira, P.M. The Macrophage Switch in Obesity Development. *Front. Immunol.* **2015**, *6*, 637. [CrossRef] [PubMed]
53. Nigro, E.; Scudiero, O.; Monaco, M.L.; Palmieri, A.; Mazzarella, G.; Costagliola, C.; Bianco, A.; Daniele, A. New insight into adiponectin role in obesity and obesity-related diseases. *BioMed Res. Int.* **2014**, *2014*, 658913. [CrossRef] [PubMed]
54. Yanai, H.; Yoshida, H. Beneficial Effects of Adiponectin on Glucose and Lipid Metabolism and Atherosclerotic Progression: Mechanisms and Perspectives. *Int. J. Mol. Sci.* **2019**, *20*, 1190. [CrossRef] [PubMed]
55. Yokota, T.; Oritani, K.; Takahashi, I.; Ishikawa, J.; Matsuyama, A.; Ouchi, N.; Kihara, S.; Funahashi, T.; Tenner, A.J.; Tomiyama, Y.; et al. Adiponectin, a new member of the family of soluble defense collagens, negatively regulates the growth of myelomonocytic progenitors and the functions of macrophages. *Blood* **2000**, *96*, 1723–1732. [PubMed]
56. Hanahan, D.; Weinberg, R.A. Hallmarks of cancer: The next generation. *Cell* **2011**, *144*, 646–674. [CrossRef] [PubMed]
57. Brakenhielm, E.; Veitonmaki, N.; Cao, R.; Kihara, S.; Matsuzawa, Y.; Zhivotovsky, B.; Funahashi, T.; Cao, Y. Adiponectin-induced antiangiogenesis and antitumor activity involve caspase-mediated endothelial cell apoptosis. *Proc. Natl. Acad. Sci. USA* **2004**, *101*, 2476–2481. [CrossRef]
58. Bergers, G.; Hanahan, D. Modes of resistance to anti-angiogenic therapy. *Nat. Rev. Cancer* **2008**, *8*, 592–603. [CrossRef]
59. Mahadev, K.; Wu, X.; Donnelly, S.; Ouedraogo, R.; Eckhart, A.D.; Goldstein, B.J. Adiponectin inhibits vascular endothelial growth factor-induced migration of human coronary artery endothelial cells. *Cardiov. Res.* **2008**, *78*, 376–384. [CrossRef]
60. Hebbard, L.W.; Garlatti, M.; Young, L.J.; Cardiff, R.D.; Oshima, R.G.; Ranscht, B. T-cadherin supports angiogenesis and adiponectin association with the vasculature in a mouse mammary tumor model. *Cancer Res.* **2008**, *68*, 1407–1416. [CrossRef]
61. Bray, F.; Ferlay, J.; Soerjomataram, I.; Siegel, R.L.; Torre, L.A.; Jemal, A. Global cancer statistics 2018: GLOBOCAN estimates of incidence and mortality worldwide for 36 cancers in 185 countries. *Cancer J. Clin.* **2018**, *68*, 394–424. [CrossRef]

62. Picon-Ruiz, M.; Morata-Tarifa, C.; Valle-Goffin, J.J.; Friedman, E.R.; Slingerland, J.M. Obesity and adverse breast cancer risk and outcome: Mechanistic insights and strategies for intervention. *Cancer J. Clin.* **2017**, *67*, 378–397. [CrossRef] [PubMed]

63. Panis, C.; Herrera, A.; Aranome, A.M.F.; Victorino, V.J.; Michelleti, P.L.; Morimoto, H.K.; Cecchini, A.L.; Simao, A.N.C.; Cecchini, R. Clinical insights from adiponectin analysis in breast cancer patients reveal its anti-inflammatory properties in non-obese women. *Mol. Cell. Endocrinol.* **2014**, *382*, 190–196. [CrossRef] [PubMed]

64. Carroll, P.A.; Healy, L.; Lysaght, J.; Boyle, T.; Reynolds, J.V.; Kennedy, M.J.; Pidgeon, G.; Connolly, E.M. Influence of the metabolic syndrome on leptin and leptin receptor in breast cancer. *Mol. Carcinog.* **2011**, *50*, 643–651. [CrossRef] [PubMed]

65. Beck, J.C.; Hosick, H.L.; Watkins, B.A. Growth of epithelium from a preneoplastic mammary outgrowth in response to mammary adipose tissue. *In Vitro Cell. Dev. Biol.* **1989**, *25*, 409–418. [CrossRef]

66. Iyengar, P.; Combs, T.P.; Shah, S.J.; Gouon-Evans, V.; Pollard, J.W.; Albanese, C.; Flanagan, L.; Tenniswood, M.P.; Guha, C.; Lisanti, M.P.; et al. Adipocyte-secreted factors synergistically promote mammary tumorigenesis through induction of anti-apoptotic transcriptional programs and proto-oncogene stabilization. *Oncogene* **2003**, *22*, 6408–6423. [CrossRef] [PubMed]

67. Dos Santos, E.; Benaitreau, D.; Dieudonne, M.N.; Leneveu, M.C.; Serazin, V.; Giudicelli, Y.; Pecquery, R. Adiponectin mediates an antiproliferative response in human MDA-MB 231 breast cancer cells. *Oncol. Rep.* **2008**, *20*, 971–977. [PubMed]

68. Arditi, J.D.; Venihaki, M.; Karalis, K.P.; Chrousos, G.P. Antiproliferative effect of adiponectin on MCF7 breast cancer cells: A potential hormonal link between obesity and cancer. *Hormone Metab. Res.* **2007**, *39*, 9–13. [CrossRef]

69. Dieudonne, M.N.; Bussiere, M.; Dos Santos, E.; Leneveu, M.C.; Giudicelli, Y.; Pecquery, R. Adiponectin mediates antiproliferative and apoptotic responses in human MCF7 breast cancer cells. *Biochem. Biophys. Res. Commun.* **2006**, *345*, 271–279. [CrossRef]

70. Miyoshi, Y.; Funahashi, T.; Kihara, S.; Taguchi, T.; Tamaki, Y.; Matsuzawa, Y.; Noguchi, S. Association of serum adiponectin levels with breast cancer risk. *Clin. Cancer Res.* **2003**, *9*, 5699–5704.

71. Macis, D.; Guerrieri-Gonzaga, A.; Gandini, S. Circulating adiponectin and breast cancer risk: A systematic review and meta-analysis. *In. J. Epidemiol.* **2014**, *43*, 1226–1236. [CrossRef]

72. Tian, Y.F.; Chu, C.H.; Wu, M.H.; Chang, C.L.; Yang, T.; Chou, Y.C.; Hsu, G.C.; Yu, C.P.; Yu, J.C.; Sun, C.A. Anthropometric measures, plasma adiponectin, and breast cancer risk. *Endocr. Cancer* **2007**, *14*, 669–677. [CrossRef] [PubMed]

73. Ye, J.; Jia, J.; Dong, S.; Zhang, C.; Yu, S.; Li, L.; Mao, C.; Wang, D.; Chen, J.; Yuan, G. Circulating adiponectin levels and the risk of breast cancer: A meta-analysis. *Eur. J. Cancer Prev.* **2014**, *23*, 158–165. [CrossRef]

74. Mantzoros, C.; Petridou, E.; Dessypris, N.; Chavelas, C.; Dalamaga, M.; Alexe, D.M.; Papadiamantis, Y.; Markopoulos, C.; Spanos, E.; Chrousos, G.; et al. Adiponectin and breast cancer risk. *J. Clin. Endocrinol. Metab.* **2004**, *89*, 1102–1107. [CrossRef]

75. Tworoger, S.S.; Eliassen, A.H.; Kelesidis, T.; Colditz, G.A.; Willett, W.C.; Mantzoros, C.S.; Hankinson, S.E. Plasma adiponectin concentrations and risk of incident breast cancer. *J. Clin. Endocrinol. Metab.* **2007**, *92*, 1510–1516. [CrossRef]

76. Cust, A.E.; Stocks, T.; Lukanova, A.; Lundin, E.; Hallmans, G.; Kaaks, R.; Jonsson, H.; Stattin, P. The influence of overweight and insulin resistance on breast cancer risk and tumour stage at diagnosis: A prospective study. *Breast Cancer Res. Treat.* **2009**, *113*, 567–576. [CrossRef] [PubMed]

77. Hancke, K.; Grubeck, D.; Hauser, N.; Kreienberg, R.; Weiss, J.M. Adipocyte fatty acid-binding protein as a novel prognostic factor in obese breast cancer patients. *Breast Cancer Res. Treat.* **2010**, *119*, 367. [CrossRef] [PubMed]

78. Macis, D.; Gandini, S.; Guerrieri-Gonzaga, A.; Johansson, H.; Magni, P.; Ruscica, M.; Lazzeroni, M.; Serrano, D.; Cazzaniga, M.; Mora, S.; et al. Prognostic effect of circulating adiponectin in a randomized 2 x 2 trial of low-dose tamoxifen and fenretinide in premenopausal women at risk for breast cancer. *J. Clin. Oncol.* **2012**, *30*, 151–157. [CrossRef]

79. Gu, L.; Cao, C.; Fu, J.; Li, Q.; Li, D.H.; Chen, M.Y. Serum adiponectin in breast cancer: A meta-analysis. *Medicine* **2018**, *97*, e11433. [CrossRef]

80. Jeong, Y.J.; Bong, J.G.; Park, S.H.; Choi, J.H.; Oh, H.K. Expression of leptin, leptin receptor, adiponectin, and adiponectin receptor in ductal carcinoma in situ and invasive breast cancer. *J. Breast Cancer* **2011**, *14*, 96–103. [CrossRef]

81. Yu, Z.; Tang, S.; Ma, H.; Duan, H.; Zeng, Y. Association of serum adiponectin with breast cancer: A meta-analysis of 27 case-control studies. *Medicine* **2019**, *98*, e14359. [CrossRef] [PubMed]

82. Liu, L.Y.; Wang, M.; Ma, Z.B.; Yu, L.X.; Zhang, Q.; Gao, D.Z.; Wang, F.; Yu, Z.G. The role of adiponectin in breast cancer: A meta-analysis. *PLoS ONE* **2013**, *8*, e73183. [CrossRef] [PubMed]

83. Silva, F.M.; de Almeida, J.C.; Feoli, A.M. Effect of diet on adiponectin levels in blood. *Nutr. Rev.* **2011**, *69*, 599–612. [CrossRef] [PubMed]

84. Lyons, A.; Coleman, M.; Riis, S.; Favre, C.; O'Flanagan, C.H.; Zhdanov, A.V.; Papkovsky, D.B.; Hursting, S.D.; O'Connor, R. Insulin-like growth factor 1 signaling is essential for mitochondrial biogenesis and mitophagy in cancer cells. *J. Biol. Chem.* **2017**, *292*, 16983–16998. [CrossRef] [PubMed]

85. Lai, A.; Sarcevic, B.; Prall, O.W.; Sutherland, R.L. Insulin/insulin-like growth factor-I and estrogen cooperate to stimulate cyclin E-Cdk2 activation and cell Cycle progression in MCF-7 breast cancer cells through differential regulation of cyclin E and p21(WAF1/Cip1). *J. Biol. Chem.* **2001**, *276*, 25823–25833. [CrossRef] [PubMed]

86. Gavrila, A.; Chan, J.L.; Yiannakouris, N.; Kontogianni, M.; Miller, L.C.; Orlova, C.; Mantzoros, C.S. Serum adiponectin levels are inversely associated with overall and central fat distribution but are not directly regulated by acute fasting or leptin administration in humans: Cross-sectional and interventional studies. *J. Clin. Endocrinol. Metab.* **2003**, *88*, 4823–4831. [CrossRef] [PubMed]

87. Georgiou, G.P.; Provatopoulou, X.; Kalogera, E.; Siasos, G.; Menenakos, E.; Zografos, G.C.; Gounaris, A. Serum resistin is inversely related to breast cancer risk in premenopausal women. *Breast* **2016**, *29*, 163–169. [CrossRef] [PubMed]

88. Guo, M.M.; Duan, X.N.; Cui, S.D.; Tian, F.G.; Cao, X.C.; Geng, C.Z.; Fan, Z.M.; Wang, X.; Wang, S.; Jiang, H.C.; et al. Circulating High-Molecular-Weight (HMW) Adiponectin Level Is Related with Breast Cancer Risk Better than Total Adiponectin: A Case-Control Study. *PLoS ONE* **2015**, *10*, e0129246. [CrossRef] [PubMed]

89. Wang, Y.; Lam, J.B.; Lam, K.S.; Liu, J.; Lam, M.C.; Hoo, R.L.; Wu, D.; Cooper, G.J.; Xu, A. Adiponectin modulates the glycogen synthase kinase-3beta/beta-catenin signaling pathway and attenuates mammary tumorigenesis of MDA-MB-231 cells in nude mice. *Cancer Res.* **2006**, *66*, 11462–11470. [CrossRef] [PubMed]

90. Grossmann, M.E.; Nkhata, K.J.; Mizuno, N.K.; Ray, A.; Cleary, M.P. Effects of adiponectin on breast cancer cell growth and signaling. *Br. J. Cancer* **2008**, *98*, 370–379. [CrossRef]

91. Nakayama, S.; Miyoshi, Y.; Ishihara, H.; Noguchi, S. Growth-inhibitory effect of adiponectin via adiponectin receptor 1 on human breast cancer cells through inhibition of S-phase entry without inducing apoptosis. *Breast Cancer Res. Treat.* **2008**, *112*, 405–410. [CrossRef] [PubMed]

92. Mauro, L.; Pellegrino, M.; De Amicis, F.; Ricchio, E.; Giordano, F.; Rizza, P.; Catalano, S.; Bonofiglio, D.; Sisci, D.; Panno, M.L.; et al. Evidences that estrogen receptor alpha interferes with adiponectin effects on breast cancer cell growth. *Cell Cycle* **2014**, *13*, 553–564. [CrossRef] [PubMed]

93. Panno, M.L.; Naimo, G.D.; Spina, E.; Ando, S.; Mauro, L. Different molecular signaling sustaining adiponectin action in breast cancer. *Curr. Opin. Pharmacol.* **2016**, *31*, 1–7. [CrossRef] [PubMed]

94. Mauro, L.; Naimo, G.D.; Gelsomino, L.; Malivindi, R.; Bruno, L.; Pellegrino, M.; Tarallo, R.; Memoli, D.; Weisz, A.; Panno, M.L.; et al. Uncoupling effects of estrogen receptor alpha on LKB1/AMPK interaction upon adiponectin exposure in breast cancer. *FASEB J.* **2018**, *32*, 4343–4355. [CrossRef] [PubMed]

95. Kang, J.H.; Lee, Y.Y.; Yu, B.Y.; Yang, B.S.; Cho, K.H.; Yoon, D.K.; Roh, Y.K. Adiponectin induces growth arrest and apoptosis of MDA-MB-231 breast cancer cell. *Archives Pharm. Res.* **2005**, *28*, 1263–1269. [CrossRef]

96. Li, Z.J.; Yang, X.L.; Yao, Y.; Han, W.Q.; Li, B.O. Circulating adiponectin levels and risk of endometrial cancer: Systematic review and meta-analysis. *Exp. Ther. Med.* **2016**, *11*, 2305–2313. [CrossRef] [PubMed]

97. Lin, T.; Zhao, X.; Kong, W.M. Association between adiponectin levels and endometrial carcinoma risk: Evidence from a dose-response meta-analysis. *BMJ open* **2015**, *5*, e008541. [CrossRef] [PubMed]

98. Zeng, F.; Shi, J.; Long, Y.; Tian, H.; Li, X.; Zhao, A.Z.; Li, R.F.; Chen, T. Adiponectin and Endometrial Cancer: A Systematic Review and Meta-Analysis. *Cell. Physiol. Biochem.* **2015**, *36*, 1670–1678. [CrossRef]

99. Zheng, Q.; Wu, H.; Cao, J. Circulating adiponectin and risk of endometrial cancer. *PLoS ONE* **2015**, *10*, e0129824. [CrossRef] [PubMed]

100. Gong, T.T.; Wu, Q.J.; Wang, Y.L.; Ma, X.X. Circulating adiponectin, leptin and adiponectin-leptin ratio and endometrial cancer risk: Evidence from a meta-analysis of epidemiologic studies. *Int. J. Cancer* **2015**, *137*, 1967–1978. [CrossRef] [PubMed]

101. Jin, J.H.; Kim, H.J.; Kim, C.Y.; Kim, Y.H.; Ju, W.; Kim, S.C. Association of plasma adiponectin and leptin levels with the development and progression of ovarian cancer. *Obstetrics Gynecol. Sci.* **2016**, *59*, 279–285. [CrossRef] [PubMed]

102. Dossus, L.; Franceschi, S.; Biessy, C.; Navionis, A.S.; Travis, R.C.; Weiderpass, E.; Scalbert, A.; Romieu, I.; Tjonneland, A.; Olsen, A.; et al. Adipokines and inflammation markers and risk of differentiated thyroid carcinoma: The EPIC study. *Int. J. Cancer* **2018**, *142*, 1332–1342. [CrossRef] [PubMed]

103. Warakomski, J.; Romuk, E.; Jarzab, B.; Krajewska, J.; Sieminska, L. Concentrations of Selected Adipokines, Interleukin-6, and Vitamin D in Patients with Papillary Thyroid Carcinoma in Respect to Thyroid Cancer Stages. *Int. J. Endocrinol.* **2018**, *2018*, 4921803. [CrossRef] [PubMed]

104. Abooshahab, R.; Yaghmaei, P.; Ghadaksaz, H.G.; Hedayati, M. Lack of Association between Serum Adiponectin/Leptin Levels and Medullary Thyroid Cancer. *Asian Pac. J. Cancer Prev.* **2016**, *17*, 3861–3864.

105. Mitsiades, N.; Pazaitou-Panayiotou, K.; Aronis, K.N.; Moon, H.S.; Chamberland, J.P.; Liu, X.; Diakopoulos, K.N.; Kyttaris, V.; Panagiotou, V.; Mylvaganam, G.; et al. Circulating adiponectin is inversely associated with risk of thyroid cancer: In vivo and in vitro studies. *J. Clin. Endocrinol. Metab.* **2011**, *96*, E2023–E2028. [CrossRef] [PubMed]

106. Liao, Q.; Long, C.; Deng, Z.; Bi, X.; Hu, J. The role of circulating adiponectin in prostate cancer: A meta-analysis. *Int. J. Biol. Markers* **2015**, *30*. [CrossRef] [PubMed]

107. Ikeda, A.; Nakagawa, T.; Kawai, K.; Onozawa, M.; Hayashi, T.; Matsushita, Y.; Tsutsumi, M.; Kojima, T.; Miyazaki, J.; Nishiyama, H. Serum adiponectin concentration in 2,939 Japanese men undergoing screening for prostate cancer. *Prostate Inte.* **2015**, *3*, 87–92. [CrossRef] [PubMed]

108. Li, H.; Stampfer, M.J.; Mucci, L.; Rifai, N.; Qiu, W.; Kurth, T.; Ma, J. A 25-year prospective study of plasma adiponectin and leptin concentrations and prostate cancer risk and survival. *Clin. Chem.* **2010**, *56*, 34–43. [CrossRef]

109. Baillargeon, J.; Platz, E.A.; Rose, D.P.; Pollock, B.H.; Ankerst, D.P.; Haffner, S.; Higgins, B.; Lokshin, A.; Troyer, D.; Hernandez, J.; et al. Obesity, adipokines, and prostate cancer in a prospective population-based study. *Cancer Epidemiol. Biomark. Prev.* **2006**, *15*, 1331–1335. [CrossRef] [PubMed]

110. Goktas, S.; Yilmaz, M.I.; Caglar, K.; Sonmez, A.; Kilic, S.; Bedir, S. Prostate cancer and adiponectin. *Urology* **2005**, *65*, 1168–1172. [CrossRef]

111. Jemal, A.; Bray, F.; Center, M.M.; Ferlay, J.; Ward, E.; Forman, D. Global cancer statistics. *Cancer J. Clin.* **2011**, *61*, 69–90. [CrossRef]

112. Orekoya, O.; Samson, M.E.; Trivedi, T.; Vyas, S.; Steck, S.E. The Impact of Obesity on Surgical Outcome in Endometrial Cancer Patients: A Systematic Review. *J. Gynecol. Surg.* **2016**, *32*, 149–157. [CrossRef]

113. Crosbie, E.J.; Zwahlen, M.; Kitchener, H.C.; Egger, M.; Renehan, A.G. Body mass index, hormone replacement therapy, and endometrial cancer risk: A meta-analysis. *Cancer Epidemiol. Biomarkers Prev.* **2010**, *19*, 3119–3130. [CrossRef] [PubMed]

114. Aarestrup, J.; Gamborg, M.; Ulrich, L.G.; Sorensen, T.I.; Baker, J.L. Childhood body mass index and height and risk of histologic subtypes of endometrial cancer. *Int. J. Obesity* **2016**, *40*, 1096–1102. [CrossRef] [PubMed]

115. van Kruijsdijk, R.C.; van der Wall, E.; Visseren, F.L. Obesity and cancer: The role of dysfunctional adipose tissue. *Cancer Epidemiol. Biomarkers Prev.* **2009**, *18*, 2569–2578. [CrossRef] [PubMed]

116. Ma, Y.; Liu, Z.; Zhang, Y.; Lu, B. Serum leptin, adiponectin and endometrial cancer risk in Chinese women. *J. Gynecol. Oncol.* **2013**, *24*, 336–341. [CrossRef] [PubMed]

117. Zhang, L.; Wen, K.; Han, X.; Liu, R.; Qu, Q. Adiponectin mediates antiproliferative and apoptotic responses in endometrial carcinoma by the AdipoRs/AMPK pathway. *Gynecol. Oncol.* **2015**, *137*, 311–320. [CrossRef]

118. Cust, A.E.; Kaaks, R.; Friedenreich, C.; Bonnet, F.; Laville, M.; Lukanova, A.; Rinaldi, S.; Dossus, L.; Slimani, N.; Lundin, E.; et al. Plasma adiponectin levels and endometrial cancer risk in pre- and postmenopausal women. *J. Clin. Endocrinol. Metab.* **2007**, *92*, 255–263. [CrossRef]

119. Rzepka-Gorska, I.; Bedner, R.; Cymbaluk-Ploska, A.; Chudecka-Glaz, A. Serum adiponectin in relation to endometrial cancer and endometrial hyperplasia with atypia in obese women. *Eur. J. Gynaecol. Oncol.* **2008**, *29*, 594–597.

120. Moon, H.S.; Chamberland, J.P.; Aronis, K.; Tseleni-Balafouta, S.; Mantzoros, C.S. Direct role of adiponectin and adiponectin receptors in endometrial cancer: In vitro and ex vivo studies in humans. *Mol. Cancer Ther.* **2011**, *10*, 2234–2243. [CrossRef]

121. Yabushita, H.; Iwasaki, K.; Obayashi, Y.; Wakatsuki, A. Clinicopathological roles of adiponectin and leptin receptors in endometrial carcinoma. *Oncol. Lett.* **2014**, *7*, 1109–1117. [CrossRef] [PubMed]

122. Romero, I.; Bast, R.C., Jr. Minireview: Human ovarian cancer: Biology, current management, and paths to personalizing therapy. *Endocrinology* **2012**, *153*, 1593–1602. [CrossRef] [PubMed]

123. Kalliala, I.; Markozannes, G.; Gunter, M.J.; Paraskevaidis, E.; Gabra, H.; Mitra, A.; Terzidou, V.; Bennett, P.; Martin-Hirsch, P.; Tsilidis, K.K.; et al. Obesity and gynaecological and obstetric conditions: Umbrella review of the literature. *BMJ* **2017**, *359*, j4511. [CrossRef] [PubMed]

124. Diaz, E.S.; Karlan, B.Y.; Li, A.J. Obesity-associated adipokines correlate with survival in epithelial ovarian cancer. *Gynecol. Oncol.* **2013**, *129*, 353–357. [CrossRef] [PubMed]

125. Slomian, G.J.; Nowak, D.; Buczkowska, M.; Glogowska-Gruszka, A.; Slomian, S.P.; Roczniak, W.; Janyga, S.; Nowak, P. The role of adiponectin and leptin in the treatment of ovarian cancer patients. *Endokr. Polska* **2019**, *70*, 57–63. [CrossRef]

126. Li, X.; Yu, Z.; Fang, L.; Liu, F.; Jiang, K. Expression of Adiponectin Receptor-1 and Prognosis of Epithelial Ovarian Cancer Patients. *Med. Sci. Monit.* **2017**, *23*, 1514–1521. [CrossRef]

127. Hoffmann, M.; Gogola, J.; Ptak, A. Adiponectin Reverses the Proliferative Effects of Estradiol and IGF-1 in Human Epithelial Ovarian Cancer Cells by Downregulating the Expression of Their Receptors. *Hormones Cancer* **2018**, *9*, 166–174. [CrossRef]

128. Haugen, B.R.; Alexander, E.K.; Bible, K.C.; Doherty, G.M.; Mandel, S.J.; Nikiforov, Y.E.; Pacini, F.; Randolph, G.W.; Sawka, A.M.; Schlumberger, M.; et al. 2015 American Thyroid Association Management Guidelines for Adult Patients with Thyroid Nodules and Differentiated Thyroid Cancer: The American Thyroid Association Guidelines Task Force on Thyroid Nodules and Differentiated Thyroid Cancer. *Thyroid* **2016**, *26*, 1–133. [CrossRef]

129. Schmid, D.; Ricci, C.; Behrens, G.; Leitzmann, M.F. Adiposity and risk of thyroid cancer: A systematic review and meta-analysis. *Obesity Rev.* **2015**, *16*, 1042–1054. [CrossRef]

130. Pappa, T.; Alevizaki, M. Obesity and thyroid cancer: A clinical update. *Thyroid* **2014**, *24*, 190–199. [CrossRef]

131. Cheng, S.P.; Liu, C.L.; Hsu, Y.C.; Chang, Y.C.; Huang, S.Y.; Lee, J.J. Expression and biologic significance of adiponectin receptors in papillary thyroid carcinoma. *Cell Biochem. Biophys.* **2013**, *65*, 203–210. [CrossRef] [PubMed]

132. Hu, M.B.; Liu, S.H.; Jiang, H.W.; Bai, P.D.; Ding, Q. Obesity affects the biopsy-mediated detection of prostate cancer, particularly high-grade prostate cancer: A dose-response meta-analysis of 29,464 patients. *PLoS ONE* **2014**, *9*, e106677. [CrossRef] [PubMed]

133. Hu, M.B.; Xu, H.; Bai, P.D.; Jiang, H.W.; Ding, Q. Obesity has multifaceted impact on biochemical recurrence of prostate cancer: A dose-response meta-analysis of 36,927 patients. *Med. Oncol.* **2014**, *31*, 829. [CrossRef] [PubMed]

134. Hu, M.B.; Xu, H.; Hu, J.M.; Zhu, W.H.; Yang, T.; Jiang, H.W.; Ding, Q. Genetic polymorphisms in leptin, adiponectin and their receptors affect risk and aggressiveness of prostate cancer: Evidence from a meta-analysis and pooled-review. *Oncotarget* **2016**, *7*, 81049–81061. [CrossRef] [PubMed]

135. Michalakis, K.; Williams, C.J.; Mitsiades, N.; Blakeman, J.; Balafouta-Tselenis, S.; Giannopoulos, A.; Mantzoros, C.S. Serum adiponectin concentrations and tissue expression of adiponectin receptors are reduced in patients with prostate cancer: A case control study. *Cancer Epidemiol. Biomarkers Prev.* **2007**, *16*, 308–313. [CrossRef] [PubMed]

136. Tan, W.; Wang, L.; Ma, Q.; Qi, M.; Lu, N.; Zhang, L.; Han, B. Adiponectin as a potential tumor suppressor inhibiting epithelial-to-mesenchymal transition but frequently silenced in prostate cancer by promoter methylation. *Prostate* **2015**, *75*, 1197–1205. [CrossRef] [PubMed]

137. Lu, J.P.; Hou, Z.F.; Duivenvoorden, W.C.; Whelan, K.; Honig, A.; Pinthus, J.H. Adiponectin inhibits oxidative stress in human prostate carcinoma cells. *Prostate Cancer Prostatic Dis.* **2012**, *15*, 28–35. [CrossRef] [PubMed]

138. Bub, J.D.; Miyazaki, T.; Iwamoto, Y. Adiponectin as a growth inhibitor in prostate cancer cells. *Biochem. Biophys. Res. Commun.* **2006**, *340*, 1158–1166. [CrossRef] [PubMed]

139. Gao, Q.; Zheng, J.; Yao, X.; Peng, B. Adiponectin inhibits VEGF-A in prostate cancer cells. *Tumour Biol.* **2015**, *36*, 4287–4292. [CrossRef] [PubMed]

140. Gao, Q.; Yao, X.; Zheng, J. MiR-323 Inhibits Prostate Cancer Vascularization Through Adiponectin Receptor. *Cellular Physiol. Biochem.* **2015**, *36*, 1491–1498. [CrossRef]

141. Rider, J.R.; Fiorentino, M.; Kelly, R.; Gerke, T.; Jordahl, K.; Sinnott, J.A.; Giovannucci, E.L.; Loda, M.; Mucci, L.A.; Finn, S.; et al. Tumor expression of adiponectin receptor 2 and lethal prostate cancer. *Carcinogenesis* **2015**, *36*, 639–647. [CrossRef] [PubMed]

142. Nguyen, P.L.; Ma, J.; Chavarro, J.E.; Freedman, M.L.; Lis, R.; Fedele, G.; Fiore, C.; Qiu, W.; Fiorentino, M.; Finn, S.; et al. Fatty acid synthase polymorphisms, tumor expression, body mass index, prostate cancer risk, and survival. *J.Clin. Oncol.* **2010**, *28*, 3958–3964. [CrossRef] [PubMed]

143. Gu, C.; Qu, Y.; Zhang, G.; Sun, L.; Zhu, Y.; Ye, D. A single nucleotide polymorphism in ADIPOQ predicts biochemical recurrence after radical prostatectomy in localized prostate cancer. *Oncotarget* **2015**, *6*, 32205–32211. [CrossRef] [PubMed]

144. Saxena, N.K.; Sharma, D. Metastasis suppression by adiponectin: LKB1 rises up to the challenge. *Cell Adhes. Migr.* **2010**, *4*, 358–362. [CrossRef] [PubMed]

145. Wu, X.; Yan, Q.; Zhang, Z.; Du, G.; Wan, X. Acrp30 inhibits leptin-induced metastasis by downregulating the JAK/STAT3 pathway via AMPK activation in aggressive SPEC-2 endometrial cancer cells. *Oncol. Rep.* **2012**, *27*, 1488–1496. [CrossRef] [PubMed]

146. Hadad, S.M.; Fleming, S.; Thompson, A.M. Targeting AMPK: A new therapeutic opportunity in breast cancer. *Crit. Rev. Oncol. Hematol.* **2008**, *67*, 1–7. [CrossRef] [PubMed]

147. Otvos, L., Jr.; Haspinger, E.; La Russa, F.; Maspero, F.; Graziano, P.; Kovalszky, I.; Lovas, S.; Nama, K.; Hoffmann, R.; Knappe, D.; et al. Design and development of a peptide-based adiponectin receptor agonist for cancer treatment. *BMC Biotech.* **2011**, *11*, 90. [CrossRef]

148. Otvos, L., Jr.; Kovalszky, I.; Olah, J.; Coroniti, R.; Knappe, D.; Nollmann, F.I.; Hoffmann, R.; Wade, J.D.; Lovas, S.; Surmacz, E. Optimization of adiponectin-derived peptides for inhibition of cancer cell growth and signaling. *Biopolymers* **2015**, *104*, 156–166. [CrossRef] [PubMed]

149. Sun, Y.; Zang, Z.; Zhong, L.; Wu, M.; Su, Q.; Gao, X.; Zan, W.; Lin, D.; Zhao, Y.; Zhang, Z. Identification of adiponectin receptor agonist utilizing a fluorescence polarization based high throughput assay. *PLoS ONE* **2013**, *8*, e63354. [CrossRef] [PubMed]

150. Maeda, N.; Takahashi, M.; Funahashi, T.; Kihara, S.; Nishizawa, H.; Kishida, K.; Nagaretani, H.; Matsuda, M.; Komuro, R.; Ouchi, N.; et al. PPARgamma ligands increase expression and plasma concentrations of adiponectin, an adipose-derived protein. *Diabetes* **2001**, *50*, 2094–2099. [CrossRef]

151. Burstein, H.J.; Demetri, G.D.; Mueller, E.; Sarraf, P.; Spiegelman, B.M.; Winer, E.P. Use of the peroxisome proliferator-activated receptor (PPAR) gamma ligand troglitazone as treatment for refractory breast cancer: A phase II study. *Breast Cancer Res. Treat.* **2003**, *79*, 391–397. [CrossRef] [PubMed]

152. Williams, R. Discontinued in 2013: Oncology drugs. *Exp. Opin. Invest. Drugs* **2015**, *24*, 95–110. [CrossRef] [PubMed]

153. Ealey, K.N.; Kaludjerovic, J.; Archer, M.C.; Ward, W.E. Adiponectin is a negative regulator of bone mineral and bone strength in growing mice. *Exper. Biol. Med.* **2008**, *233*, 1546–1553. [CrossRef] [PubMed]

154. Holland, W.L.; Scherer, P.E. Cell Biology. Ronning after the adiponectin receptors. *Science* **2013**, *342*, 1460–1461. [CrossRef] [PubMed]

155. Kriketos, A.D.; Gan, S.K.; Poynten, A.M.; Furler, S.M.; Chisholm, D.J.; Campbell, L.V. Exercise increases adiponectin levels and insulin sensitivity in humans. *Diabetes Care* **2004**, *27*, 629–630. [CrossRef] [PubMed]

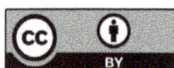

International Journal of
Molecular Sciences

MDPI

Review

Adiponectin, Obesity, and Cancer: Clash of the Bigwigs in Health and Disease

Sheetal Parida *,†, Sumit Siddharth *,† and Dipali Sharma *

Department of Oncology, Johns Hopkins University School of Medicine and the Sidney Kimmel Comprehensive Cancer Center at Johns Hopkins, Baltimore, MD 21231, USA
* Correspondence: sparida1@jhu.edu (S.P.); ssiddha2@jhmi.edu (S.S.); dsharma7@jhmi.edu (D.S.);
  Tel.: +1-410-455-1345 (D.S.); Fax: +1-410-614-4073 (D.S.)
† These authors contributed equally to this work.

Received: 1 May 2019; Accepted: 17 May 2019; Published: 22 May 2019

Abstract: Adiponectin is one of the most important adipocytokines secreted by adipocytes and is called a "guardian angel adipocytokine" owing to its unique biological functions. Adiponectin inversely correlates with body fat mass and visceral adiposity. Identified independently by four different research groups, adiponectin has multiple names; Acrp30, apM1, GBP28, and AdipoQ. Adiponectin mediates its biological functions via three known receptors, AdipoR1, AdipoR2, and T-cadherin, which are distributed throughout the body. Biological functions of adiponectin are multifold ranging from anti-diabetic, anti-atherogenic, anti-inflammatory to anti-cancer. Lower adiponectin levels have been associated with metabolic syndrome, type 2 diabetes, insulin resistance, cardiovascular diseases, and hypertension. A plethora of experimental evidence supports the role of obesity and increased adiposity in multiple cancers including breast, liver, pancreatic, prostrate, ovarian, and colorectal cancers. Obesity mediates its effect on cancer progression via dysregulation of adipocytokines including increased production of oncogenic adipokine leptin along with decreased production of adiponectin. Multiple studies have shown the protective role of adiponectin in obesity-associated diseases and cancer. Adiponectin modulates multiple signaling pathways to exert its physiological and protective functions. Many studies over the years have shown the beneficial effect of adiponectin in cancer regression and put forth various innovative ways to increase adiponectin levels.

Keywords: adiponectin; obesity; cancer

---

1. Discovery of a Guardian Angel Adipocytokine

White adipose tissue (WAT), once regarded as the major site of energy storage and homeostasis, is now known to be an endocrine organ producing numerous biologically active molecules and hormones, one of the most important being adiponectin. Mainly secreted by adipocytes, adiponectin is also produced to some extent by bone marrow, osteoblasts, fetal tissue, myocytes, cardiomyocytes, and salivary gland epithelial cells [1,2]. The first report on adiponectin was published in 1995, where it was denoted as an adipocyte complement related protein of 30 kDa (Acrp30), specifically expressed in the adipose tissues and differentiated adipocytes [3]. Another group identified mouse adiponectin and referred to it as AdipoQ using an mRNA differential display technique. They reported 247 amino acids polypeptide coded by adipoQ cDNA specifically in adipose tissues of mice and rats. Importantly, they also showed the reduction of adipoQ mRNA in obese mice and humans [4]. These two pioneering papers indicated the function of adiponectin in energy homeostasis. The next few years observed a revolutionary rise in the exploration of adiponectin. In 1996, another research group discerned adiponectin as the most abundant transcript in the cDNA library of human adipose tissue, which was termed as adipose most abundant gene transcript1 (*apM1*) [5]. In the same year, yet another group isolated adiponectin from human plasma using affinity chromatography, followed by protein sequencing and referred to as gelatin-binding protein of 28 kDa (GBP28) [6]. Adiponectin is a small protein composed of 224 amino acids, present in circulating concentrations as high as 2 to 10 µg/mL in humans. The protein encompasses a signal domain followed by a variable domain which is species specific, a collagen domain, and a globular domain.

Berg and colleagues and Yamauchi and colleagues were the first to identify the physiological importance of adiponectin and highlighted the adiponectin axis as a possible therapeutic field for the treatment of diabetes [7,8]. Enhanced circulating levels of adiponectin inhibits gluconeogenesis [9]. They concluded that reduced adiponectin in obese- and adipose-tissue-deficient mice serve as a responsible factor for the development of insulin resistance [9]. The work of Yamauchi et al. [8] reported decreased adiponectin in insulin resistance and altered insulin-sensitive mice models. In the continuation work, Yamauchi et al. showed that in skeletal muscle, both globular as well as full-length adiponectin are able to induce AMP activated protein kinase (AMPK), while only full-length adiponectin can stimulate AMPK in liver cells [10]. Ahima and co-workers [11] demonstrated that intravenous injections of adiponectin lead to an increase in the adiponectin level in cerebrospinal fluid. Intracerebroventricular administration of adiponectin in leptin-induced obese mice caused enhanced thermogenesis, weight loss, and decrease in serum glucose and serum lipid levels [11]. The second decade of the 21st century observed the rediscovery of the physiological role of adiponectin. Holland et al. [12] observed increased ceramide content in the liver of obese mice (ob/ob mice or high-fat diet mice). An increase in ceramide is associated with insulin resistance, cell death, and atherosclerosis [13]. Holland et al. [12] reported that adiponectin enhances the ceramide catabolism in the liver via the ceramidase activity of its receptors, AdipoR1 and AdipoR2, which was independent of AMPK activation. Xia et al. reported a decrease in the ceramide level in transgenic mice with genetically induced acid ceramidase activity in the hepatic cells or in adipose tissues [14]. The contribution of adiponectin is not only restricted to liver, but also extends to other major organs. Rutkowski et al. showed that overexpression of adiponectin recovered the kidney podocytes rapidly and demonstrated low intestinal fibrosis. But the lack of adiponectin caused irreparable albuminuria and damage in kidney podocytes [15]. Adiponectin enhances the myocyte enhancer factor-2 (MEF2) induction in cardiomyocytes via p38 MAPK (mitogen-activated protein kinases) signaling [16].

Adiponectin works by AdipoR1 and AdipoR2 receptors, which are unique and universally expressed. AdipoR1 is most abundantly found in skeletal muscle whereas AdipoR2 is predominantly present in liver [17]. AdipoR1 exhibits higher affinity for globular adiponectin, whereas AdipoR2 shows higher affinity for full-length adiponectin [17]. Both AdipoR1 and AdipoR2 accumulate in homodimeric and heterodimeric complexes once bound by adiponectin [17]. Hug et al. [18] identified T-cadherin, a member of the cadherin superfamily, as an effective receptor of hexamers and of high molecular weight (HMW) adiponectin oligomers. Adiponectin can exert its biological functions by directly interacting with its specific receptors that provide some organ and functional specificity to adiponectin. In addition, multiple regulatory mechanisms tightly regulate adiponectin and further control its biological impact on various organs in normal as well as disease state.

2. Tight Regulation of Adiponectin at Multiple Levels

2.1. The Role of Coactivators in Transcriptional Regulation of Adiponectin

Peroxisome proliferator-activated receptor gamma is an important transcription factor belonging to the PPAR family, is a positive regulator of adiponectin transcription, and is widely expressed in adipose tissue. Lower adiponectin levels have been associated with the P12A mutation in PPARγ. The Thiazolidinedione class of medications (TZDs) are PPARγ agonists that stimulate adiponectin production and are used as antidiabetics. Its efficacy has been shown in vitro as well as in vivo studies [19–21] but could be limited by a mutation at a putative PPARγ-recognizing PPAR response element (PPRE) site [19]. However, some reports demonstrate an increase in high molecular weight (HMW) adiponectin biosynthesis in response to TZDs without changing adiponectin mRNA levels indicating a predominantly translational regulation of adiponectin synthesis. Forkhead box protein O1 (FoxO1) is another key regulator of adipocyte differentiation which is known to positively regulate adiponectin transcription [22]. Biological functions and cellular localization of this transcription factor is regulated by NAD-dependent deacetylase Sirt1 (sirtuin 1) and by additional post-translational modifications including phosphorylation and acetylation. It complexes with CCAAT-enhancer-binding proteins (C/EBPα) which in turn is stimulated by Sirt1 overexpression, consequently, activating adiponectin promoter [23]. However, FoxO1 activity could be controlled by multiple upstream events that can in turn regulate adiponectin levels. C/EBPα interacts with the CCAAT motif of the adiponectin promoter recruiting co-activators, in turn stimulating transcriptional activity. Co-expression of PPARγ and C/EBPα are known to significantly increase adiponectin expression [24,25]. Sterol regulatory element-binding proteins (SERBPs) are membrane-bound precursors that interact with the nuclear envelope or ER (endoplasmic reticulum) membranes. Sterol regulatory element-binding proteins regulate the transcription of lipid-metabolizing enzymes. Binding of SREBP to the SERBP response element (SRE) on adiponectin promoter amplifies adiponectin expression. Adiponectin promoter is also transactivated by SREBP-1c and is prevented in case there is a mutation in the SRE motif. Adenovirus-mediated overexpression of SREBP-1c is known to elevate adiponectin levels in 3T3-L1 adipocytes [26].

2.2. Involvement of Multiple Co-Factors in Transcriptional Repression of Adiponectin

cAMP response element-binding protein (CREB) is a master regulator of adipogenesis and has been associated with systemic insulin resistance in obese state [27]. Camp response element-binding protein indirectly represses adiponectin transcription by upregulating transcription factor ATF3 (activating transcription factor 3), which binds to the AP-1 (activator protein-1) site next to the NFAT (nuclear factor of activated T-cells) binding site of adiponectin promoter [28]. Nuclear factor of activated T-cell proteins are calcium-sensitive proteins associated with immune functions and have been detected in 3T3-L1 adipocytes [29]. Overexpressed in obesity and diabetes, they have been associated with WAT activity but the exact mechanism of NFAT in adiponectin regulation is unclear. Nuclear factor of activated T-cell binding site deletion in adiponectin promoter [27] enhances adiponectin expression while overexpression of NFAT diminishes adiponectin transcription. Additional transcription factors involved in downregulation of adiponectin transcription include AP-2β (activating enhancer binding protein-2β), IGFBP-3 (IGF-1-binding protein 3), and Id3 (inhibitor of differentiation-3) [30]. Fat accumulation in obese state induces a hypoxic microenvironment, which is known to inhibit adiponectin transcription via hypoxia inducible factor 1 alpha (HIF1α). Obesity-induced chronic inflammation leads to overexpression of TNFα (tumor necrosis factor alpha), IL6 (interleukin 6), IL18 (interleukin 18), and other pro-inflammatory cytokines that are also known to inhibit adiponectin. Tumor necrosis factor alpha suppresses transcription activator PPARγ via JNK (c-Jun N-terminal kinases)-mediated phosphorylation which reduces its DNA binding [31]. Tumor necrosis factor alpha also promotes IGFBP-3 inhibiting adiponectin transcription and conferring insulin resistance [32]. Tumor necrosis factor alpha has also been shown to inhibit FoxO1 and C/EBPα [30,32]. Interleukin 6 suppresses adiponectin transcription in 3T3-L1 adipocytes via p44/42 MAPK pathway [33]. Interleukin 18, on the other hand, phosphorylates and activates NFATc4, a repressor of adiponectin transcription in a ERK (extracellular-signal-regulated kinase) 1/2 dependent manner [28].

2.3. Control of Adiponectin Expression via Post-Translational Modifications

Post-translational modifications are the most important determinants of adiponectin functionality since different isoforms (trimeric, hexameric, and HMW multimeric forms) of adiponectin exhibit different biological activities. While trimeric and hexameric forms mostly regulate food intake [34], HMW forms of adiponectin mostly regulate insulin sensitivity, hepatic gluconeogenesis, and other metabolic functions [35]. Other forms also mediate some metabolic functions. Since different forms of adiponectin function differently, activity of adiponectin can be modulated by changing the ratios of different isoforms of adiponectin in serum. For example, activity of thiazolidinediones, statins, and angiotensin receptor blockers depend on increasing the proportion of HMW adiponectin [30]. There is very little evidence to support the notion that adiponectin isoforms can interconvert after secretion indicating that modulation of intracellular processes guiding multimerization of adiponectin is important. Multimerization of adiponectin into HMW complexes is a complicated and active area of research. Structurally, adiponectin has an N-terminal variable domain, a collagenous domain, and a C-terminal globular domain. Production and secretion of HMW adiponectin is dependent on hydroxylation and glycosylation of lysine residues of the collagenous domain [36–39]. Substitution of lysine residues for arginine completely abolishes HMW adiponectin synthesis. Multimerization also requires proline hydroxylation [39]. Inhibiting prolyl and lysyl hydroxylases using 2,20-dipyridyl can completely impair adiponectin multimerization [39]. ER retention of folded adiponectin molecules without being secreted leads to ER stress. It is very common in obese state and it is a major factor causing low circulating adiponectin levels. ER retention of adiponectin is maintained by thiol-mediated retention via (ER) chaperone protein 44 (ERp44) [40]. Thiol bond-reducing agents induce a 7- to 8-fold increase in secretion of adiponectin in 3T3-L1 adipocytes. Thiol-bond formation is also the determinant of adiponectin folding and assembly prior to secretion [40]. Another important factor in multimerization and release is intermolecular disulfide bond exchange by ER chaperone Ero-1La [41]. Increased expression of Ero-1La or inhibition of SIRT1, suppressor of Ero-1La results in increased assembly and release of HMW adiponectin [41]. Similarly, ERp44 inhibition using TZDs may be utilized to prevent ER retention of adiponectin and increase its circulatory levels [42]. DsbA-L (disulfide-bond A oxidoreductase-like protein) is yet another ER chaperone known to directly bind to adiponectin and aid HMW multimerization [43]. Though the mechanism is not completely understood, PPARα agonists are known to upregulate DsbA-L [43]. Hence, a combination of molecular events at the transcriptional and translational level regulate adiponectin (Figure 1).

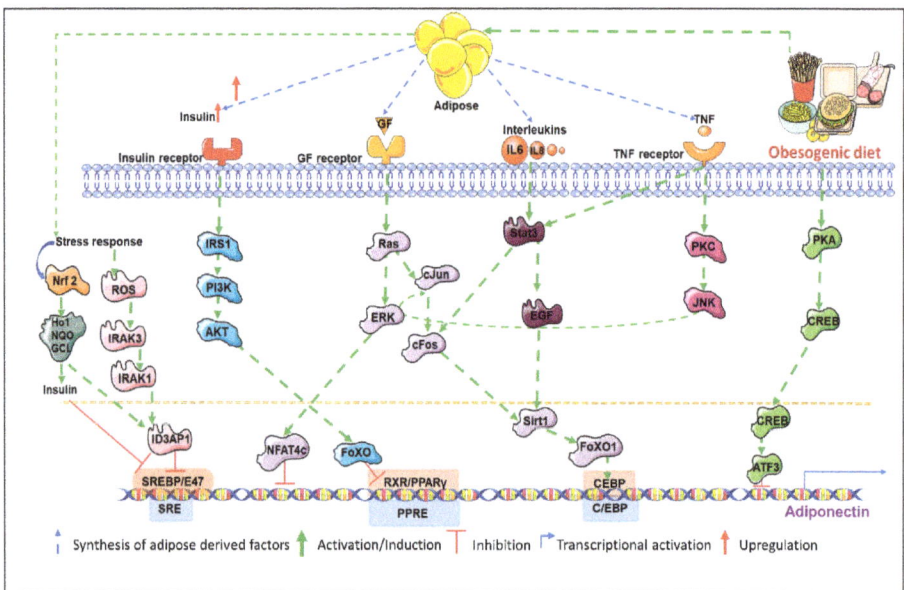

Figure 1. Multiple signaling networks converge to regulate adiponectin.

3. Physiological Functions of Adiponectin

3.1. A Central Role in the Reproductive System

Similar to other adipokines like leptin, resistin, and ghrelin, adiponectin plays a central role in reproductive functions. Circulating levels of adiponectin are known to be higher in females compared to males; testosterone exposure has been shown to reduce serum adiponectin levels. In the ovaries, adiponectin receptors 1 and 2 have been found to be expressed in granulosa cells, oocytes, and corpus luteum [44]. Adiponectin induces expression of cyclooxygenase 2 (COX2), vascular endothelial growth factor (VEGF), and prostaglandin E synthase (PGES) in granulosa cells in a porcine model [1]. Similarly, increased adiponectin and *AdipoR1* gene expression was observed in immature rat ovaries in response to human chorionic gonadotropin (hCG) [45]. Some studies also suggest a role of adiponectin in ovarian steroidogenesis, while additional studies showed species-specific variable results. Gene expression changes induced by adiponectin in the ovaries have been demonstrated to be modulated by AMPK (AMP activated protein kinase) or ERK1/2-MAPK dependent pathway [45]. Adiponectin-induced AMPK has been shown to regulate the energy requirement for follicular growth. AMPK phosphorylates PPARγ, which structurally resembles steroid hormone receptors, repressing its transactivation [45]. PPARγ is known to influence steroidogenesis, ovulation, oocyte maturation, and maintenance of corpus luteum [45]. AMPK and PPARγ, therefore, cooperatively regulate the energy balance in the ovary, thus, ensuring optimum growth of ovarian follicles [46,47]. However, mice lacking functional AdipoR1 or AdipoR2 do not demonstrate defective reproduction suggesting that adiponectin is not indispensable for reproductive functions and evidence suggests adiponectin's effect on the ovaries is by virtue of its insulin sensitizing efficiency [46,47]. The essential role of adiponectin has been explained in the early stages of fetal development [48]. Adiponectin receptor expression is higher in the endometrial epithelium of women in the mid-secretory phase of the menstrual cycle indicating a role of adiponectin in the endometrial changes associated with embryo implantation [49]. Additionally, adiponectin inhibits IL-1β-mediated inflammatory response via AMPK [49] in the stromal cells of endometrium. Adiponectin has also been detected in early developmental stages of rabbits, pigs, and mice embryos, and improves development of pig embryo by accelerating meiosis in a p38MAPK dependent manner. During developmental stages, adiponectin is not confined to adipose tissue but is also expressed in epidermis, smooth muscle fibers, small intestine wall, major arterial vessels, and ocular lens suggesting multifold functions of the hormone that remain to be understood. Gestational diabetes, a common pregnancy-related complication is also correlated with plasma adiponectin levels. Women who develop gestational diabetes during late pregnancy exhibit lower adiponectin levels in early pregnancy [1]. Hypoadiponectinemia has also been associated with polycystic ovary syndrome (PCOS), a major cause of anovulatory infertility, though reports have been inconsistent. Polycystic ovary syndrome is known to have a strong genetic association and it has been reported that single nucleotide polymorphism (SNP) in the adiponectin gene might be associated with increased risk of PCOS. Polycystic ovary syndrome patients are susceptible to glucose intolerance, insulin resistance, hypertension, and hyperlipidemia with evidently low circulating adiponectin levels [1].

3.2. Regulation of Insulin Sensitivity and Protection against Fatty Liver

Adiponectin is shown to be protective against fatty liver disease and a low circulating adiponectin has been observed in patients with chronic hepatitis and liver steatosis; inverse quantitative correlation between circulating adiponectin and grade of hepatic steatosis has been found. Some studies also suggest a SNP variation in adiponectin and mutation in AdipoR2 receptor to be associated with hepatic steatosis and fibrosis [50,51]. The most important known biological role of adiponectin is the regulation of insulin sensitivity in muscle cells, which makes it a central player in type 2 diabetes mellitus (T2DM) and metabolic syndrome. In humans, adiponectin is also known to be secreted by the skeletal muscles where it regulates lipid metabolism via AMPK, p38MAPK, and PPARα pathways [52,53] resulting in more efficient glucose metabolism via glucose transporter type 4 (GLUT4) receptor and fatty acid oxidation, thus maintaining insulin sensitivity [54,55]. Though both AdipoR1 and AdipoR2 have been detected in the skeletal muscles, the relative levels of the two receptors appear to be regulated by insulin levels, fasting–feeding cycles, and other pathophysiological situations; potentially via a PI3K/FoxO1 mediated pathway [56]. Direct role of adiponectin in regulating insulin sensitivity and the fact that adiponectin deficient mice are insulin resistant accompanied by lower insulin production in response to glucose intake suggests a potential role of adiponectin in regulation of insulin production by the β-cells which express both AdipoR1 and AdipoR2 [57]. Adiponectin receptor levels are also lower in pancreas of genetically obese mice. Consistently, adiponectin administration increases insulin secretion in response to glucose in experimental mice [58,59]. In vitro, adiponectin has been shown to prevent free fatty acid induced programed cell death in β-cell lines [59]. Adiponectin, thus, plays an important role in survival and functions of the pancreas protecting it from physiological damage, which in turn regulates the levels of insulin in the body that is central to most metabolic processes. In fact, Zyromski et al. [60] elegantly demonstrated that increasing circulating adiponectin in obese rodents by cannabinoid receptor-1 antagonist leads to recovery of acute pancreatitis.

3.3. Adiponectin in the Central Nervous System

Adiponectin receptors have been detected throughout the central nervous system including the hypothalamus and brainstem and can stimulate neuroendocrine and autonomic responses in the central nervous system (CNS) [61]. While some studies suggest that intracerebroventricular administration of adiponectin results in elevated energy expenditure and promotes weight loss without effecting appetite, some other studies show adiponectin induces increased food intake and reduced energy expenditure. While these results are conflicting, it also draws attention to the fact that adipokines by nature are neuromodulators that signal the brain to regulate food intake and energy expenditure in a context specific manner. Adiponectin receptors have been detected in the pituitary gland of humans suggesting a direct role in regulation of pituitary functions. Using in vitro models, adiponectin has been demonstrated to inhibit growth hormone (GH) and luteinizing hormone (LH) production by rat pituitary cells [62,63]. Yet other studies have indicated a cerebro-protective role of adiponectin via endothelial nitric oxide synthase (eNOS)-mediated pathway as well as migraine-associated inflammation and vasodilation, though more detailed studies are required [63]. In addition to playing important roles in normal physiology, an imbalance in adiponectin levels is associated with multiple pathophysiological states.

4. Perturbations in Adiponectin Levels Manifest in Disease States

4.1. Association of Adiponectin with Inflammation

In contrast to most other adipokines, adiponectin is a well-known anti-inflammatory agent. Using in vitro systems, it has been demonstrated to inhibit B cells differentiation from bone marrow and elevate expression of anti-inflammatory cytokines IL10, IL6, TNFα, and IFNγ in monocyte-derived cell types by inhibiting NFκB (nuclear factor kappa light-chain-enhancer of activated B cells) pathway [64–66]. However, the response is variable depending on the isoforms of the hormone and the cell type targeted, for example, while low molecular weight adiponectin can inhibit LPS-induced IL6 and elevate IL10 in differentiated TH1 macrophages, the multimers of the adipokine do not modulate the abovementioned cytokines [64]. The HMW adiponectin elicit IL6 secretion from monocytes and THP-1 macrophages [64]. Reciprocal regulation of adiponectin by pro-inflammatory cytokines is equally well known. Obesity is a chronic state of low-grade inflammation with sustained and significantly higher level of inflammatory cytokines like TNFα that is known to directly inhibit adiponectin transcription. A large body of research suggests that a higher level of circulating adiponectin in lean humans induces a resistance to inflammatory stimulus in the macrophages. The context specific role of adiponectin in inflammatory processes is also implicated by the fact that higher levels of adiponectin in serum and synovial fluid of rheumatoid arthritis (RA) patients where a sustained inflammatory environment results in degradation of joints and disease severity is directly proportional to circulating adiponectin levels [67,68]. Both adiponectin and adiponectin receptors have been detected in synovial fibroblast of RA patients indicating a local paracrine signaling event [67,68]. In these synovial fibroblasts, adiponectin induces IL6 and pro-matrix metalloproteinase-1 (pro-MMP1) synthesis via p38MAPK and NFκB pathways without influencing other cytokines [69]. It has also been reported to escalate IL8 production which can be attenuated by inhibiting AdipoR2 using RNA interference but not via AdipoR1 [69].

4.2. Adiponectin in Cardiovascular Diseases

Cardiovascular diseases (CVDs) strongly correlate with visceral adiposity which in turn associates with lower circulating adiponectin, verifiable in patients with cardiovascular disease [70]. Similar to other physiological scenarios, CVD dependence on adiponectin levels is context specific. Lower levels of HMW adiponectin correlate with incidence of CVD [71]. Hypoadiponectinemia has been associated with severity of myocardial infraction with elevated levels of TNFα and increased apoptotic death in myocytes and stromal cells [72]; adiponectin administration attenuates these complications and reduces severity of infraction via the COX-2/EP4 pathway mediated by AMPK [73]. Adiponectin regulates the cardioprotective COX-2 signaling via sphingosine kinase (SphK) signaling [73,74]. Additionally, adiponectin has also been studied in the context of atherosclerosis. In injured blood vessels, adiponectin has been reported to bind collagen type I, III, and V, suggesting a role in repair of vasculature [1]. It suppresses vascular cell adhesion protein-1 (VCAM-1) expression in monocytes resulting in suppression of TNFα synthesis, thus preventing them from adhering to the aortic endothelial cells [75]. Adiponectin also inhibits the class A macrophage scavenger receptor in macrophages preventing them from being converted into foam cells, the culprits of atherosclerosis. It has also been proposed that adiponectin gene variation can be used as a predictor of coronary heart disease risk since T/T homozygotes of the adiponectin gene were at lower risk of developing coronary artery disease compared to G/G or G/T genotype individuals [50].

5. Obese State and Adiponectin—An Inverse Relation

In contrast to other known adipokines, adiponectin is inversely related to body mass index (BMI) and central adiposity; the strongest negative correlation has been observed with waist-to-hip ratio [76]. Undoubtedly, a feedback loop regulates it at transcriptional, translational or post-translational level. A similar trend in downregulation of its receptors AdipoR1 and AdipoR2 have also been observed [77]. Normal levels of adiponectin as well as its receptors are re-established post weight/fat loss. Though a number of mechanisms have been proposed, none of them precisely explain the feedback mechanism in adiponectin regulation. An obese state is a situation of chronic inflammation in the body characterized by a marked increase in the levels of inflammatory cytokines IL6, IL8, TNFα, and leptin, which are directly known to inhibit adiponectin transcription. In addition, the most important and well-understood role of adiponectin is insulin sensitization in the skeletal muscles. Increase in visceral fat mass lowers systemic adiponectin levels creating insulin resistance in the skeletal muscle while glucose signaling in response to food intake stimulates elevated insulin secretion by the pancreas that is free from adiponectin's regulatory control due to its lower circulating concentrations. As a result, there is increased conversion of glucose and glycogen into fats, which is then taken up by the skeletal muscles leading to intramuscular fat accumulation, typical of type 2 diabetes. Consequently, a vicious cycle is initiated where increased adiposity causes a drop in adiponectin levels that in turn results in fat accumulation in muscles and vital organs like liver that further lowers adiponectin levels giving way to cardiovascular diseases and atherosclerosis. Again, gender specific differences are evident since lower adiponectin levels have been recorded in diabetic men compared to women which has been partially attributed to higher testosterone levels in men.

Though both total and HMW adiponectin are downregulated, HMW adiponectin is a better predictor of insulin resistance [78,79]. As such, individuals harboring mutations for adiponectin multimerization are more susceptible to type II diabetes [78]. Lipoatrophic mice lacking circulating adiponectin were found to be hyperglycemic as well as had higher levels of insulin, both of which could be reverted by continuous adiponectin administration. In light of genetic association, +45 G-allele of the adiponectin gene has been shown to regulate glucose tolerance and insulin sensitivity [50,80]. Similarly, AdipoR1 −3882 T > C polymorphism has been shown to be responsible for lower insulin resistance and fasting glucose levels [50,80]. Adiponectin has been shown to have a direct and immediate effect on blood pressure and lower circulating adiponectin levels can be considered a predictor of hypertension risk. Experimentally, angiotensin II administration decreases circulatory adiponectin while angiotensin II receptor blockade results in increase in its plasma concentrations [81,82]. Adiponectin has been widely studied in the context of lipoprotein metabolism, a dysregulation of which is termed as dyslipidemia. Obesity is often characterized by increased triglycerides, free fatty acids and low-density lipoprotein (LDL), and a decrease in high-density lipoprotein (HDL). Circulatory adiponectin positively correlates with HDL and size density of LDL, and negatively correlates with plasma triglycerides [83,84]. Hypoadiponectinemia often associates with an atherosclerotic lipid profile. The positive correlation between HDL and adiponectin is known to be regulated by apolipoprotein A-I (apoA-I) [85]. Metabolic syndrome is defined as the physiological state of complete metabolic dysfunction characterized by hyperglycemia, insulin resistance, hypertension, dyslipidemia, and obesity. All these conditions are strongly associated with lower adiponectin levels, particularly, HMW adiponectin [86,87]. It has also been shown to be a predictor of metabolic syndrome in a 6-year follow-up study in Japan [87]. Though few studies have been successfully conducted, the physiological relevance of adiponectin in eating disorders like bulimia and anorexia nervosa is still unclear, since both upregulation and downregulation of the adipokines in these conditions have been reported. More detailed analyses with special attention to the confounding factors is required to clearly delineate the inverse relationship between obesity and adiponectin.

6. Adiponectin- and Obesity-Associated Disorders

Deregulated adiponectin production in obesity may be the leading cause of endometrial impairment, hypertension, myocardial infarction, and other complexities of metabolic syndrome along with cancer initiation and progression (Table 1).

Table 1. Obesity-related diseases associated with hypoadiponectinemia.

Diseases	Findings
Hypertension	Obese patients suffering from hypertension display lower adiponectin.
Atherosclerosis	Higher incidences of cardiovascular events are associated with lower hypoadiponectinemia.
Obstructive sleep apnea syndrome	OSAS (Obstructive sleep apnea syndrome) patients revealed lower expression level of adiponectin compared to control patients.
Diabetic retinopathy	T2DM patients with diabetic retinopathy have lower levels of adiponectin compared to T2DM patients without diabetic retinopathy.
Cancer	Multiple evidences suggest low adiponectin levels are associated with the threat of developing several types of cancers.
Metabolic syndrome	Metabolic syndrome represents a group of complications like obesity, hypertension, dyslipidemia, hyperglycemia, and insulin resistance. Enhancement of metabolic syndrome components is associated with a decrease in adiponectin concentration in plasma [88].
Dyslipidemia	Disorder of lipid metabolism leading to high levels of LDL, serum triglycerides, and decreased levels of HDL. Inverse association exists between adiponectin level with LDL and serum triglycerides with a positive association with HDL levels [89].
Hepatic disease non-alcoholic fat	Inverse association exists between adiponectin level in liver with non-alcoholic fatty liver disease as well as non-alcoholic steatohepatitis [90].

6.1. Hypertension

Several factors contribute to the association of obesity and hypertension including sympathetic activation of the nervous system, endothelial dysfunction (due to an increase in free fatty acids and oxidative stress), and an abnormal adipokine production [88]. Adults with hypertension display lower levels of adiponectin [89]. Total adiponectin levels were found to be lower in obese individuals suffering from hypertension in comparison to lean and normotensive individuals [90]. Adiponectin coordinates blood pressure by mechanisms regulated by brain and endothelium [91,92]. Studies reveal that adiponectin suppresses TNFα and inhibits foam cell transformation of macrophages [93]. Adiponectin prevents the atheroma formation by nitric oxide (NO) production via phosphoinositide 3-kinase (PI3K) and AMPK pathways in endothelial cells [91,92]. Adiponectin also reduces the proliferation of smooth muscle cells and TNF-α in macrophages [93].

6.2. Atherosclerosis

There are multiple mechanisms linking obesity to cardiovascular diseases [94,95]. Several adipokines facilitate the cross-talk between adipose tissue, heart, and vessels in the "adipo-cardiovascular axis". A prothrombotic state is stimulated by the altered release of adipokines that leads to cardiovascular disease and atherosclerosis [96,97]. Reduced levels of serum adiponectin are interpreters of atherosclerosis and myocardial infarction. Additionally, there is a strong correlation between hypoadiponectinemia and coronary heart diseases well supported by clinical trials which confirm that higher incidences of cardiovascular events are associated with lower levels of adiponectin [98]. Reports suggest HMW adiponectin to be a better independent risk factor than the total adiponectin for cardiovascular diseases [99,100]. In vivo studies using adiponectin deficient mice reveal severely injured arteries while adiponectin supplementation impaired neointimal proliferation. In vitro culture studies demonstrate that platelet-derived growth factor (PDGF), heparin-binding epidermal growth factor (HB-EGF), basic fibroblast growth factor (BFGF), and epidermal growth factor (EGF)-induced DNA synthesis, cell proliferation and cell migration are impaired by adiponectin [101]. Adiponectin reduces inflammatory cytokines and adhesion molecules in endothelial cells. Apart from inhibiting the conversion of macrophages into foam cells, adiponectin also decreases TNF-alpha production as well as induces the production of the anti-inflammatory cytokine, IL-10 [102].

6.3. Obstructive Sleep Apnea Syndrome

Obstructive sleep apnea syndrome (OSAS) is a condition characterized by recurrent respiratory disorders during sleep [103]. The level of adiponectin is undoubtedly lower in OSAS patients. A study by Hargens et al. [104] confirmed lower adiponectin levels in OSAS patients in comparison to controls. Yet, there are some studies which suggest that patients suffering from OSAS do not show alteration in adiponectin levels. Intermittent hypoxia resulting in a decrease of total and HMW adiponectin is argued to be the major cause of the reduction of adiponectin in OSAS [105,106].

6.4. Diabetic Retinopathy

One of the major risk factors for diabetic microvascular complications is obesity. Increased levels of glucose in T2DM are thought to be a risk for microvascular (retinopathy, nephropathy and neuropathy) and macrovascular (coronary heart disease, stroke and peripheral vascular disease) complications [107]. The most common complication of diabetic microvascular disease is diabetic retinopathy which affects 30–50% of all diabetics [107]. Both obesity and T2DM patients display decreased adiponectin levels in circulation. Additionally, T2DM patients with diabetic retinopathy (non-proliferative and proliferative) have reduced levels of adiponectin compared to patients without retinopathy [108].

7. Obesity, Adiponectin, and Cancer: Interplay of Bigwigs

Multiple epidemiological evidences associate obesity with the risk of cancer development. The study conducted by the American Cancer Society comparing individuals with a body mass index (BMI) over 30 kg/m^2 with individuals over 25 kg/m^2 concluded that the relative risk of colorectal cancer is at 1.8 for obese males and 1.2 for obese females [109]. A meta-analysis of 11 studies indicated the probability of 6% increase in the risk of kidney cancer in men and 7% in women per unit BMI increase with an average 36% higher risk in overweight individuals (BMI > 25 kg/m^2) and 84% higher risk in obese individuals (BMI > 30 kg/m^2) [109]. Lagergren et al. reported a positive correlation of esophageal carcinoma with increased BMI (>25.6 kg/m^2 in males and >24.2 kg/m^2 in females) along with a higher risk in individuals with a BMI greater than 30 kg/m^2 [109]. According to the International Agency for Research on Cancer and the World Cancer Research Fund (WCRF), obesity is strongly associated with endometrial cancer, adenocarcinoma of the esophagus, colorectal cancer, postmenopausal breast, prostate, and renal cancer. Leukemia, non-Hodgkin's lymphoma, multiple myeloma, malignant melanoma, and thyroid tumors represent some lesser common malignancies associated with obesity [89,110,111]. The strongest correlation between obesity and cancer risk has been observed in the case of breast cancer. Approximately 80% of the breast is composed of adipose tissue or fat. The mammary epithelial cells are therefore in close contact with a cocktail of adipokines produced by the adipose tissue and any imbalance in the hormonal milieu renders the breast susceptible to tumorigenesis. Reduced levels of total and HMW adiponectin have been shown be associated with breast cancers irrespective of age, BMI, hormone status, and other factors which was first reported by Noguchi and group [112,113]. Adiponectin and its receptors are known to be expressed in breast epithelial as well as myoepithelial cells of the breast. Cytoplasmic expression of both the AdiopRs is known in normal breast epithelial and breast cancer cells but breast cancer tissue exhibits a higher expression of AdipoR2 which also significantly and positively correlates with vascular and lymphovascular invasion in breast cancer. Adiponectin receptors are known to be expressed on most breast cancer cell lines including MCF7, T47D, MDA-MB-231, MDA-MB-361, and SKBR3. While MDA-MB-231, T47D, and MCF-7 showed higher expression of AdipoR1, MDA-MB-361 had higher expression of AdipoR2. Adiponectin protein distribution also varied between cell lines. Insulin, insulin-like growth factor-1 (IGF1), leptin, adiponectin, steroid hormones, and cytokines are some host factors associated with obesity that not only influences the initiation and progression of breast cancer, but also affects its response to therapies [114]. Reports reveal decreased adiponectin in breast and endometrial cancer and vice versa in non-small cell lung cancer, pancreatic, liver, prostate, gastric, renal cell carcinoma, and colon cancer [115–118]. Wei et al. [119] performed a meta-analysis of 107 studies in a random effect model to analyze the levels of circulating adiponectin in cancer patients versus controls. They found that the circulating adiponectin levels were significantly downregulated in cancer patients compared to control patients with a pooled SMD of −0.334 µg/mL. Further analysis of eight different studies showed that the circulating levels of HMW adiponectin was lower in cancer cases than control cases with a pooled standard mean differences (SMD) of −0.502 µg/mL (Table 2).

Table 2. Studies showing circulating HMW adiponectin and its association with cancer risk. RIA: radioimmunoassay; ELISA: enzyme linked immunosorbent assay.

Cancer Type	Ethnicity	Sample	Cases/Control	Method	Reference
Breast cancer	Caucasian	Serum sample	74/76	RIA	[120]
Liver cancer	Asian	Serum sample	59/334	ELISA	[121]
Liver cancer	Asian	Serum sample	97/97	ELISA	[122]
Colorectal cancer	Asian	Plasma sample	165/102	ELISA	[123]
Colorectal cancer	Caucasian	Serum sample	1206/1206	ELISA	[124]
Multiple myeloma	Caucasian	Plasma sample	174/348	ELISA	[125]
Endometrial cancer	Caucasian	Serum sample	62/124	ELISA	[126]
Breast cancer	Asian	Serum sample	66/66	Other method	[127]

8. Adiponectin Orchestrates Multiple Biological Functions to Inhibit Cancer Progression

8.1. Inhibition of Angiogenesis

Tumor growth and metastasis are high-energy expenditure processes requiring constant supply of growth factors and nutrients, which is ensured by profusely leaky tumor vasculature. Adipocytes as well as pre-adipocytes are known to synthesize proangiogenic factors including leptin, TNFα, IL6, HGF (hepatocyte growth factor), and bFGF. Vasculogenesis requires fibroblast growth factor-2 (FGF-2) for proliferation of endothelial cells followed by migration of the endothelial cells and tubulogenesis that is facilitated by the vascular endothelial growth factor, VEGF. Using culture-based studies, it has been demonstrated that adiponectin is capable of inhibiting endothelial cell proliferation induced by FGF2 as well as migration of endothelial cells by VEGF. In a mouse fibrocarcinomas model, intratumoral administration of adiponectin resulted in disruption of tumor vasculature and caspase-3-mediated intratumoral apoptosis, possibly by nutrient deprivation of tumor cells, resulting in over 60% tumor regression. Adiponectin inhibits in vitro proliferation of human umbilical vein endothelial cells (HUVECs) and subsequent vessel formation. Adiponectin null mice have also been shown to exhibit retarded tumor growth, diminished vascularization, and inhibition of pulmonary metastasis [128]. However, contradictory results have also been observed in literature and regulation of vasulogenesis by adiponectin warrants further investigation.

8.2. Inhibition of Growth and Proliferation

Adiponectin has been shown to inhibit cell proliferation via ERK1/2-MAPK pathway in T47D cells. In MDA-MB-231 xenografts, recombinant as well as adenovirus-mediated adiponectin overexpression, regressed tumor development, inhibited secondary tumor development in adjacent fat pads, and prevented lung metastasis via the GSK3β/βcatenin signaling pathway [113,129]. Kang et al. [130] reported that inhibitory effects (growth arrest as well as apoptosis) of adiponectin have been more pronounced in the mesenchymal-like cell line MDA-MB-231 compared to the luminal-like cell line T47D by inducing G0/G1 cell cycle arrest. Adiponectin is thought to enhance Bax and p53 expression while downregulating CyclinD1, blocking JNK signaling, and inducing PARP cleavage via AdipoRs [113] Another proposed mechanism of adiponectin-induced growth inhibition and apoptosis in MCF7, T47D, SK-BR3, and MCF10A is AMPK activation as a result of adiponectin binding to AdipoRs resulting in p42/p44MAPK inhibition which consequently modulates p53, Bax, Bcl-2, c-myc, and cyclin D1 [113]. Grossman et al. further explain that estrogen receptor alpha (ERα) positive cell lines MCF7 and T47D cells could be inhibited even with low concentrations of adiponectin, but to achieve similar results in ERα negative cell line SKBR3, much higher concentrations of the adipokines are necessary. They further investigated the role of ER in adiponectin-mediated inhibition by expressing estrogen receptor in MDA-MB-231 which resulted in cells being responsive to adiponectin-induced growth inhibition via a blockade of JNK2 signaling [113]. Adiponectin has also been shown to inhibit leptin-induced cell proliferation in MDA-MB-231, MDA-MB-361, SK-BR-3, MCF-7, and T47D cells at varying doses [120]. Genetic variations in adiponectin and its receptor has also been suggested to be associated with breast cancer risk. One study found that the women who had adiponectin rs2241766 (+45 T → G) TG genotype, the genotype associated with higher circulatory adiponectin, were at 39% lower risk of developing breast cancer where as those with adiponectin rs1501299 (+276 G → T) TG and GG genotypes, low adiponectin genotypes, were at 59% and 80% higher risk of developing breast cancer, respectively. AdipoR1 rs7539542 (+10225 C → G) CC and CG genotypes were also predicted to carry a lower breast cancer risk.

In a Chinese case control study, prostate cancer patients exhibited significantly lower levels of adiponectin in circulation. To demonstrate the role of adiponectin in prostate cancer incidence and progression they developed stable transfects of prostate cancer cell lines deficient for adiponectin receptor. Adiponectin administration to parent cell line suppressed cell migration, tube formation, and induced cell cycle arrest, while adiponectin deficiency enhanced the proliferative, migratory, and pro-angiogenic potential of these cells [121]. Gao et al. [122] in 2015 demonstrated that adiponectin overexpression in prostate cancer cells results in depletion of VEGFA and vice versa via an AMPK/TSC2 mediated mechanism. Recently, Shrestha et al. demonstrated the critical role of transcription factor FoxO3A in adiponectin-mediated growth arrest and apoptosis in cancer cells. Globular adiponectin induces p27 but inhibits Cyclin D1 in breast cancer cell lines MCF7 and hepatic cancer cell line HepG2 along with caspase 3/7 activation and FasL expression. Silencing FoxO3A using siRNA inhibited p27 and activated CyclinD1 while preventing caspase and FasL activation suggesting FoxO3A-mediated growth arrest in these cells. On silencing AMPK, however, they observed an inhibition of nuclear translocation of FoxO3A along with inhibition of adiponectin-induced cell cycle arrest and apoptosis. AMPK, thus, acts upstream of FoxO3A in regulating adiponectin cytotoxicity in cancer cells [123]. Another study using HepG2 and Huh7 cell lines elaborates adiponectin-induced inhibition of hepatocellular carcinoma through JNK and mTOR pathway modulation, though upstream regulation remains to be determined. Adiponectin-induced cell death in these cell lines is accompanied by intracellular reactive oxygen species (ROS) accumulation and adiponectin's effects were inhibited by N-acetylcysteine. Levels of thioredoxin proteins, Trx1 and 2 were altered while overexpression of either of the proteins rescued adiponectin's effect [124].

High circulating adiponectin has also been shown to be associated with 50% lower risk of endometrial cancer irrespective of BMI, hence, it can be considered an independent predictor of endometrial cancer risk. Similarly, adiponectin receptors have been detected in prostate cancer cell lines and in patients. Adiponectin in circulation was evaluated to be negatively correlated with histological grade prostate cancer. Consistently, full-length adiponectin also inhibited growth of prostate cancer cell lines in vitro. In models of CRC, adiponectin knockdown resulted in increased multiplicity of colorectal polyps which were also more aggressive and metastatic with higher COX2 levels compared to their wild-type counterparts suggesting that higher levels of circulating adiponectin could be associated with better prognosis of colorectal cancer as well. In adiponectin-deficient mice, adiponectin inhibited tumor progression and angiogenesis when fed an obesogenic diet but not with normal diet [125–127]. Adiponectin deficiency also aggravated azoxymethane-induced (carcinogen-induced) colon cancer in C57BL/6J mice [131]. A series of studies by Saxena et al. demonstrated that adiponectin conferred protection against inflammation-induced colon cancers by preventing apoptosis in the goblet cells and promoting differentiation of epithelial cells to goblet cells [132,133]. In HCT116, HT29, and LoVo CRC cell lines, adiponectin induces G1/S cell cycle arrest with concurrent overexpression of p21 and p27 via AMPK phosphorylation; inhibition of adiponectin receptors freed the cells of adiponectin-induced growth arrest [134]. Moreover, adiponectin rs266729 (−11365 C → G) GG and GC genotypes have been reported to be at 27% lower risk of encountering colorectal cancer compared to individuals with CC genotype, though results in this regard have been inconsistent [135].

8.3. Inhibition of Invasion, Migration, and Metastasis

Owing to its strong negative association with multiple cancers and its role in tumor angiogenesis and vasculature development, many research groups have studied the involvement of adiponectin in cancer invasion and metastasis. However, not many studies have specifically examined the role of adiponectin in cancer metastasis. Adipokine leptin is a strong predictor of poor outcome in breast cancer. Adiponectin has been shown to counteract the effect of leptin by inhibiting leptin-induced migration and invasion in breast cancer in addition to leptin-induced clonogenicity and anchorage independent cell growth. Adiponectin pretreatment suppresses leptin-induced ERK and Akt signaling. Additionally, it amplifies the protein tyrosine phosphatase 1B (PTP1B) expression and activity, physiological leptin inhibitor and PTP1B inhibition restores leptin activity. Adenoviral adiponectin treatment retards tumor progression in xenograft [136]. In endometrial cancer cell line SPEC-2, adiponectin reverses its metastatic phenotype. Adiponectin inhibits leptin-induced proliferation as well as invasion potential of the SPEC2 cells. Mechanistically, adiponectin prevents leptin-induced invasion by inhibiting signal transducer and activator of transcription 3 (STAT3) phosphorylation and MAPK-mediated nuclear translocation [137]. In liver cancer xenografts, adiponectin inhibits tumor progression and reduces lung metastasis. Adiponectin inhibits hepatic stellate cell activation, intratumoral macrophage infiltration, and diminishes tumor vascularization by downregulating ROCK/IP10/VEGF signaling and inhibition of lamellipodia formation [138]. In non-small cell lung carcinoma (NSCLC), adiponectin prevents migration and invasion of cancer cells by inhibiting epithelial-to-mesenchymal transition (EMT). Adiponectin upregulates epithelial marker expression and decreases mesenchymal markers which could be reversed by knocking down Twist, AdipoR1, and AdipoR2 [139]. Though compelling experimental evidence support metastasis inhibitory effects of adiponectin, results across studies are still inconsistent and more detailed investigation is warranted.

9. Molecular Mechanisms Mediating Adiponectin's Effects in Cancer

The literature clearly suggests that adiponectin can activate several pathways like AMPK, MAPK and PI3K/AKt. AMPK affects cell growth via mammalian target of rapamycin (mTOR), thereby inhibiting the induction of tumor formation. Adiponectin induces growth arrest and apoptosis by activating AMPK in various cell lines in a p53 and p21 dependent manner. In vitro studies of adiponectin on several colon cancer cell lines (HCT116, HT29, and LoVo) show that adiponectin inhibits colon cancer cell proliferation and impairs the cell cycle at G1/S transition phase by inducing p21 and p27 [134]. Adiponectin induces the tumor suppressor gene, *LKB1*, thereby resulting in AMPK activation and inhibition of cell adhesion, invasion and migration in breast cancer cell lines [140,141]. Adiponectin-mediated LKB1 upregulation is also involved in the induction of cytotoxic autophagy leading to tumor inhibition [142]. The role of adiponectin on MAPK signaling remains debatable. The study by Daniele et al. reveal higher adiponectin in the serum samples of chronic obstructive pulmonary disease (COPD) patients compared to control subjects [143]. Adiponectin treatment downregulates ERK1/2 signaling leading to reduction of cell viability in breast and endometrial cancer cell lines [144,145]. Adiponectin-treated MCF7 cells reveal a decrease in the expression level of c-myc, cyclin-D1, and Bcl2 with an increased expression of p52 and Bax, thereby leading to cell cycle arrest [145]. JNK, a member of MAP kinases, has a role in tumor development by regulating cell proliferation and apoptosis [146]. It is also involved in obesity and insulin resistance [146,147]. Similarly, STAT3 (signal transducer and activator of transcription 3) is also involved in cell survival and proliferation and the deregulation of STAT3 leads to tumor progression and metastasis. Saxena et al. reported that adiponectin treatment enhances JNK activation and causes apoptosis in hepatocellular carcinoma cell line in a caspase-3 dependent manner [148]. Reports reveal that adiponectin treatment reduces STAT3 and Akt phosphorylation in liver and prostate cancer cell lines [149]. Adiponectin-treated breast and colorectal cancer cell lines reveal a decrease in PI3K and Akt phosphorylation [150]. At the same time, adiponectin also induces AMPK and inhibits mammalian target of rapamycin (mTOR) cascade in colorectal cancer cell lines [151]. The Wnt signaling pathway plays a proven role in self-renewal and differentiation in different cancer models. The binding of WNT ligand to frizzled activates the signaling cascade by inhibiting glycogen synthase kinase 3 beta (GSK-3β) which is a negative regulator of β-Catenin. The inhibition of GSK-3β promotes the nuclear translocation of β-Catenin, thus, activating WNT signaling. Wang et al. reported that adiponectin inhibits GSK-3β phosphorylation and prevents β-Catenin nuclear translocation in MDA-MB-231 triple-negative breast cancer cells [129]. Liu et al. showed that adiponectin treatment induces Wnt inhibitory factor 1 (WIF1) in a time-dependent manner and results in the decrease of cell proliferation, nuclear translocation of β-Catenin, and reduces expression of cyclin-D1 in breast cancer cells [152]. One of the major anti-apoptotic pathways is the NF-Kβ pathway. Ouchi et al. reported that human aortic endothelial cells pre-incubated with adiponectin show reduced phosphorylation of TNF-alpha-induced Ikappaβ-α, thereby suppressing NFKβ activation via cAMP accumulation. This effect is blocked in the presence of adenylate cyclase or protein kinase A (PKA) inhibitor [153]. Adiponectin modulates various signaling mechanisms to inhibit cancer growth and progression (Figure 2).

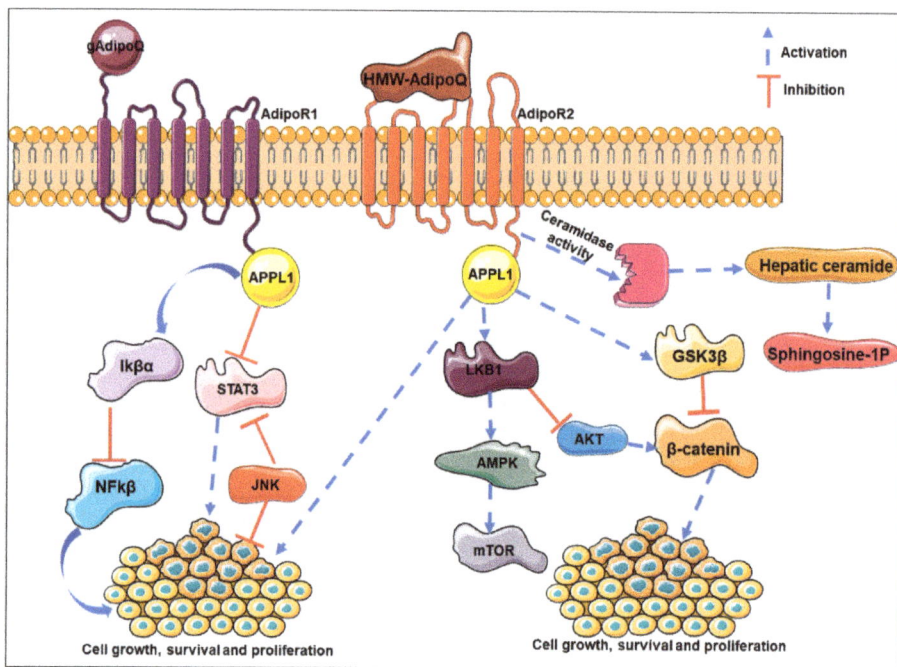

Figure 2. Adiponectin modulates various signaling mechanisms to inhibit caner growth.

10. Potential Therapeutic Modulation of Adiponectin

Obesity and metabolic syndrome have grown to be the root cause of most life-threatening diseases ranging from type 2 diabetes, cardiovascular diseases, and cancer. Obesity leads to hormonal dysregulation and insulin resistance which initiates a cascade of events leading to failure of the metabolic machinery of the body, hence morbidity. Therapeutic regulation of adiponectin may be achieved either by administration of exogenous recombinant adiponectin or using pharmacological agents to induce increased production of exogenous adiponectin [36]. However, similar to most biologics, mass production of functional adiponectin is challenging since within the biological system it is under intense post-transcriptional and post-translational modifications which are hard to mimic in vitro [36,154]. Bacterial systems lack mammalian protein synthesis machinery and fail to produce functionally active adiponectin. Exploitation of the mammalian culture system for mass production is not a scalable process. In addition, adiponectin has a short half-life in circulation making exogenous administration of recombinant adiponectin a non-feasible approach [36,155]. The only practical mode of adiponectin therapy is, therefore, to induce increased production of endogenous adiponectin using either natural means or pharmacological interventions. The most natural means of boosting adiponectin production is weight loss since adiponectin is the hormone secreted by the lean adipose tissue and is suppressed by leptin and other inflammatory cytokines produced by obese adipose. Multiple effective interventions of weight loss, discussed later, have been strategized in recent years but weight loss remains to be a difficult hurdle. The most feasible method of adiponectin therapy would therefore be the use of pharmacological intervention to enhance adiponectin biosynthesis, bioavailability and bioactivity. The key to designing adiponectin enhancing therapies is to understand its transcriptional and translational regulation. The adiponectin promoter is known to bind a number of transcription factors capable of modulating its activity [30]. It is composed of a PPAR responsive element [19], a CCAAT box [156], multiple C/EBPα enhancers and a sterol regulator element or SRE [157]. Several pharmacological agents have been developed to target or modulate adiponectin machinery.

10.1. Pharmacological Agents

Though results from clinical trials are conflicting, statins including pravastatin [158], simvastatin [159], rosuvastatin [160], and atorvastatin [161] have been reported to be effective in increasing circulating adiponectin. Statins function by releasing cellular oxidative stress resulting in increased multimerization and release. These include ramipril [162], Quinapril [163], Losartan [164], Telmisartan [164,165], Irbesartan [165,166], and Candesartan [166], all of which have shown promising results in clinical trials. They function by enhancing adiponectin secretion via PPARγ, though some are also known to induce transcription. Pioglitazone and Rosiglitazone are known to enhance circulating adiponectin levels 2–4 fold [167,168]. TZDs function by inducing transcription of adiponectin via PPARγ. They have also been found to enhance secretion of folded adiponectin by inhibiting ERp44 and upregulating Ero1-La and DsbA-L. Other potential drugs include non-statin anti-hyperlipidemic drugs like Fenofibrate and Zetia, non-TZD anti-diabetic drugs, such as Acarbose [36] and the sulfonylurea Glimepiride [169] and Sulfonylureas. Androgen blockers have also been proven to be effective at increasing HMW adiponectin and can be used in cases of prostate cancers.

10.2. Weight Loss Interventions

Caloric restriction has been the most commonly implemented intervention for weight loss. It creates an energy deficit forcing the body to utilize energy stored in adipose tissue to fuel basal metabolic activities. However, with the surge in obesity research and better understanding of hormonal regulation of metabolic processes, the therapeutic significance of caloric restriction has been questioned. It has been observed that with constant intake of low energy food, the body activates a coping mechanism by lowering the basal metabolic rate and develops resistance to fat catabolism. As a result, the metabolic processes do not switch, they merely slow down; consequently, there is no change in hormonal milieu of the body. In addition, only recently have we started to fully appreciate the hormone central to all metabolic processes, insulin. It is now believed that an obesogenic diet is one with higher glycemic index rather than caloric density and insulin responds to a spike in blood glucose by directing cells to store energy in the form of fat. The glycemic index of food is determined by its macronutrient composition, precisely the ratio of carbohydrates, fat, protein, and fiber (a form of complex carbohydrate). While caloric restriction may promote some weight loss, it does not seem to have therapeutic benefit.

In recent years, intermittent fasting and ketogenic diets have been shown to have immense health benefits and have also been utilized as therapeutic regimens. Intermittent fasting refers to a form of diet when food is consumed within small windows of time of a few hours followed by long hours of fasting without calorie restriction. As a result, insulin levels remain constant for long time intervals with a limited period of insulin spike preventing fat storage. During periods of fasting, fat metabolism is induced resulting in weight loss. This mode of feeding has been shown to improve metabolic functions, improve insulin sensitivity, and restore hormonal balance. A recent study suggests that intermittent fasting induces beiging of white adipose tissue via microbiome modulation [170], such change could probably induce adiponectin synthesis and lower leptin levels. Ketogenic diet, on the other hand, relies on dietary fat as a major energy source. It is composed of 60–80% fat, 20% proteins, and only 5–10% carbohydrates most of which is dietary fiber. It works on the principle of insulin response; the glycemic index of macronutrients varies in the order of carbohydrates (minus fibers) > protein > fat. Since fats are the main energy source, insulin response to the diet is minimal, shutting down the process of fat storage. Utilizing fat as the source of energy, the body adapts to fat utilization rather than depending on glycogen stores in hours of need, thus it results in fat loss. Fats and proteins are known to induce high levels of satiety resulting in appetite reduction which also promotes weight loss. A combination of intermittent fasting and a ketogenic diet has been shown to be most effective in promoting weight loss and rewiring metabolic dysfunctions. Body fat loss and increased insulin sensitivity are the most effective and natural methods of reversing obesity-associated inflammation and leptin downregulation, and thus, adiponectin upregulation. Physical activity and exercising is another reliable method of weight loss and is known to reduce inflammation [171]. A recent meta-analysis comprising 2996 individuals investigated metabolic regulation in diabetes patients and how it is affected by exercise [172]. Of all exercise modalities, only aerobic exercise was found to increase adiponectin and decrease leptin levels [172]. Collectively, these studies indicate that combination regimens of diet, exercise, and fasting can help boost adiponectin levels in hypoadiponectinemia.

11. Conclusions

Adiponectin, an important adipocytokine mainly produced by lean adipocytes, is considered a guardian angel adipocytokine owing to its protective functions against various disease states associated with obesity. Adiponectin inversely correlates with obesity and is under tight regulation at transcriptional and translational levels. Though important in most chronic diseases including CVD and T2DM, the role of adiponectin in cancers is most critical. Women who are genetically wired to have lower levels of circulating adiponectin live with a significantly higher risk of breast cancer irrespective of BMI and adiposity. Similar associations have also been observed in other cancers including CRC, prostrate, and hepatic malignancies. Modulation of adipose-secreted hormones regulates metabolic functions of the body, and therefore have direct consequences on cancers which survive by hijacking host metabolic machinery. However, as detailed in this review, adiponectin works in concert with other important hormones including insulin, leptin, and various cytokines making its pharmacological exploitation more difficult. Various strategies have been developed to modulate adiponectin levels in disease state to harness its beneficial effects including pharmacological agents functioning at transcriptional and post-translational levels as well as weight loss strategies. Evidently, adiponectin intervention alone is not sufficient to confront these chronic conditions; it definitely plays an important supportive role in these pathologic states and deserves attention. While pharmacological interventions can prove helpful in treatment of patients genetically deficient in adiponectin, weight management strategies including aerobic exercise and ketogenic diets could be effective in conjunction with other systemic therapies and medications.

Funding: This work was supported by NCI NIH R01CA204555 and the Breast Cancer Research Foundation (BCRF) 90047965 (to D.S.).

Acknowledgments: All figures have been constructed with the help of smart images from Servier medical art (https://smart.servier.com/).

Conflicts of Interest: The authors declare no conflict of interest.

Abbreviations

Acrp30	Adipocyte complement related protein of 30 kDa
apM1	Adipose most abundant gene transcript1
GBP28	Gelatin-binding protein of 28 kDa
AdipoR1	Adiponectin receptor 1
AdipoR2	Adiponectin receptor 2
PPARγ	Peroxisome proliferator-activated receptor gamma
TZD	Thiazolidinedione
PPRE	PPAR response element
HMW adiponectin	High molecular weight adiponectin
FoxO1	Forkhead box protein O1
Sirt1	Sirtuin 1
C/EBPα	CCAAT-enhancer-binding proteins
SERBP	Sterol regulatory element-binding proteins
SRE	SERBP response element
CREB	cAMP response element-binding protein
ATF3	Activating transcription factor 3

NFAT	Nuclear factor of activated T-cells
AP-2β	Activating enhancer binding protein-2β
IGFBP-3	IGF-1-binding protein 3
Id3	Inhibitor of differentiation-3
HIF1α	Hypoxia inducible factor alpha
TNFα	Tumor necrosis factor alpha
IFNγ	Interferon gamma
IL	Interleukin
JNK	c-Jun N-terminal kinases
ERK	Extracellular-signal-regulated kinase
MAPK	Mitogen-activated protein kinases
ERp44	ER chaperone protein 44
Ero-1La	ERO1-like protein alpha
DsbA-L	Disulfide-bond A oxidoreductase-like protein
COX2	Cyclooxygenase 2
VEGF	Vascular endothelial growth factor
PGES	Prostaglandin E synthase
hCG	Human chorionic gonadotropin
AMPK	AMP activated protein kinase
PCOS	Polycystic ovary syndrome
SNP	Single nucleotide polymorphism
GLUT4	Glucose transporter type 4
CNS	Central nervous system
GH	Growth hormone
LH	Luteinizing hormone
eNOS	Endothelial NOS
NFκB	Nuclear factor kappa-light-chain-enhancer of activated B cells
MMP	Matrix metalloproteinase
CVD	Cardiovascular disease
EP4	Prostaglandin E2 receptor 4
SphK	Sphingosine kinase
VCAM-1	Vascular cell adhesion protein 1
BMI	Body mass index
LDL	Low density lipoprotein
HDL	High density lipoprotein
apoA-I	Apolipoprotein A-I
NO	Nitric oxide
PI3K	Phosphoinositide 3-kinase
PDGF	Platelet-derived growth factor
HB-EGF	Heparin-binding epidermal growth factor
BFGF	Basic fibroblast growth factor
EGF	Epidermal growth factor
OSAS	Obstructive sleep apnea syndrome
T2DM	Type 2 diabetes mellitus
IARC	International agency for research on cancer
WCRF	World cancer research fund
SMD	Standard mean differences
RIA	Radioimmunoassay
ELISA	Enzyme linked immunosorbent assay
HGF	Hepatocyte growth factor
bFGF	Basic fibroblast growth factor
FGF-2	Fibroblast growth factor-2
HUVEC	Human Umbilical Vein Endothelial Cells

mTOR	Mammalian target of rapamycin
ROS	Reactive oxygen species
Trx	Thioredoxin
CRC	Colorectal cancer
PTP1B	Protein tyrosine phosphatase 1B
NSCLC	Non-small cell lung carcinoma
EMT	Epithelial to mesenchymal transition
PKA	Protein kinase A
IGF1	Insulin like growth factor-1
COPD	Chronic Obstructive Pulmonary Disease
STAT3	Signal transducer and activator of transcription 3
GSK3β	Glycogen synthase kinase 3 beta
DsbA-L	Disulfide-bond A oxidoreductase-like protein

References

1. Brochu-Gaudreau, K.; Rehfeldt, C.; Blouin, R.; Bordignon, V.; Murphy, B.D.; Palin, M.-F. Adiponectin action from head to toe. *Endocrine* **2010**, *37*, 11–32. [CrossRef]
2. Wang, G.-X.; Zhao, X.-Y.; Lin, J.D. The brown fat secretome: Metabolic functions beyond thermogenesis. *Trends Endocrinol. Metab. TEM* **2015**, *26*, 231–237. [CrossRef] [PubMed]
3. Scherer, P.E.; Williams, S.; Fogliano, M.; Baldini, G.; Lodish, H.F. A novel serum protein similar to C1q, produced exclusively in adipocytes. *J. Biol. Chem.* **1995**, *270*, 26746–26749. [CrossRef] [PubMed]
4. Hu, E.; Liang, P.; Spiegelman, B.M. AdipoQ is a novel adipose-specific gene dysregulated in obesity. *J. Biol. Chem.* **1996**, *271*, 10697–10703. [CrossRef] [PubMed]
5. Maeda, K.; Okubo, K.; Shimomura, I.; Funahashi, T.; Matsuzawa, Y.; Matsubara, K. cDNA cloning and expression of a novel adipose specific collagen-like factor, apM1 (AdiPose Most abundant Gene transcript 1). *Biochem. Biophys. Res. Commun.* **1996**, *221*, 286–289. [CrossRef] [PubMed]
6. Nakano, Y.; Tobe, T.; Choi-Miura, N.H.; Mazda, T.; Tomita, M. Isolation and characterization of GBP28, a novel gelatin-binding protein purified from human plasma. *J. Biochem.* **1996**, *120*, 803–812. [CrossRef]
7. Berg, A.H.; Combs, T.P.; Du, X.; Brownlee, M.; Scherer, P.E. The adipocyte-secreted protein Acrp30 enhances hepatic insulin action. *Nat. Med.* **2001**, *7*, 947–953. [CrossRef]
8. Yamauchi, T.; Kamon, J.; Waki, H.; Terauchi, Y.; Kubota, N.; Hara, K.; Mori, Y.; Ide, T.; Murakami, K.; Tsuboyama-Kasaoka, N.; et al. The fat-derived hormone adiponectin reverses insulin resistance associated with both lipoatrophy and obesity. *Nat. Med.* **2001**, *7*, 941–946. [CrossRef]
9. Combs, T.P.; Berg, A.H.; Obici, S.; Scherer, P.E.; Rossetti, L. Endogenous glucose production is inhibited by the adipose-derived protein Acrp30. *J. Clin. Investig.* **2001**, *108*, 1875–1881. [CrossRef]
10. Yamauchi, T.; Kamon, J.; Minokoshi, Y.; Ito, Y.; Waki, H.; Uchida, S.; Yamashita, S.; Noda, M.; Kita, S.; Ueki, K.; et al. Adiponectin stimulates glucose utilization and fatty-acid oxidation by activating AMP-activated protein kinase. *Nat. Med.* **2002**, *8*, 1288–1295. [CrossRef]
11. Qi, Y.; Takahashi, N.; Hileman, S.M.; Patel, H.R.; Berg, A.H.; Pajvani, U.B.; Scherer, P.E.; Ahima, R.S. Adiponectin acts in the brain to decrease body weight. *Nat. Med.* **2004**, *10*, 524–529. [CrossRef] [PubMed]
12. Holland, W.L.; Miller, R.A.; Wang, Z.V.; Sun, K.; Barth, B.M.; Bui, H.H.; Davis, K.E.; Bikman, B.T.; Halberg, N.; Rutkowski, J.M.; et al. Receptor-mediated activation of ceramidase activity initiates the pleiotropic actions of adiponectin. *Nat. Med.* **2011**, *17*, 55–63. [CrossRef] [PubMed]
13. Chaurasia, B.; Summers, S.A. Ceramides—Lipotoxic Inducers of Metabolic Disorders. *Trends Endocrinol. Metab.* **2015**, *26*, 538–550. [CrossRef]
14. Xia, J.Y.; Holland, W.L.; Kusminski, C.M.; Sun, K.; Sharma, A.X.; Pearson, M.J.; Sifuentes, A.J.; McDonald, J.G.; Gordillo, R.; Scherer, P.E. Targeted Induction of Ceramide Degradation Leads to Improved Systemic Metabolism and Reduced Hepatic Steatosis. *Cell Metab.* **2015**, *22*, 266–278. [CrossRef]
15. Rutkowski, J.M.; Wang, Z.V.; Park, A.S.; Zhang, J.; Zhang, D.; Hu, M.C.; Moe, O.W.; Susztak, K.; Scherer, P.E. Adiponectin promotes functional recovery after podocyte ablation. *J. Am. Soc. Nephrol.* **2013**, *24*, 268–282. [CrossRef]

16. Dadson, K.; Turdi, S.; Hashemi, S.; Zhao, J.; Polidovitch, N.; Beca, S.; Backx, P.H.; McDermott, J.C.; Sweeney, G. Adiponectin is required for cardiac MEF2 activation during pressure overload induced hypertrophy. *J. Mol. Cell Cardiol.* **2015**, *86*, 102–109. [CrossRef] [PubMed]

17. Kadowaki, T.; Yamauchi, T. Adiponectin and adiponectin receptors. *Endocr. Rev.* **2005**, *26*, 439–451. [CrossRef]

18. Hug, C.; Wang, J.; Ahmad, N.S.; Bogan, J.S.; Tsao, T.S.; Lodish, H.F. T-cadherin is a receptor for hexameric and high-molecular-weight forms of Acrp30/adiponectin. *Proc. Natl. Acad. Sci. USA* **2004**, *101*, 10308–10313. [CrossRef]

19. Iwaki, M.; Matsuda, M.; Maeda, N.; Funahashi, T.; Matsuzawa, Y.; Makishima, M.; Shimomura, I. Induction of Adiponectin, a Fat-Derived Antidiabetic and Antiatherogenic Factor, by Nuclear Receptors. *Diabetes* **2003**, *52*, 1655–1663. [CrossRef]

20. Yu, J.G.; Javorschi, S.; Hevener, A.L.; Kruszynska, Y.T.; Norman, R.A.; Sinha, M.; Olefsky, J.M. The Effect of Thiazolidinediones on Plasma Adiponectin Levels in Normal, Obese, and Type 2 Diabetic Subjects. *Diabetes* **2002**, *51*, 2968–2974. [CrossRef] [PubMed]

21. Kanatani, Y.; Usui, I.; Ishizuka, K.; Bukhari, A.; Fujisaka, S.; Urakaze, M.; Haruta, T.; Kishimoto, T.; Naka, T.; Kobayashi, M. Effects of Pioglitazone on Suppressor of Cytokine Signaling 3 Expression. *Potential Mech. Its Eff. Insul. Sensit. Adiponectin Expr.* **2007**, *56*, 795–803.

22. Nakae, J.; Kitamura, T.; Kitamura, Y.; Biggs, W.H.; Arden, K.C.; Accili, D. The Forkhead Transcription Factor Foxo1 Regulates Adipocyte Differentiation. *Dev. Cell* **2003**, *4*, 119–129. [CrossRef]

23. Qiao, L.; Shao, J. SIRT1 Regulates Adiponectin Gene Expression through Foxo1-C/Enhancer-binding Protein α Transcriptional Complex. *J. Biol. Chem.* **2006**, *281*, 39915–39924. [CrossRef]

24. Park, B.-H.; Qiang, L.; Farmer, S.R. Phosphorylation of C/EBPβ at a Consensus Extracellular Signal-Regulated Kinase/Glycogen Synthase Kinase 3 Site Is Required for the Induction of Adiponectin Gene Expression during the Differentiation of Mouse Fibroblasts into Adipocytes. *Mol. Cell. Biol.* **2004**, *24*, 8671–8680. [CrossRef]

25. Gustafson, B.; Jack, M.M.; Cushman, S.W.; Smith, U. Adiponectin gene activation by thiazolidinediones requires PPARγ2, but not C/EBPα—Evidence for differential regulation of the aP2 and adiponectin genes. *Biochem. Biophys. Res. Commun.* **2003**, *308*, 933–939. [CrossRef]

26. Seo, J.B.; Moon, H.M.; Noh, M.J.; Lee, Y.S.; Jeong, H.W.; Yoo, E.J.; Kim, W.S.; Park, J.; Youn, B.-S.; Kim, J.W.; et al. Adipocyte Determination- and Differentiation-dependent Factor 1/Sterol Regulatory Element-binding Protein 1c Regulates Mouse Adiponectin Expression. *J. Biol. Chem.* **2004**, *279*, 22108–22117. [CrossRef]

27. Zhang, J.-W.; Klemm, D.J.; Vinson, C.; Lane, M.D. Role of CREB in Transcriptional Regulation of CCAAT/Enhancer-binding Protein β Gene during Adipogenesis. *J. Biol. Chem.* **2004**, *279*, 4471–4478. [CrossRef]

28. Kim, H.B.; Kong, M.; Kim, T.M.; Suh, Y.H.; Kim, W.-H.; Lim, J.H.; Song, J.H.; Jung, M.H. NFATc4 and ATF3 Negatively Regulate Adiponectin Gene Expression in 3T3-L1 Adipocytes. *Diabetes* **2006**, *55*, 1342–1352. [CrossRef]

29. Ho, I.-C.; Kim, J.H.-J.; Rooney, J.W.; Spiegelman, B.M.; Glimcher, L.H. A potential role for the nuclear factor of activated T cells family of transcriptional regulatory proteins in adipogenesis. *Proc. Natl. Acad. Sci. USA* **1998**, *95*, 15537–15541. [CrossRef]

30. Liu, M.; Liu, F. Transcriptional and post-translational regulation of adiponectin. *Biochem. J.* **2010**, *425*, 41–52. [CrossRef]

31. Lim, J.-Y.; Kim, W.H.; Park, S.I. GO6976 prevents TNF-α-induced suppression of adiponectin expression in 3T3-L1 adipocytes: Putative involvement of protein kinase C. *FEBS Lett.* **2008**, *582*, 3473–3478. [CrossRef]

32. Zappalà, G.; Rechler, M.M. IGFBP-3, hypoxia and TNF-α inhibit adiponectin transcription. *Biochem. Biophys. Res. Commun.* **2009**, *382*, 785–789. [CrossRef]

33. Fasshauer, M.; Kralisch, S.; Klier, M.; Lossner, U.; Bluher, M.; Klein, J.; Paschke, R. Adiponectin gene expression and secretion is inhibited by interleukin-6 in 3T3-L1 adipocytes. *Biochem. Biophys. Res. Commun.* **2003**, *301*, 1045–1050. [CrossRef]

34. Kusminski, C.M.; McTernan, P.G.; Schraw, T.; Kos, K.; O'Hare, J.P.; Ahima, R.; Kumar, S.; Scherer, P.E. Adiponectin complexes in human cerebrospinal fluid: Distinct complex distribution from serum. *Diabetologia* **2007**, *50*, 634–642. [CrossRef]

35. Kadowaki, T.; Yamauchi, T.; Kubota, N.; Hara, K.; Ueki, K.; Tobe, K. Adiponectin and adiponectin receptors in insulin resistance, diabetes, and the metabolic syndrome. *J. Clin. Investig.* **2006**, *116*, 1784–1792. [CrossRef]

36. Phillips, S.A.; Kung, J.T. Mechanisms of adiponectin regulation and use as a pharmacological target. *Curr. Opin. Pharmacol.* **2010**, *10*, 676–683. [CrossRef]
37. Berg, A.H.; Combs, T.P.; Scherer, P.E. ACRP30/adiponectin: An adipokine regulating glucose and lipid metabolism. *Trends Endocrinol. Metab.* **2002**, *13*, 84–89. [CrossRef]
38. Wang, Y.; Lam, K.S.L.; Chan, L.; Chan, K.W.; Lam, J.B.B.; Lam, M.C.; Hoo, R.C.L.; Mak, W.W.N.; Cooper, G.J.S.; Xu, A. Post-translational Modifications of the Four Conserved Lysine Residues within the Collagenous Domain of Adiponectin Are Required for the Formation of Its High Molecular Weight Oligomeric Complex. *J. Biol. Chem.* **2006**, *281*, 16391–16400. [CrossRef]
39. Richards, A.A.; Macdonald, G.A.; Charlton, H.K.; Prins, J.B.; Stephens, T.; Whitehead, J.P.; Jones, A. Adiponectin Multimerization Is Dependent on Conserved Lysines in the Collagenous Domain: Evidence for Regulation of Multimerization by Alterations in Posttranslational Modifications. *Mol. Endocrinol.* **2006**, *20*, 1673–1687. [CrossRef]
40. Wang, Z.V.; Schraw, T.D.; Kim, J.-Y.; Khan, T.; Rajala, M.W.; Follenzi, A.; Scherer, P.E. Secretion of the Adipocyte-Specific Secretory Protein Adiponectin Critically Depends on Thiol-Mediated Protein Retention. *Mol. Cell. Biol.* **2007**, *27*, 3716–3731. [CrossRef]
41. Qiang, L.; Wang, H.; Farmer, S.R. Adiponectin Secretion Is Regulated by SIRT1 and the Endoplasmic Reticulum Oxidoreductase Ero1-Lα. *Mol. Cell. Biol.* **2007**, *27*, 4698–4707. [CrossRef]
42. Phillips, S.A.; Kung, J.; Ciaraldi, T.P.; Choe, C.; Christiansen, L.; Mudaliar, S.; Henry, R.R. Selective regulation of cellular and secreted multimeric adiponectin by antidiabetic therapies in humans. *Am. J. Physiol. Endocrinol. Metab.* **2009**, *297*, E767–E773. [CrossRef] [PubMed]
43. Liu, M.; Zhou, L.; Xu, A.; Lam, K.S.L.; Wetzel, M.D.; Xiang, R.; Zhang, J.; Xin, X.; Dong, L.Q.; Liu, F. A disulfide-bond A oxidoreductase-like protein (DsbA-L) regulates adiponectin multimerization. *Proc. Natl. Acad. Sci. USA* **2008**, *105*, 18302–18307. [CrossRef] [PubMed]
44. Mitchell, M.; Armstrong, D.T.; Robker, R.L.; Norman, R.J. Adipokines: Implications for female fertility and obesity. *Reproduction* **2005**, *130*, 583. [CrossRef] [PubMed]
45. Chabrolle, C.; Tosca, L.; Dupont, J.L. Regulation of adiponectin and its receptors in rat ovary by human chorionic gonadotrophin treatment and potential involvement of adiponectin in granulosa cell steroidogenesis. *Reproduction* **2007**, *133*, 719. [CrossRef] [PubMed]
46. Leff, T. AMP-activated protein kinase regulates gene expression by direct phosphorylation of nuclear proteins. *Biochem. Soc. Trans.* **2003**, *31*, 224–227. [CrossRef]
47. Dupont, J.; Chabrolle, C.; Ramé, C.; Tosca, L.; Coyral-Castel, S. Role of the peroxisome proliferator-activated receptors, adenosine monophosphate-activated kinase, and adiponectin in the ovary. *Ppar Res.* **2008**, *2008*, 176275. [CrossRef]
48. Archanco, M.; Gómez-Ambrosi, J.; Tena-Sempere, M.; Frühbeck, G.; Burrell, M.A. Expression of Leptin and Adiponectin in the Rat Oviduct. *J. Histochem. Cytochem.* **2007**, *55*, 1027–1037. [CrossRef]
49. Morimoto, C.; Koga, K.; Harada, M.; Yoshino, O.; Hirata, T.; Hirota, Y.; Taketani, Y.; Takemura, Y.; Osuga, Y.; Yano, T.; et al. Expression of Adiponectin Receptors and Its Possible Implication in the Human Endometrium. *Endocrinology* **2006**, *147*, 3203–3210.
50. Breitfeld, J.; Stumvoll, M.; Kovacs, P. Genetics of adiponectin. *Biochimie* **2012**, *94*, 2157–2163. [CrossRef]
51. Tokushige, K.; Hashimoto, E.; Noto, H.; Yatsuji, S.; Taniai, M.; Torii, N.; Shiratori, K. Influence of adiponectin gene polymorphisms in Japanese patients with non-alcoholic fatty liver disease. *J. Gastroenterol.* **2009**, *44*, 976–982. [CrossRef]
52. Yoon, M.J.; Lee, G.Y.; Chung, J.-J.; Ahn, Y.H.; Hong, S.H.; Kim, J.B. Adiponectin Increases Fatty Acid Oxidation in Skeletal Muscle Cells by Sequential Activation of AMP-Activated Protein Kinase, p38 Mitogen-Activated Protein Kinase, and Peroxisome Proliferator–Activated Receptor α. *Diabetes* **2006**, *55*, 2562–2570. [CrossRef]
53. Tomas, E.; Tsao, T.-S.; Saha, A.K.; Murrey, H.E.; Zhang, C.c.; Itani, S.I.; Lodish, H.F.; Ruderman, N.B. Enhanced muscle fat oxidation and glucose transport by ACRP30 globular domain: Acetyl–CoA carboxylase inhibition and AMP-activated protein kinase activation. *Proc. Natl. Acad. Sci. USA* **2002**, *99*, 16309–16313. [CrossRef]
54. Ceddia, R.B.; Somwar, R.; Maida, A.; Fang, X.; Bikopoulos, G.; Sweeney, G. Globular adiponectin increases GLUT4 translocation and glucose uptake but reduces glycogen synthesis in rat skeletal muscle cells. *Diabetologia* **2005**, *48*, 132–139. [CrossRef]

55. Fang, X.; Palanivel, R.; Zhou, X.; Liu, Y.; Xu, A.; Wang, Y.; Sweeney, G. Hyperglycemia- and hyperinsulinemia-induced alteration of adiponectin receptor expression and adiponectin effects in L6 myoblasts. *J. Mol. Endocrinol.* **2005**, *35*, 465–476. [CrossRef]

56. Tsuchida, A.; Yamauchi, T.; Ito, Y.; Hada, Y.; Maki, T.; Takekawa, S.; Kamon, J.; Kobayashi, M.; Suzuki, R.; Hara, K.; et al. Insulin/Foxo1 Pathway Regulates Expression Levels of Adiponectin Receptors and Adiponectin Sensitivity. *J. Biol. Chem.* **2004**, *279*, 30817–30822. [CrossRef]

57. Kharroubi, I.; Rasschaert, J.; Eizirik, D.L.; Cnop, M. Expression of adiponectin receptors in pancreatic β cells. *Biochem. Biophys. Res. Commun.* **2003**, *312*, 1118–1122. [CrossRef]

58. Gu, W.; Li, X.; Liu, C.; Yang, J.; Ye, L.; Tang, J.; Gu, Y.; Yang, Y.; Hong, J.; Zhang, Y.; et al. Globular adiponectin augments insulin secretion from pancreatic Islet β cells at high glucose concentrations. *Endocrine* **2006**, *30*, 217–221. [CrossRef]

59. Okamoto, M.; Ohara-Imaizumi, M.; Kubota, N.; Hashimoto, S.; Eto, K.; Kanno, T.; Kubota, T.; Wakui, M.; Nagai, R.; Noda, M.; et al. Adiponectin induces insulin secretion in vitro and in vivo at a low glucose concentration. *Diabetologia* **2008**, *51*, 827–835. [CrossRef]

60. Zyromski, N.J.; Mathur, A.; Pitt, H.A.; Wade, T.E.; Wang, S.; Swartz-Basile, D.A.; Prather, A.D.; Lillemoe, K.D. Cannabinoid Receptor-1 Blockade Attenuates Acute pancreatitis in Obesity by An adiponectin Mediated Mechanism. *J. Gastrointest. Surg.* **2009**, *13*, 831. [CrossRef]

61. Bloemer, J.; Pinky, P.D.; Govindarajulu, M.; Hong, H.; Judd, R.; Amin, R.H.; Moore, T.; Dhanasekaran, M.; Reed, M.N.; Suppiramaniam, V. Role of Adiponectin in Central Nervous System Disorders. *Neural Plast.* **2018**, *2018*, 4593530. [CrossRef]

62. Martinez-Fuentes, A.J.; Rodriguez-Pacheco, F.; Castaño, J.P.; Pinilla, L.; Tena-Sempere, M.; Malagon, M.a.M.; Dieguez, C.; Tovar, S. Regulation of Pituitary Cell Function by Adiponectin. *Endocrinology* **2007**, *148*, 401–410.

63. Nishimura, M.; Izumiya, Y.; Higuchi, A.; Shibata, R.; Qiu, J.; Kudo, C.; Shin, H.K.; Moskowitz, M.A.; Ouchi, N. Adiponectin Prevents Cerebral Ischemic Injury Through Endothelial Nitric Oxide Synthase–Dependent Mechanisms. *Circulation* **2008**, *117*, 216–223. [CrossRef]

64. Neumeier, M.; Weigert, J.; Schäffler, A.; Wehrwein, G.; Müller-Ladner, U.; Schölmerich, J.; Wrede, C.; Buechler, C. Different effects of adiponectin isoforms in human monocytic cells. *J. Leukoc. Biol.* **2006**, *79*, 803–808. [CrossRef] [PubMed]

65. Wulster-Radcliffe, M.C.; Ajuwon, K.M.; Wang, J.; Christian, J.A.; Spurlock, M.E. Adiponectin differentially regulates cytokines in porcine macrophages. *Biochem. Biophys. Res. Commun.* **2004**, *316*, 924–929. [CrossRef]

66. Wolf, A.M.; Wolf, D.; Rumpold, H.; Enrich, B.; Tilg, H. Adiponectin induces the anti-inflammatory cytokines IL-10 and IL-1RA in human leukocytes. *Biochem. Biophys. Res. Commun.* **2004**, *323*, 630–635. [CrossRef]

67. Šenolt, L.; Pavelka, K.; Housa, D.; Haluzík, M. Increased adiponectin is negatively linked to the local inflammatory process in patients with rheumatoid arthritis. *Cytokine* **2006**, *35*, 247–252. [CrossRef]

68. Ebina, K.; Fukuhara, A.; Ando, W.; Hirao, M.; Koga, T.; Oshima, K.; Matsuda, M.; Maeda, K.; Nakamura, T.; Ochi, T.; et al. Serum adiponectin concentrations correlate with severity of rheumatoid arthritis evaluated by extent of joint destruction. *Clin. Rheumatol.* **2009**, *28*, 445–451. [CrossRef]

69. Ehling, A.; Schäffler, A.; Herfarth, H.; Tarner, I.H.; Anders, S.; Distler, O.; Paul, G.; Distler, J.; Gay, S.; Schölmerich, J.; et al. The Potential of Adiponectin in Driving Arthritis. *J. Immunol.* **2006**, *176*, 4468–4478. [CrossRef]

70. Nakamura, T.; Tokunaga, K.; Shimomura, I.; Nishida, M.; Yoshida, S.; Kotani, K.; Islam, A.H.M.W.; Keno, Y.; Kobatake, T.; Nagai, Y.; et al. Contribution of visceral fat accumulation to the development of coronary artery disease in non-obese men. *Atherosclerosis* **1994**, *107*, 239–246. [CrossRef]

71. Kobayashi, H.; Ouchi, N.; Kihara, S.; Walsh, K.; Kumada, M.; Abe, Y.; Funahashi, T.; Matsuzawa, Y. Selective Suppression of Endothelial Cell Apoptosis by the High Molecular Weight Form of Adiponectin. *Circ. Res.* **2004**, *94*, e27–e31. [CrossRef]

72. Otsuka, F.; Sugiyama, S.; Kojima, S.; Maruyoshi, H.; Funahashi, T.; Matsui, K.; Sakamoto, T.; Yoshimura, M.; Kimura, K.; Umemura, S.; et al. Plasma Adiponectin Levels Are Associated with Coronary Lesion Complexity in Men with Coronary Artery Disease. *J. Am. Coll. Cardiol.* **2006**, *48*, 1155–1162. [CrossRef]

73. Shibata, R.; Sato, K.; Pimentel, D.R.; Takemura, Y.; Kihara, S.; Ohashi, K.; Funahashi, T.; Ouchi, N.; Walsh, K. Adiponectin protects against myocardial ischemia-reperfusion injury through AMPK- and COX-2–dependent mechanisms. *Nat. Med.* **2005**, *11*, 1096. [CrossRef]

74. Ikeda, Y.; Ohashi, K.; Shibata, R.; Pimentel, D.R.; Kihara, S.; Ouchi, N.; Walsh, K. Cyclooxygenase-2 induction by adiponectin is regulated by a sphingosine kinase-1 dependent mechanism in cardiac myocytes. *FEBS Lett.* **2008**, *582*, 1147–1150. [CrossRef]

75. Ouchi, N.; Kihara, S.; Arita, Y.; Maeda, K.; Kuriyama, H.; Okamoto, Y.; Hotta, K.; Nishida, M.; Takahashi, M.; Nakamura, T.; et al. Novel Modulator for Endothelial Adhesion Molecules. *Circulation* **1999**, *100*, 2473–2476. [CrossRef]

76. Cnop, M.; Havel, P.J.; Utzschneider, K.M.; Carr, D.B.; Sinha, M.K.; Boyko, E.J.; Retzlaff, B.M.; Knopp, R.H.; Brunzell, J.D.; Kahn, S.E. Relationship of adiponectin to body fat distribution, insulin sensitivity and plasma lipoproteins: Evidence for independent roles of age and sex. *Diabetologia* **2003**, *46*, 459–469. [CrossRef]

77. Rasmussen, M.S.; Lihn, A.S.; Pedersen, S.B.; Bruun, J.M.; Rasmussen, M.; Richelsen, B. Adiponectin Receptors in Human Adipose Tissue: Effects of Obesity, Weight Loss, and Fat Depots. *Obesity* **2006**, *14*, 28–35. [CrossRef]

78. Spranger, J.; Kroke, A.; Möhlig, M.; Bergmann, M.M.; Ristow, M.; Boeing, H.; Pfeiffer, A.F.H. Adiponectin and protection against type 2 diabetes mellitus. *Lancet* **2003**, *361*, 226–228. [CrossRef]

79. Hara, K.; Horikoshi, M.; Yamauchi, T.; Yago, H.; Miyazaki, O.; Ebinuma, H.; Imai, Y.; Nagai, R.; Kadowaki, T. Measurement of the High–Molecular Weight Form of Adiponectin in Plasma Is Useful for the Prediction of Insulin Resistance and Metabolic Syndrome. *Diabetes Care* **2006**, *29*, 1357–1362. [CrossRef]

80. Ruchat, S.-M.; Loos, R.J.F.; Rankinen, T.; Vohl, M.-C.; Weisnagel, S.J.; Després, J.-P.; Bouchard, C.; Pérusse, L. Associations between glucose tolerance, insulin sensitivity and insulin secretion phenotypes and polymorphisms in adiponectin and adiponectin receptor genes in the Quebec Family Study. *Diabet. Med.* **2008**, *25*, 400–406. [CrossRef]

81. Wang, Z.V.; Scherer, P.E. Adiponectin, Cardiovascular Function, and Hypertension. *Hypertension* **2008**, *51*, 8–14. [CrossRef]

82. Kurukulasuriya, L.R.; Stas, S.; Lastra, G.; Manrique, C.; Sowers, J.R. Hypertension in Obesity. *Endocrinol. Metab. Clin. N. Am.* **2008**, *37*, 647–662. [CrossRef]

83. Kantartzis, K.; Rittig, K.; Balletshofer, B.; Machann, J.; Schick, F.; Porubska, K.; Fritsche, A.; Häring, H.-U.; Stefan, N. The Relationships of Plasma Adiponectin with a Favorable Lipid Profile, Decreased Inflammation, and Less Ectopic Fat Accumulation Depend on Adiposity. *Clin. Chem.* **2006**, *52*, 1934–1942. [CrossRef]

84. Okada, T.; Saito, E.; Kuromori, Y.; Miyashita, M.; Iwata, F.; Hara, M.; Harada, K. Relationship between serum adiponectin level and lipid composition in each lipoprotein fraction in adolescent children. *Atherosclerosis* **2006**, *188*, 179–183. [CrossRef] [PubMed]

85. Vergès, B.; Petit, J.M.; Duvillard, L.; Dautin, G.; Florentin, E.; Galland, F.; Gambert, P. Adiponectin Is an Important Determinant of ApoA-I Catabolism. *Arteriosclerosis. Thrombosis. Vasc. Biol.* **2006**, *26*, 1364–1369. [CrossRef] [PubMed]

86. Seino, Y.; Hirose, H.; Saito, I.; Itoh, H. High-molecular-weight adiponectin is a predictor of progression to metabolic syndrome: A population-based 6-year follow-up study in Japanese men. *Metabolism* **2009**, *58*, 355–360. [CrossRef]

87. Lara-Castro, C.; Luo, N.; Wallace, P.; Klein, R.L.; Garvey, W.T. Adiponectin Multimeric Complexes and the Metabolic Syndrome Trait Cluster. *Diabetes* **2006**, *55*, 249–259. [CrossRef]

88. Demirci, H.; Nuhoglu, C.; Ursavas, I.S.; Isildak, S.; Basaran, E.O.; Kilic, M.Y. Obesity and asymptomatic hypertension among children aged 6–13 years living in Bursa, Turkey. *Fam. Pr.* **2013**, *30*, 629–633. [CrossRef]

89. Kim, N.H.; Cho, N.H.; Yun, C.H.; Lee, S.K.; Yoon, D.W.; Cho, H.J.; Ahn, J.H.; Seo, J.A.; Kim, S.G.; Choi, K.M.; et al. Association of obstructive sleep apnea and glucose metabolism in subjects with or without obesity. *Diabetes Care* **2013**, *36*, 3909–3915. [CrossRef]

90. Ouchi, N.; Kihara, S.; Funahashi, T.; Matsuzawa, Y.; Walsh, K. Obesity, adiponectin and vascular inflammatory disease. *Curr. Opin. Lipidol.* **2003**, *14*, 561–566. [CrossRef] [PubMed]

91. Iwashima, Y.; Katsuya, T.; Ishikawa, K.; Ouchi, N.; Ohishi, M.; Sugimoto, K.; Fu, Y.; Motone, M.; Yamamoto, K.; Matsuo, A.; et al. Hypoadiponectinemia is an independent risk factor for hypertension. *Hypertension* **2004**, *43*, 1318–1323. [CrossRef]

92. di Chiara, T.; Licata, A.; Argano, C.; Duro, G.; Corrao, S.; Scaglione, R. Plasma adiponectin: A contributing factor for cardiac changes in visceral obesity-associated hypertension. *Blood Press* **2014**, *23*, 147–153. [CrossRef]

93. Ouchi, N.; Kihara, S.; Arita, Y.; Nishida, M.; Matsuyama, A.; Okamoto, Y.; Ishigami, M.; Kuriyama, H.; Kishida, K.; Nishizawa, H.; et al. Adipocyte-derived plasma protein, adiponectin, suppresses lipid accumulation and class A scavenger receptor expression in human monocyte-derived macrophages. *Circulation* **2001**, *103*, 1057–1063. [CrossRef]

94. Avogaro, A.; de Kreutzenberg, S.V. Mechanisms of endothelial dysfunction in obesity. *Clin. Chim. Acta* **2005**, *360*, 9–26. [CrossRef]

95. Shimamoto, Y.; Mizukoshi, M.; Kuroi, A.; Imanishi, T.; Takeshita, T.; Terada, M.; Akasaka, T. Is visceral fat really a coronary risk factor? A multi-detector computed tomography study. *Int. Heart J.* **2013**, *54*, 273–278. [CrossRef]

96. Choi, S.H.; Hong, E.S.; Lim, S. Clinical implications of adipocytokines and newly emerging metabolic factors with relation to insulin resistance and cardiovascular health. *Front. Endocrinol.* **2013**, *4*, 97. [CrossRef]

97. Rega-Kaun, G.; Kaun, C.; Wojta, J. More than a simple storage organ: Adipose tissue as a source of adipokines involved in cardiovascular disease. *Thromb. Haemost.* **2013**, *110*, 641–650. [CrossRef]

98. Diaz-Melean, C.M.; Somers, V.K.; Rodriguez-Escudero, J.P.; Singh, P.; Sochor, O.; Llano, E.M.; Lopez-Jimenez, F. Mechanisms of adverse cardiometabolic consequences of obesity. *Curr. Atheroscler Rep.* **2013**, *15*, 364. [CrossRef]

99. Villarreal-Molina, M.T.; Antuna-Puente, B. Adiponectin: Anti-inflammatory and cardioprotective effects. *Biochimie* **2012**, *94*, 2143–2149. [CrossRef]

100. Matsuda, M.; Shimomura, I. Roles of adiponectin and oxidative stress in obesity-associated metabolic and cardiovascular diseases. *Rev. Endocr. Metab. Disord.* **2014**, *15*, 1–10. [CrossRef]

101. Matsuda, M.; Shimomura, I.; Sata, M.; Arita, Y.; Nishida, M.; Maeda, N.; Kumada, M.; Okamoto, Y.; Nagaretani, H.; Nishizawa, H.; et al. Role of adiponectin in preventing vascular stenosis. The missing link of adipo-vascular axis. *J. Biol. Chem.* **2002**, *277*, 37487–37491. [CrossRef]

102. Ouchi, N.; Walsh, K. Cardiovascular and metabolic regulation by the adiponectin/C1q/tumor necrosis factor-related protein family of proteins. *Circulation* **2012**, *125*, 3066–3068. [CrossRef]

103. Mathew, J.L.; Narang, I. Sleeping too close together: Obesity and obstructive sleep apnea in childhood and adolescence. *Paediatr. Respir Rev.* **2014**, *15*, 211–218. [CrossRef]

104. Hargens, T.A.; Guill, S.G.; Kaleth, A.S.; Nickols-Richardson, S.M.; Miller, L.E.; Zedalis, D.; Gregg, J.M.; Gwazdauskas, F.; Herbert, W.G. Insulin resistance and adipose-derived hormones in young men with untreated obstructive sleep apnea. *Sleep Breath* **2013**, *17*, 403–409. [CrossRef]

105. Nakagawa, Y.; Kishida, K.; Kihara, S.; Yoshida, R.; Funahashi, T.; Shimomura, I. Nocturnal falls of adiponectin levels in sleep apnea with abdominal obesity and impact of hypoxia-induced dysregulated adiponectin production in obese murine mesenteric adipose tissue. *J. Atheroscler. Thromb.* **2011**, *18*, 240–247. [CrossRef]

106. Magalang, U.J.; Cruff, J.P.; Rajappan, R.; Hunter, M.G.; Patel, T.; Marsh, C.B.; Raman, S.V.; Parinandi, N.L. Intermittent hypoxia suppresses adiponectin secretion by adipocytes. *Exp. Clin. Endocrinol. Diabetes* **2009**, *117*, 129–134. [CrossRef]

107. Klein, B.E. Overview of epidemiologic studies of diabetic retinopathy. *Ophthalmic Epidemiol.* **2007**, *14*, 179–183. [CrossRef] [PubMed]

108. Yilmaz, M.I.; Sonmez, A.; Acikel, C.; Celik, T.; Bingol, N.; Pinar, M.; Bayraktar, Z.; Ozata, M. Adiponectin may play a part in the pathogenesis of diabetic retinopathy. *Eur. J. Endocrinol.* **2004**, *151*, 135–140. [CrossRef]

109. Vainio, H.; Bianchini, F. (Eds.) *IARC Handbook of Cancer Prevention*; IARC Press: Lyon, France, 2002; Volume 6.

110. Iskander, K.; Farhour, R.; Ficek, M.; Ray, A. Obesity-related complications: Few biochemical phenomena with reference to tumorigenesis. *Malays. J. Pathol.* **2013**, *35*, 1–15.

111. Kwan, M.L.; John, E.M.; Caan, B.J.; Lee, V.S.; Bernstein, L.; Cheng, I.; Gomez, S.L.; Henderson, B.E.; Keegan, T.H.; Kurian, A.W.; et al. Obesity and mortality after breast cancer by race/ethnicity: The California Breast Cancer Survivorship Consortium. *Am. J. Epidemiol.* **2014**, *179*, 95–111. [CrossRef]

112. Miyoshi, Y.; Funahashi, T.; Kihara, S.; Taguchi, T.; Tamaki, Y.; Matsuzawa, Y.; Noguchi, S. Association of Serum Adiponectin Levels with Breast Cancer Risk. *Clin. Cancer Res.* **2003**, *9*, 5699–5704.

113. Chen, X.; Wang, Y. Adiponectin and breast cancer. *Med. Oncol.* **2011**, *28*, 1288–1295. [CrossRef] [PubMed]

114. Surmacz, E. Leptin and adiponectin: Emerging therapeutic targets in breast cancer. *J. Mammary Gland Biol. Neoplasia* **2013**, *18*, 321–332. [CrossRef] [PubMed]

115. Ohbuchi, Y.; Suzuki, Y.; Hatakeyama, I.; Nakao, Y.; Fujito, A.; Iwasaka, T.; Isaka, K. A lower serum level of middle-molecular-weight adiponectin is a risk factor for endometrial cancer. *Int. J. Clin. Oncol.* **2014**, *19*, 667–673. [CrossRef]

116. Kerenidi, T.; Lada, M.; Tsaroucha, A.; Georgoulias, P.; Mystridou, P.; Gourgoulianis, K.I. Clinical significance of serum adipokines levels in lung cancer. *Med. Oncol.* **2013**, *30*, 507. [CrossRef] [PubMed]

117. Kosova, F.; Coskun, T.; Kaya, Y.; Kara, E.; Ari, Z. Adipocytokine levels of colon cancer patients before and after treatment. *Bratisl. Lek. Listy* **2013**, *114*, 394–397. [CrossRef] [PubMed]

118. Liao, L.M.; Schwartz, K.; Pollak, M.; Graubard, B.I.; Li, Z.; Ruterbusch, J.; Rothman, N.; Davis, F.; Wacholder, S.; Colt, J.; et al. Serum leptin and adiponectin levels and risk of renal cell carcinoma. *Obesity* **2013**, *21*, 1478–1485. [CrossRef] [PubMed]

119. Wei, T.; Ye, P.; Peng, X.; Wu, L.L.; Yu, G.Y. Circulating adiponectin levels in various malignancies: An updated meta-analysis of 107 studies. *Oncotarget* **2016**, *7*, 48671–48691. [CrossRef] [PubMed]

120. Sun, Y.; Chen, X. Effect of adiponectin on apoptosis: Proapoptosis or antiapoptosis? *BioFactors* **2010**, *36*, 179–186. [CrossRef]

121. Fu, S.; Xu, H.; Liu, C.; Gu, M.; Wang, Q.; Zhou, J.; Wang, Z. Role of adiponectin in prostate cancer: A preliminary study. *Zhonghua Nan Ke Xue Natl. J. Androl.* **2017**, *23*, 975–981.

122. Gao, Q.; Zheng, J.; Yao, X.; Peng, B. Adiponectin inhibits VEGF-A in prostate cancer cells. *Tumor Biol.* **2015**, *36*, 4287–4292. [CrossRef]

123. Shrestha, A.; Nepal, S.; Kim, M.J.; Chang, J.H.; Kim, S.-H.; Jeong, G.-S.; Jeong, C.-H.; Park, G.H.; Jung, S.; Lim, J.; et al. Critical Role of AMPK/FoxO3A Axis in Globular Adiponectin-Induced Cell Cycle Arrest and Apoptosis in Cancer Cells. *J. Cell. Physiol.* **2016**, *231*, 357–369. [CrossRef] [PubMed]

124. Xing, S.-Q.; Zhang, C.-G.; Yuan, J.-F.; Yang, H.-M.; Zhao, S.-D.; Zhang, H. Adiponectin induces apoptosis in hepatocellular carcinoma through differential modulation of thioredoxin proteins. *Biochem. Pharmacol.* **2015**, *93*, 221–231. [CrossRef] [PubMed]

125. Otani, K.; Ishihara, S.; Yamaguchi, H.; Murono, K.; Yasuda, K.; Nishikawa, T.; Tanaka, T.; Kiyomatsu, T.; Hata, K.; Kawai, K.; et al. Adiponectin and colorectal cancer. *Surg. Today* **2017**, *47*, 151–158. [CrossRef] [PubMed]

126. Fujisawa, T.; Endo, H.; Tomimoto, A.; Sugiyama, M.; Takahashi, H.; Saito, S.; Inamori, M.; Nakajima, N.; Watanabe, M.; Kubota, N.; et al. Adiponectin suppresses colorectal carcinogenesis under the high-fat diet condition. *Gut* **2008**, *57*, 1531–1538. [CrossRef] [PubMed]

127. Moon, H.-S.; Liu, X.; Nagel, J.M.; Chamberland, J.P.; Diakopoulos, K.N.; Brinkoetter, M.T.; Hatziapostolou, M.; Wu, Y.; Robson, S.C.; Iliopoulos, D.; et al. Salutary effects of adiponectin on colon cancer: In vivo and in vitro studies in mice. *Gut* **2013**, *62*, 561–570. [CrossRef] [PubMed]

128. Bråkenhielm, E.; Veitonmäki, N.; Cao, R.; Kihara, S.; Matsuzawa, Y.; Zhivotovsky, B.; Funahashi, T.; Cao, Y. Adiponectin-induced antiangiogenesis and antitumor activity involve caspase-mediated endothelial cell apoptosis. *Proc. Natl. Acad. Sci. USA* **2004**, *101*, 2476–2481. [CrossRef]

129. Wang, Y.; Lam, J.B.; Lam, K.S.L.; Liu, J.; Lam, M.C.; Hoo, R.L.C.; Wu, D.; Cooper, G.J.S.; Xu, A. Adiponectin Modulates the Glycogen Synthase Kinase-3β/β-Catenin Signaling Pathway and Attenuates Mammary Tumorigenesis of MDA-MB-231 Cells in Nude Mice. *Cancer Res.* **2006**, *66*, 11462–11470. [CrossRef]

130. Kang, J.H.; Lee, Y.Y.; Yu, B.Y.; Yang, B.-S.; Cho, K.-H.; Yoon, D.K.; Roh, Y.K. Adiponectin induces growth arrest and apoptosis of MDA-MB-231 breast cancer cell. *Arch. Pharmacal. Res.* **2005**, *28*, 1263–1269. [CrossRef]

131. Mutoh, M.; Teraoka, N.; Takasu, S.; Takahashi, M.; Onuma, K.; Yamamoto, M.; Kubota, N.; Iseki, T.; Kadowaki, T.; Sugimura, T.; et al. Loss of Adiponectin Promotes Intestinal Carcinogenesis in Min and Wild-type Mice. *Gastroenterology* **2011**, *140*, 2000–2008.e2002. [CrossRef]

132. Saxena, A.; Chumanevich, A.; Fletcher, E.; Larsen, B.; Lattwein, K.; Kaur, K.; Fayad, R. Adiponectin deficiency: Role in chronic inflammation induced colon cancer. *Biochim. Biophys. Acta* **2012**, *1822*, 527–536. [CrossRef]

133. Saxena, A.; Baliga, M.S.; Ponemone, V.; Kaur, K.; Larsen, B.; Fletcher, E.; Greene, J.; Fayad, R. Mucus and adiponectin deficiency: Role in chronic inflammation-induced colon cancer. *Int. J. Colorectal Dis.* **2013**, *28*, 1267–1279. [CrossRef]

134. Kim, A.Y.; Lee, Y.S.; Kim, K.H.; Lee, J.H.; Lee, H.K.; Jang, S.-H.; Kim, S.-E.; Lee, G.Y.; Lee, J.-W.; Jung, S.-A.; et al. Adiponectin represses colon cancer cell proliferation via AdipoR1- and -R2-mediated AMPK activation. *Mol. Endocrinol.* **2010**, *24*, 1441–1452. [CrossRef]

135. Guo, X.; Liu, J.; You, L.; Li, G.; Huang, Y.; Li, Y. Association between adiponectin polymorphisms and the risk of colorectal cancer. *Genet. Test. Mol. Biomark.* **2015**, *19*, 9–13. [CrossRef]

136. Taliaferro-Smith, L.; Nagalingam, A.; Knight, B.B.; Oberlick, E.; Saxena, N.K.; Sharma, D. Integral role of PTP1B in adiponectin-mediated inhibition of oncogenic actions of leptin in breast carcinogenesis. *Neoplasia* **2013**, *15*, 23–38. [CrossRef]

137. Wu, X.; Zhang, Z.; Du, G.; Wan, X. Acrp30 inhibits leptin-induced metastasis by downregulating the JAK/STAT3 pathway via AMPK activation in aggressive SPEC-2 endometrial cancer cells. *Oncol. Rep.* **2012**, *27*, 1488–1496.

138. Man, K.; Ng, K.T.P.; Xu, A.; Cheng, Q.; Lo, C.M.; Xiao, J.W.; Sun, B.S.; Lim, Z.X.H.; Cheung, J.S.; Wu, E.X.; et al. Suppression of Liver Tumor Growth and Metastasis by Adiponectin in Nude Mice through Inhibition of Tumor Angiogenesis and Downregulation of Rho Kinase/IFN-Inducible Protein 10/Matrix Metalloproteinase 9 Signaling. *Clin. Cancer Res.* **2010**, *16*, 967–977. [CrossRef]

139. Cui, E.; Guo, H.; Shen, M.; Yu, H.; Gu, D.; Mao, W.; Wang, X. Adiponectin inhibits migration and invasion by reversing epithelial-mesenchymal transition in non-small cell lung carcinoma. *Oncol. Rep.* **2018**, *40*, 1330–1338. [CrossRef]

140. Taliaferro-Smith, L.; Nagalingam, A.; Zhong, D.; Zhou, W.; Saxena, N.K.; Sharma, D. LKB1 is required for adiponectin-mediated modulation of AMPK-S6K axis and inhibition of migration and invasion of breast cancer cells. *Oncogene* **2009**, *28*, 2621–2633. [CrossRef]

141. Saxena, N.K.; Sharma, D. Metastasis suppression by adiponectin: LKB1 rises up to the challenge. *Cell Adh Migr* **2010**, *4*, 358–362. [CrossRef]

142. Chung, S.J.; Nagaraju, G.P.; Nagalingam, A.; Muniraj, N.; Kuppusamy, P.; Walker, A.; Woo, J.; Gyorffy, B.; Gabrielson, E.; Saxena, N.K.; et al. ADIPOQ/adiponectin induces cytotoxic autophagy in breast cancer cells through STK11/LKB1-mediated activation of the AMPK-ULK1 axis. *Autophagy* **2017**, *13*, 1386–1403. [CrossRef]

143. Daniele, A.; de Rosa, A.; Nigro, E.; Scudiero, O.; Capasso, M.; Masullo, M.; de Laurentiis, G.; Oriani, G.; Sofia, M.; Bianco, A. Adiponectin oligomerization state and adiponectin receptors airway expression in chronic obstructive pulmonary disease. *Int. J. Biochem. Cell Biol.* **2012**, *44*, 563–569. [CrossRef]

144. Cong, L.; Gasser, J.; Zhao, J.; Yang, B.; Li, F.; Zhao, A.Z. Human adiponectin inhibits cell growth and induces apoptosis in human endometrial carcinoma cells, HEC-1-A and RL95 2. *Endocr. Relat. Cancer* **2007**, *14*, 713–720. [CrossRef]

145. Dieudonne, M.N.; Bussiere, M.; Santos, E.D.; Leneveu, M.C.; Giudicelli, Y.; Pecquery, R. Adiponectin mediates antiproliferative and apoptotic responses in human MCF7 breast cancer cells. *Biochem. Biophys. Res. Commun.* **2006**, *345*, 271–279. [CrossRef]

146. Davis, R.J. Signal transduction by the JNK group of MAP kinases. *Cell* **2000**, *103*, 239–252. [CrossRef]

147. Hirosumi, J.; Tuncman, G.; Chang, L.; Gorgun, C.Z.; Uysal, K.T.; Maeda, K.; Karin, M.; Hotamisligil, G.S. A central role for JNK in obesity and insulin resistance. *Nature* **2002**, *420*, 333–336. [CrossRef]

148. Saxena, N.K.; Fu, P.P.; Nagalingam, A.; Wang, J.; Handy, J.; Cohen, C.; Tighiouart, M.; Sharma, D.; Anania, F.A. Adiponectin modulates C-jun N-terminal kinase and mammalian target of rapamycin and inhibits hepatocellular carcinoma. *Gastroenterology* **2010**, *139*, 1762–1773. [CrossRef]

149. Sharma, D.; Wang, J.; Fu, P.P.; Sharma, S.; Nagalingam, A.; Mells, J.; Handy, J.; Page, A.J.; Cohen, C.; Anania, F.A.; et al. Adiponectin antagonizes the oncogenic actions of leptin in hepatocellular carcinogenesis. *Hepatology* **2010**, *52*, 1713–1722. [CrossRef]

150. Vara, J.A.F.; Casado, E.; de Castro, J.; Cejas, P.; Belda-Iniesta, C.; Gonzalez-Baron, M. PI3K/Akt signalling pathway and cancer. *Cancer Treat. Rev.* **2004**, *30*, 193–204. [CrossRef]

151. Sugiyama, M.; Takahashi, H.; Hosono, K.; Endo, H.; Kato, S.; Yoneda, K.; Nozaki, Y.; Fujita, K.; Yoneda, M.; Wada, K.; et al. Adiponectin inhibits colorectal cancer cell growth through the AMPK/mTOR pathway. *Int. J. Oncol.* **2009**, *34*, 339–344.

152. Liu, J.; Lam, J.B.; Chow, K.H.; Xu, A.; Lam, K.S.; Moon, R.T.; Wang, Y. Adiponectin stimulates Wnt inhibitory factor-1 expression through epigenetic regulations involving the transcription factor specificity protein 1. *Carcinogenesis* **2008**, *29*, 2195–2202. [CrossRef]

153. Ouchi, N.; Kihara, S.; Arita, Y.; Okamoto, Y.; Maeda, K.; Kuriyama, H.; Hotta, K.; Nishida, M.; Takahashi, M.; Muraguchi, M.; et al. Adiponectin, an adipocyte-derived plasma protein, inhibits endothelial NF-kappaB signaling through a cAMP-dependent pathway. *Circulation* **2000**, *102*, 1296–1301. [CrossRef]

154. Wang, Y.; Xu, A.; Knight, C.; Xu, L.Y.; Cooper, G.J.S. Hydroxylation and Glycosylation of the Four Conserved Lysine Residues in the Collagenous Domain of Adiponectin: POTENTIAL ROLE IN THE MODULATION OF ITS INSULIN-SENSITIZING ACTIVITY. *J. Biol. Chem.* **2002**, *277*, 19521–19529. [CrossRef]

155. Halberg, N.; Schraw, T.D.; Wang, Z.V.; Kim, J.-Y.; Yi, J.; Hamilton, M.P.; Luby-Phelps, K.; Scherer, P.E. Systemic Fate of the Adipocyte-Derived Factor Adiponectin. *Diabetes* **2009**, *58*, 1961–1970. [CrossRef]

156. Das, K.; Lin, Y.; Widen, E.; Zhang, Y.; Scherer, P.E. Chromosomal Localization, Expression Pattern, and Promoter Analysis of the Mouse Gene Encoding Adipocyte-Specific Secretory Protein Acrp30. *Biochem. Biophys. Res. Commun.* **2001**, *280*, 1120–1129. [CrossRef]

157. Kita, A.; Yamasaki, H.; Kuwahara, H.; Moriuchi, A.; Fukushima, K.; Kobayashi, M.; Fukushima, T.; Takahashi, R.; Abiru, N.; Uotani, S.; et al. Identification of the promoter region required for human adiponectin gene transcription: Association with CCAAT/enhancer binding protein-β and tumor necrosis factor-α. *Biochem. Biophys. Res. Commun.* **2005**, *331*, 484–490. [CrossRef]

158. Kai, T.; Arima, S.; Taniyama, Y.; Nakabou, M.; Kanamasa, K. Comparison of the Effect of Lipophilic and Hydrophilic Statins on Serum Adiponectin Levels in Patients with Mild Hypertension and Dyslipidemia: Kinki Adiponectin Interventional (KAI) Study. *Clin. Exp. Hypertens.* **2008**, *30*, 530–540. [CrossRef]

159. Hu, Y.; Tong, G.; Xu, W.; Pan, J.; Ryan, K.; Yang, R.; Shuldiner, A.R.; Gong, D.-W.; Zhu, D. Anti-inflammatory effects of simvastatin on adipokines in type 2 diabetic patients with carotid atherosclerosis. *Diabetes Vasc. Dis. Res.* **2009**, *6*, 262–268. [CrossRef]

160. Tsutamoto, T.; Yamaji, M.; Kawahara, C.; Nishiyama, K.; Fujii, M.; Yamamoto, T.; Horie, M. Effect of simvastatin vs. rosuvastatin on adiponectin and haemoglobin A1c levels in patients with non-ischaemic chronic heart failure. *Eur. J. Heart Fail.* **2009**, *11*, 1195–1201. [CrossRef]

161. Qu, H.-Y.; Xiao, Y.-W.; Jiang, G.-H.; Wang, Z.-Y.; Zhang, Y.; Zhang, M. Effect of Atorvastatin Versus Rosuvastatin on Levels of Serum Lipids, Inflammatory Markers and Adiponectin in Patients with Hypercholesterolemia. *Pharm. Res.* **2009**, *26*, 958–964. [CrossRef]

162. Koh, K.K.; Quon, M.J.; Han, S.H.; Ahn, J.Y.; Jin, D.K.; Kim, H.S.; Kim, D.S.; Shin, E.K. Vascular and Metabolic Effects of Combined Therapy with Ramipril and Simvastatin in Patients with Type 2 Diabetes. *Hypertension* **2005**, *45*, 1088–1093. [CrossRef]

163. Nagamia, S.; Pandian, A.; Cheema, F.; Natarajan, R.; Khan, Q.A.; Patel, A.D.; Merchant, N.; Sola, S.; Khan, B.V. The Role of Quinapril in the Presence of a Weight Loss Regimen: Endothelial Function and Markers of Obesity in Patients with the Metabolic Syndrome. *Prev. Cardiol.* **2007**, *10*, 204–209. [CrossRef]

164. Koh, K.K.; Quon, M.J.; Han, S.H.; Chung, W.-J.; Ahn, J.Y.; Seo, Y.-H.; Kang, M.H.; Ahn, T.H.; Choi, I.S.; Shin, E.K. Additive Beneficial Effects of Losartan Combined with Simvastatin in the Treatment of Hypercholesterolemic, Hypertensive Patients. *Circulation* **2004**, *110*, 3687–3692. [CrossRef]

165. Negro, R.; Formoso, G.; Hassan, H. The effects of irbesartan and telmisartan on metabolic parameters and blood pressure in obese, insulin resistant, hypertensive patients. *J. Endocrinol. Investig.* **2006**, *29*, 957–961. [CrossRef]

166. Furuhashi, M.; Ura, N.; Higashiura, K.; Murakami, H.; Tanaka, M.; Moniwa, N.; Yoshida, D.; Shimamoto, K. Blockade of the Renin-Angiotensin System Increases Adiponectin Concentrations in Patients with Essential Hypertension. *Hypertension* **2003**, *42*, 76–81. [CrossRef]

167. Yang, W.-S.; Jeng, C.-Y.; Wu, T.-J.; Tanaka, S.; Funahashi, T.; Matsuzawa, Y.; Wang, J.-P.; Chen, C.-L.; Tai, T.-Y.; Chuang, L.-M. Synthetic Peroxisome Proliferator-Activated Receptor-γ Agonist, Rosiglitazone, Increases Plasma Levels of Adiponectin in Type 2 Diabetic Patients. *Diabetes Care* **2002**, *25*, 376–380. [CrossRef]

168. Tonelli, J.; Li, W.; Kishore, P.; Pajvani, U.B.; Kwon, E.; Weaver, C.; Scherer, P.E.; Hawkins, M. Mechanisms of Early Insulin-Sensitizing Effects of Thiazolidinediones in Type 2 Diabetes. *Diabetes* **2004**, *53*, 1621–1629. [CrossRef]

169. Araki, T.; Emoto, M.; Konishi, T.; Ikuno, Y.; Lee, E.; Teramura, M.; Motoyama, K.; Yokoyama, H.; Mori, K.; Koyama, H.; et al. Glimepiride increases high-density lipoprotein cholesterol via increasing adiponectin levels in type 2 diabetes mellitus. *Metabolism* **2009**, *58*, 143–148. [CrossRef]

170. Li, G.; Xie, C.; Lu, S.; Nichols, R.G.; Tian, Y.; Li, L.; Patel, D.; Ma, Y.; Brocker, C.N.; Yan, T.; et al. Intermittent Fasting Promotes White Adipose Browning and Decreases Obesity by Shaping the Gut Microbiota. *Cell Metab.* **2017**, *26*, 672–685.e674. [CrossRef]

171. Sirico, F.; Bianco, A.; D'Alicandro, G.; Castaldo, C.; Montagnani, S.; Spera, R.; di Meglio, F.; Nurzynska, D. Effects of Physical Exercise on Adiponectin, Leptin, and Inflammatory Markers in Childhood Obesity: Systematic Review and Meta-Analysis. *Child. Obes. (Print)* **2018**, *14*, 207–217. [CrossRef]

172. Becic, T.; Studenik, C.; Hoffmann, G. Exercise Increases Adiponectin and Reduces Leptin Levels in Prediabetic and Diabetic Individuals: Systematic Review and Meta-Analysis of Randomized Controlled Trials. *Med. Sci.* **2018**, *6*, 97. [CrossRef]

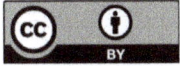

International Journal of
Molecular Sciences

MDPI

Review

The Emerging Role of Adiponectin in Female Malignancies

Luca Gelsomino [1,†], Giuseppina Daniela Naimo [1,†], Stefania Catalano [1], Loredana Mauro [1,*,‡] and Sebastiano Andò [1,2,*,‡]

[1] Department of Pharmacy, Health and Nutritional Sciences, University of Calabria,
   87036 Arcavacata di Rende (CS), Italy; lugelso@gmail.com (L.G.);
   giuseppinadanielanaimo@gmail.com (G.D.N.); stefcatalano@libero.it (S.C.)
[2] Centro Sanitario, University of Calabria, Via Pietro Bucci, 87036 Arcavacata di Rende (CS), Italy
*   Correspondence: loredana.mauro@unical.it (L.M.); sebastiano.ando@unical.it (S.A.);
   Tel.: +39-0984-492928 (L.M.); +39-0984-496201 (S.A.)
†   These authors contribute equally to this work.
‡   Joint senior authors.

Received: 4 April 2019; Accepted: 28 April 2019; Published: 30 April 2019

Abstract: Obesity, characterized by excess body weight, is now accepted as a hazardous health condition and an oncogenic factor. In different epidemiological studies obesity has been described as a risk factor in several malignancies. Some biological mechanisms that orchestrate obesity–cancer interaction have been discovered, although others are still not completely understood. The unbalanced secretion of biomolecules, called "adipokines", released by adipocytes strongly influences obesity-related cancer development. Among these adipokines, adiponectin exerts a critical role. Physiologically adiponectin governs glucose levels and lipid metabolism and is fundamental in the reproductive system. Low adiponectin circulating levels have been found in obese patients, in which its protective effects were lost. In this review, we summarize the epidemiological, in vivo and in vitro data in order to highlight how adiponectin may affect obesity-associated female cancers.

Keywords: obesity; adipokines; adiponectin; breast cancer; ovarian cancer; endometrial cancer; cervix cancer; estrogen receptor

1. Introduction

Worldwide, obesity is spreading and is reaching epidemic proportion, thus becoming a critical public health issue. Today, the World Health Organization (WHO) reported that people with a body mass index (BMI) greater than 30 kg/m^2 (30.0–34.9, grade I; 35.0–39.9, grade II; and ≥40, grade III) includes almost 1.9 billion adults and this number is rising fast [1]. This pandemic condition is associated with various metabolic disorders, cardiovascular diseases, type 2 diabetes and several cancers [2–5]. Meta-analyses and several epidemiological studies defined the fitted connection between cancer development and obesity [6–11]. In 2011, it has been described that in the United States 85,000 persons per year affected by obesity experienced cancer [10]. Obesity could be considered a risk factor for cervical, ovarian, endometrial and breast cancer, and it has been reported to be responsible for 88% mortality rates in females [7,12]. Insulin resistance and altered insulin-like growth factor-1 (IGF-1) pathway activation, changes in bioavailability of sex hormones and a chronic inflammatory state related to obesity conditions have been recognized to induce cancer development and progression [12–14]. Furthermore, obesity alters the secretion of several molecules released by adipocytes, known as adipokines. Among adipose tissue-derived factors, it has been well documented that adiponectin exerts a critical role in the pathogenesis of obesity-associated disorders. It has been reported that adiponectin circulating levels are dramatically decreased in obese patients [15,16] (Figure 1). Indeed, adiponectin expression and secretion is negatively correlated to the BMI, even though the mechanisms responsible for this down-regulation are not yet completely elucidated [17–19]. Low circulating levels of adiponectin in overweight women may be related to the blunted chronic inflammatory status in obesity. The enhanced production of tumor necrosis factor α (TNFα) and Interleukin-6 (IL-6), concomitant with the hypoxic status in adipose tissue, represent a possible mechanism involved in the adiponectin down-regulation in obese subjects [20,21]. Many epidemiologic studies established a correlation between hypoadiponectinemia and an enhanced risk of obesity-related disorders [15,22–26].

Nevertheless, there are still hidden molecular mechanisms involved in this relationship that need to be explored. In this review, we will discuss the association of this adipokine with obesity and different female cancers, in which low adiponectin levels confer altered risk and influence progression in affected women.

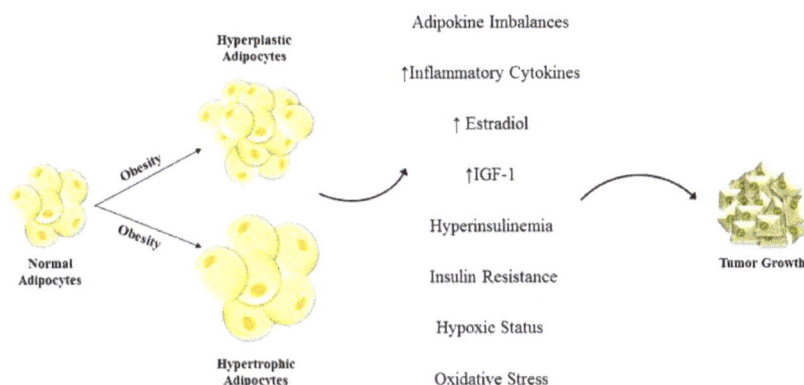

Figure 1. Unraveled mechanisms linking obesity and cancers. Hyperplastic and hypertrophic adipocytes are one of the main features of obesity. This dis-regulation of fat cells leads to change in adipokine and inflammatory cytokine secretion, enhanced insulin-like growth factor-1 (IGF-1) and estradiol production, and to hyperinsulinemia, insulin resistance, hypoxic status and oxidative stress. These alterations in the tumor microenvironment deeply impact the phenotype of the surrounding cells inducing severe modifications in cell behavior that contribute to tumor development and progression.

2. Adiponectin Structure and Biology

Adiponectin is the most abundant adipokine detected in circulating plasma, wherein its concentration ranges from 3 to 30 μg/mL [22,27,28]. Adiponectin is mainly produced and secreted by white adipose tissue and in lower amounts by other tissues such as brown adipose tissue, placenta, fetal tissue, colon, skeletal muscle, salivary glands, and liver [27–36]. Structurally, adiponectin is a 244 amino acid-long polypeptide with four domains: An N-terminal region, a variable sequence, a collagen-like motif, and a C-terminal globular domain [22,30,37,38]. Adiponectin belongs to the C1q-like protein family, sharing a high sequence homology with the complement factor C1q in the C-terminus domain, which mediates the interaction with its specific receptors [39,40]. Adiponectin is synthetized as a 30 kDa full-length monomer (fAd), detected only in the adipocytes cytoplasm, that assembles into different oligomeric complexes before secretion [22,41]. The basic form of adiponectin complexes is a trimer (low molecular weight, LMW), which in turn can oligomerize, through disulphide bonds formation, into hexamers (middle molecular weight, MMW) and multimers (high molecular weight, HMW), consisting of 12–18 monomers [42–45]. In human plasma, adiponectin exists also as a proteolytic cleavage fragment (globular adiponectin, gAd), produced by leukocyte elastase activity, corresponding to the globular domain of the full-length protein [46,47]. Particularly, globular adiponectin has been found in serum only as a trimer, with increased potency compared to other isoforms [48,49]. Circulating adiponectin levels are regulated by different physiological, environmental, and pharmacological factors such as hormonal production, inflammatory processes, genetic polymorphisms, nutritional status, and drug administration [21]. Typically, in women adiponectin levels are significantly higher than in men, with peaks of secretion in the morning and reduced production during the night [50,51]. Some reports have widely demonstrated that the different estrogens/androgens production may influence adiponectin expression [50,51]. Particularly, in vitro and in vivo evidences showed that testosterone decreased adiponectin secretion [27,50]. Plasma adiponectin levels are also closely correlated to the circulating concentrations of other hormones. Interestingly, it has been reported as having an inverse association with adiponectin levels and fasting plasma insulin [25]. Furthermore, growth hormone (GH), glucocorticoids, prolactin down-regulated adiponectin gene expression [52]. In addition, different studies addressed pro-inflammatory cytokines released from adipose tissue, such as tumor necrosis factor α (TNFα) and IL-6, as inhibitors of adiponectin synthesis [20]. Pharmacological therapies with anti-diabetic drugs, including peroxisome proliferator-activated receptor gamma (PPAR-γ) agonists belonging to the thiazolidinedione's class and metformin, can also modulate serum adiponectin concentrations, enhancing its expression and secretion [53–57]. Moreover, meta-analysis of association-studies correlated different single nucleotide polymorphisms (SNPs) in the gene encoding adiponectin, *ADIPOQ*, with reduced levels of this adipokine [58,59]. Many evidences suggested that the several active circulating forms of adiponectin exert different biological functions in specific tissues [16,38,41,60–62]. Adiponectin biological effects are mediated by membrane receptors. To date three different receptor subtypes have been cloned: Two classical adiponectin receptors, adiponectin receptor 1 (AdipoR1), adiponectin receptor (AdipoR2), and a non-classical third receptor, T-cadherin [28,38]. Structurally, AdipoR1 and AdipoR2 consist of seven transmembrane domains, with an opposite orientation of the C-terminus and N-terminus compared to the G-protein coupled receptors [63]. Both receptor subtypes are expressed ubiquitously, even though the levels of one always prevail over the other. AdipoR1 is abundant in endothelial cells and skeletal muscle, with AdipoR2 being more expressed in hepatocytes, and both mediate different adiponectin effects [48]. Despite a very high sequence homology of about 67%, the two classical receptor subtypes exhibit a different affinity for the several adiponectin circulating isoforms [28]. Specifically, it is well recognized that AdipoR1 displays a higher affinity for the gAd and lower affinity for the full-length molecule, while the HMW (fAd) adiponectin binds mainly AdipoR2 [64]. Contrariwise to AdipoR1 and AdipoR2, T-cadherin is a cell-surface receptor lacking a transmembrane domain. T-cadherin is predominantly expressed in endothelial cells, smooth muscle cells and in cardiomyocytes and displays affinity for the MMW and HMW but not for trimeric and globular forms of adiponectin [65–67]. The role of this receptor in adiponectin action has not yet been fully clarified, even though its involvement in cell adhesion and calcium-mediated signaling has been demonstrated. The lack of the intracellular domain suggested that T-cadherin acts as a co-receptor, probably competing with AdipoR1 and AdipoR2 for adiponectin binding [68]. Moreover, T-cadherin has been detected in tumor-associated endothelial cells, proposing a possible role of this receptor in tumor angiogenesis. Particularly in a mouse transgenic mammary cancer model, T-cadherin has been highlighted as a crucial factor in the cross-talk between tumor cells and the stromal compartment [69]. It is well documented that adiponectin exerts a plethora of biological effects in different target tissues, including anti-atherogenic, cardioprotective, anti-inflammatory, insulin-sensitizing, and anti-neoplastic actions. Furthermore, adiponectin regulates energy homeostasis through a direct effect on lipid metabolism and hepatic glucose output, and increasing insulin sensitivity [70]. Recent studies also highlighted that adiponectin plays a pivotal role in cell proliferation, angiogenesis, and tissue remodeling [71].

3. Adiponectin-Mediated Signaling Pathways

The various physiological effects of adiponectin depend on the several circulating isoforms of this adipokine. Nevertheless, adiponectin exerts its effects mainly by employing the Liver Kinase B 1/AMP-activated protein Kinase (LKB1/AMPK) pathway, in particular in the management of insulin in the body. Adiponectin controls glucose levels governing pancreatic β-cell proliferation and augmenting fatty acid oxidation. Moreover, adiponectin, promoting APPL-1/AMPK interaction, increased glucose uptake through glucose transporter 4 (GLUT4) [62,72,73]. It has been largely documented that insulin resistance is one of the hallmark of obese patients and low adiponectin serum levels partially contribute to this pathological state [74]. AMPK inhibits crucial signaling pathways involved in cell cycle initiation, cell growth and survival such as extracellular signal-regulated kinases 1/2 (ERK1/2), phosphatidylinositol 3-kinases (PI3K)/Protein Kinase B (Akt), c-Jun N-terminal kinase (cJNK) and signal transducer and activator of transcription 3 (STAT3) [75–77]. The AMPK pathway is also crucial for cell growth through the regulation of Akt/mTOR/S6K signaling. Particularly, AMPK is an upstream of tuberous sclerosis complex 2 (TSC2), a potent inhibitor of mTOR signaling. The decreased phosphorylation of AMPK results in stimulation of cell proliferation [64,78]. This adipokine also directly modulates the expression of different proteins involved in cell cycle and apoptosis (i.e., up-regulation of p53 and Bax, down-regulation of c-myc, cyclin D1 and Bcl-2) [79]. Adiponectin is also considered an anti-inflammatory cytokine for its ability to suppress the phosphorylation of nuclear factor k B (NF-kB), a transcription factor involved in several processes that regulates the activity of various pro-inflammatory mediators [80]. Furthermore, adiponectin shows anti-migratory effects through an inhibition of Wnt/β-catenin signaling pathway, fundamental for cancer progression [81].

4. Adiponectin and Female Cancers

Among the different identified adipokines, adiponectin has been largely studied for its role in influencing cancer development and progression [82,83]. Particularly, several studies reported a correlation between low levels of adiponectin in obese women and an increased risk of development and progression of several female tumors, such as cervical, ovarian, endometrial, and breast cancers. All epidemiological, in vivo and in vitro studies have been reported for each tumor.

5. Adiponectin in Female Cancers

5.1. Cervical Cancer and Adiponectin

Cervical cancer is the fourth most common cancer in women both for incidence and mortality. According to WHO in 2018, 569,847 new cases are diagnosed worldwide, and 311,365 deaths [84]. The major risk factor for cervical cancer is infection with the human papillomavirus (HPV), particularly HPV16 or HPV18 [85], even though other factors may also play a role [86]. Recently obesity has been reported to increase the risk of development and progression of cervical cancer [87]. Some studies evidenced a positive association between obesity and increased risk of cervical adenocarcinoma but not squamous cell carcinoma. The increased estrogens production, due to the greater aromatase activity in adipose tissue (particularly in post-menopausal women), may explain the higher incidence of the cervical adenocarcinoma, which represents the more hormonally responsive cervical cancer type [88–91]. Although some evidences suggest that low circulating adiponectin levels related to obesity conditions may be linked to cervical malignancy, nevertheless few studies describe the molecular mechanisms though which adiponectin influences cervical cancer growth [7,92]. Noteworthy in HeLa cells, AdipoR2 mRNA expression was higher than AdipoR1, which was significantly increased in adiponectin-treated cells (10μg/mL) [93]. Xie et al. reported that low adiponectin levels inhibited the proliferation of HeLa cells, as evidenced by a significant increase in the cell population in G0/G1 phase, concomitant with a reduction of cell number in S and G2/M phases. Moreover, a down-regulation of cell cycle regulators has been reported, such as cyclin D1 and c-myc, and an activation of apoptosis, mediated by the enhanced expression of p21, p53 and Bax and the reduced level of Bcl-2 [93] (Figure 2).

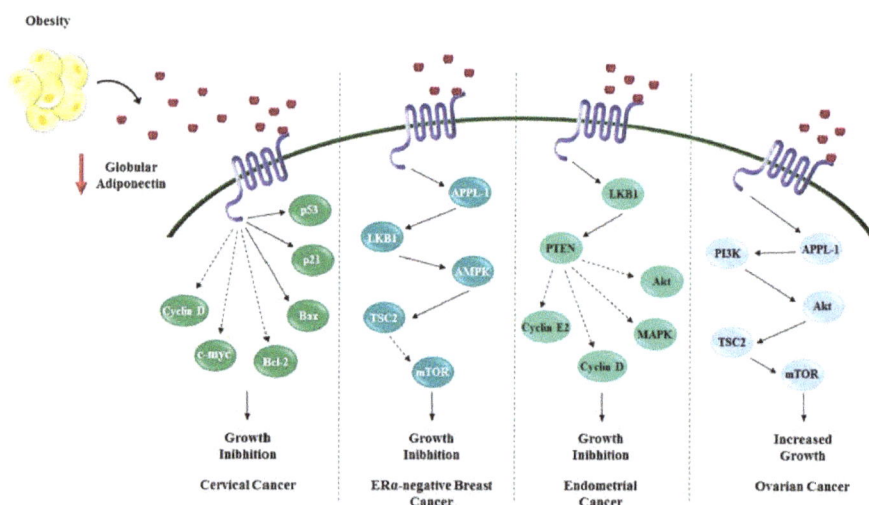

Figure 2. Role of adiponectin in influencing female cancers. Adiponectin, the most abundant secreted adipokine, heavily impacts the proliferation of cancer cells through several mechanisms that seem to be tumor-specific. Mainly adiponectin exerts its effects regulating cell cycle and apoptosis. The red ↓ indicates a reduction of globular adiponectin concentration. Dotted arrows show inhibition of downstream protein activation. Solid arrows mark activation of downstream proteins.

5.2. Ovarian Cancer and Adiponectin

Ovarian cancer affects 1.6% of whole female population, according to GLOBOCAN published data in 2018 [84]. Despite a lower variability of the incidence rates compared to other gynecological malignancies, ovarian cancer remains a fatal disease, with an estimated 184,799 annual deaths [84]. Since it is asymptomatic and has not yet had specific biomarkers identified for early detection, diagnosis of most ovarian cancer cases occurs at advanced stages [84,94]. The ovary is composed of three major cell types, namely, epithelial, stromal, and germ cells, which may undergo neoplastic transformation, generating the main forms of ovarian cancer. Particularly, 80–90% of ovarian tumors originate from epithelial cells on the surface of the ovary, while stromal and germ cell cancer account only for 7 and 5% of ovarian malignancies, respectively [95]. Recently, the relationship between obesity and ovarian tumor development has become increasingly evident, particularly in post-menopausal women. Many epidemiological studies addressed obesity as an important risk factor for ovarian cancer even though the mechanisms involved in the tumorigenesis have not been fully clarified [96–100]. Aberrant production of hormonal factors, adipokines and cytokines, and adipose related inflammatory reactions associated with obesity may affect ovarian cancer development [101–105]. Interestingly, several studies linked low plasma levels of adiponectin with ovarian tumorigenesis [105–107]. A Kaplan–Meier survival analysis provided evidences that, in a large cohort of women affected by ovarian cancer, high leptin/adiponectin ratio correlated with a poor outcome [108]. AdipoR1 is an emerging prognostic factor for this malignancy, since many reports evidenced its down-regulation, particularly in the epithelial ovarian cancer cells [109,110]. Indeed, AdipoR1 and AdipoR2 expression is generally lower in epithelial ovarian cancer cells, such as COV434, OVCAR-3 and SKOV-3 cells, compared to granulosa tumor cells, making prognosis worse for this tumor type [109]. Abnormal activation of PI3K/Akt/mTOR cascade is well documented in ovarian cancers, and it is associated with a more aggressive phenotype [71,111]. Low adiponectin levels may favor the aberrant ovarian cancer growth, induced by the persistent activation of PI3K/Akt/mTOR signaling. Thus, it is reasonable to speculate that the increase of adiponectin levels may support the conventional ovarian cancer therapies [71,111] (Figure 2). In vitro experiments demonstrated that adiponectin inhibited growth and reversed E$_2$- and IGF-1-induced cells proliferation in epithelial ovarian carcinoma. In addition, it has been demonstrated that 25 µg/mL adiponectin reduced estrogen receptor alpha (ERα), insulin growth factor 1 receptor (IGF1R), progesterone receptor (PR) mRNA, and protein expression, suggesting the functional interaction between such receptors and adiponectin signaling in epithelial ovarian cancer cells [109].

5.3. Endometrial Cancer

Endometrial cancer is the sixth most common cancer in women, with 382,069 new cases and approximately 89,929 deaths estimated worldwide in 2018 [84]. Unlike most female tumors, endometrial cancer shows a higher incidence in premenopausal women, generally nulliparous, than postmenopausal women [71]. Most of the cases are diagnosed at an early stage and surgery alone can be already effective. Nevertheless, some patients experienced disease recurrence despite adjuvant therapy [112]. Obesity is a well-recognized risk factor for endometrial carcinoma [113]. Indeed, all several bioactive molecules produced by adipose tissue, as sex steroids, insulin, insulin-like growth factors (IGFs) and the activation of their signaling sustain endometrial cancer [114,115]. Mainly, several groups investigated the correlation between adiponectin and endometrial cancer. Petridou's group conducted the first reported case-control study in 84 women with diagnosed and histologically confirmed endometrial cancer. They suggested that in younger women (<65 years) adiponectin serum levels were inversely correlated with endometrial cancer. Moreover, they evidenced that low adiponectin concentrations correlated with high level of estrogens, insulin and IGF, molecules that sustain endometrial tumorigenesis [24]. Another study further supported these results, recognizing adiponectin as a predictive marker for endometrial cancer independently associated with obesity [116]. Also in endometrial cancer, the leptin/adiponectin ratio is recognized as a more appropriate risk marker. In fact, as described in Ashizawa's work, higher leptin/adiponectin ratio were significantly linked with an increased probability of developing endometrial cancer. They found that the Odds Ratio (ORs) of the leptin/adiponectin ratios were higher than those of the two adipokines alone [117]. Three more recent meta-analyses have reported that adiponectin levels and leptin/adiponectin ratio are considered as predictive and prognostic biomarkers in order to guarantee early diagnosis and disease monitoring of endometrial cancer, especially in postmenopausal women [118–121].

Moon et al. found AdipoR1 and AdipoR2 expression in all stages of endometrial cancer as well as in non-neoplastic tissue, mainly detected in epithelial cells compared to stromal cells [122]. Moreover, both receptors have been also identified in three different established endometrial cancer cell lines, HEC-1-A, RL95-2, and KLE [122,123]. These studies reported anti-proliferative effects of adiponectin in all cell lines. At all pharmacological doses tested (ranging from 10 µg/mL to 50 µg/mL) adiponectin decreased cell growth and proliferation in a dose dependent manner (from ~20% to ~45% of reduction from low to high dose used). Cong and Moon's groups showed that the adiponectin effects were mediated by both AdipoR1 and AdipoR2 through the activation of its canonical signaling pathway, LKB1/AMPK. Particularly, adiponectin treatment reduced ERK1/2 phosphorylation in RL95-2 cells, while it abrogated AKT phosphorylation in KLE and HEC-1-A cells depending on PTEN expression and activity. The anti-proliferative effects of adiponectin were also related to significant increase at G1/G0-phase and to a simultaneous diminution of S-phase of the treated cells [122,123]. Furthermore, adiponectin inhibited the expression of two important positive regulators of cell cycle, Cyclin D1, in KLE and HEC-1A cells, and Cyclin E2, in the RL95-2 cell line [122,123] (Figure 2). In addition, Cong et al. using an Annexin-V-FITC assay evidenced that adiponectin increased the percentage of apoptotic cells [123]. Although an important role of adiponectin in blocking endometrial cancer cell growth has been defined, and this adipokine has been suggested as a potential useful agent in the management of this neoplasia, more studies are still needed to better clarify its action.

5.4. Breast Cancer

Worldwide, breast cancer is the most common malignancy diagnosed among women (2.1 million newly cases in 2018) and it still remains one of the major causes of death for cancer in over 100 countries [84]. Several epidemiological studies reported that obesity is related with breast cancer development, progression, and poor survival [124–126]. Particularly it has been described that carcinoma of the breast is a complex disease in which epithelial cell-tumor microenvironment interactions play a pivotal role [127]. In this context, adipokines secreted from adipose tissue have been recognized to influence breast tumorigenesis. Among them, adiponectin is a crucial mediator in obesity-related breast cancer, since its level dramatically decreased in this pathological condition [128]. In 2003, it was reported that low serum levels of adiponectin correlates with increased breast cancer risk and contributes to a more aggressive tumor phenotype [129]. Later, several epidemiological studies and meta-analyses confirmed these findings, primarily in postmenopausal women [23,129–132]. Moreover, adiponectin levels significantly decrease with the progression of the disease while its circulating levels were not related to stage I and II of breast cancer [133]. Nevertheless, though the role of adiponectin has been well elucidated in the other female malignancies, the contribution of this adipokine in breast cancer development and progression is still controversial and under investigation. Most of the studies recognized adiponectin as a negative regulator of cancer growth in ERα-negative breast cancers; while adiponectin at relatively low concentrations might sustain tumor development and progression in ERα-positive breast cancers [81,134–142]. Notably, in Lam's work it has been described that adiponectin haplodeficient tumors showed similar features to basal-like subtype tumors in terms of high proliferative activity and poor prognosis. Using MMTV–PyVT mice, they demonstrated that a decreased production of adiponectin in the tumor microenvironment contributes to induce genomic and phenotypic changes in mammary epithelial cells, in particular impacting PI3K/Akt/GSK-β-catenin signaling, a fundamental pathway that supports tumor development and progression [143]. Low serum–adiponectin levels negatively affect PTEN activation, contributing to a de-regulated PI3K/Akt/GSK-β-catenin signaling activation, confirmed in xenograft models. MDA-MB-231 cells treated with adiponectin, through a diminished Akt and GSK3-β phosphorylation, showed a reduction in breast tumorigenesis [81]. Moreover, it has been described that adiponectin interferes with Akt activation not only affecting PTEN but also through AMPK signaling. In another murine mammary tumor model it has been shown that adiponectin increased AMPK/PP2A activation that leads to dephosphorylation of Akt negatively regulating in vivo tumorgenicity [144]. Recent findings from Mauro et al. also correlate with these data; indeed, they found that in MDA-MB-231 xenograft models the pre-treatment with adiponectin (1, 5 and 30 μg/mL) reduced tumor growth at all doses tested amplifying AMPK signaling and reducing cyclin D1 expression [139,141]. Most of these results have been also described in vitro in ERα-negative breast cancer cells where adiponectin mainly serves to induce cell growth arrest and apoptosis regulating several proteins that govern cell cycle (i.e., p53, Bax, Bcl-2, c-myc and cyclin D1) [81,134,135,137,140,144–146] (Figure 2). Even though a large amount of authors also confirmed this pro-apoptotic role of adiponectin in ERα-positive breast cancer cells, others discovered that this adipokine might sustain tumor growth in this cell subtype. It has been reported that adiponectin fuels cell survival, migration, and differentiation of endothelial cells, and affects inflammatory cell behavior acting as a pro-angiogenic factor that contributes to breast tumor growth and progression [16,147,148]. Moreover, Mauro et al. reported that adiponectin (1 and 5 μg/mL) in MCF-7 xenografts mainly increased tumor volume concomitantly with an elevated expression of cyclin D1, high level of MAPK phosphorylation and a reduced AMPK activation [141]. Pfeleir et al. found that the combination of adiponectin and 17-β estradiol increased MCF-7 cell growth [142]. Recently, Mauro et al. in other studies fully elucidated the cross-talk between adiponectin and ERα. Firstly, they demonstrated that the multiprotein complex including AdipoR1/APPL1/c-Src/ERα/IGF-IR led to MAPK activation, in addition to adiponectin induced cyclin D1 expression at transcriptional level [140,141]. Recently they argued that this adipokine has to be considered a growth factor in

ERα-positive breast cancer cells since adiponectin might impair LKB1/AMPK interaction, inducing a rapid activation of ERα and MAPK [139–141] (Figure 3).

Noteworthy, it has been evidenced that adiponectin may differently modulate ERα-negative and ERα-positive breast cancer cell metabolism, an established hallmark of cancer. Cancer cells adopt "Warburg" like metabolism (i.e., anaerobic glycolysis) sustained by key regulators such as fatty acid synthase (FASN) and ACC [149,150]. LKB1/AMPK is also crucial pathway in regulating energy homeostasis, such as glucose uptake, glycolysis, fatty acid oxidation and mitochondrial biogenesis [149,151,152]. In ERα-negative breast cancer cells, adiponectin, activating AMPK/ACC, inhibits fatty acid synthesis, while in ERα-positive breast cancer cells it isn't able to modify this process [139,141].

Adiponectin has been also found in the exosome, as small lipid bilayer membrane vesicles secreted by adipocytes [153], that have been recognized as important mediators of cell-to-cell communication in the complex tumor microenvironment. By transferring proteins, mRNAs, microRNAs, DNAs, lipids and transcriptional factors may induce deep changes in recipient cell's behavior [154]. Particularly, exosomes from human adipose-derived mesenchymal stem cells (ADSCs) induce proliferation and migration in breast cancer [155] and exosomes secreted by preadipocytes also regulate breast tumor stem cell formation and migration [156]. It has been reported that adiponectin enhances exosome biogenesis and release, and although exosome cargoes adiponectin [153,157,158], more studies are still warranted to fully explain the role of this adipokine in circulating exosomes in breast cancer.

All these evidences attempt to clarify the role of adiponectin as a mediator of breast tumorigenesis, but how adiponectin may orchestrate breast cancer is still a controversial issue that needs to be solved.

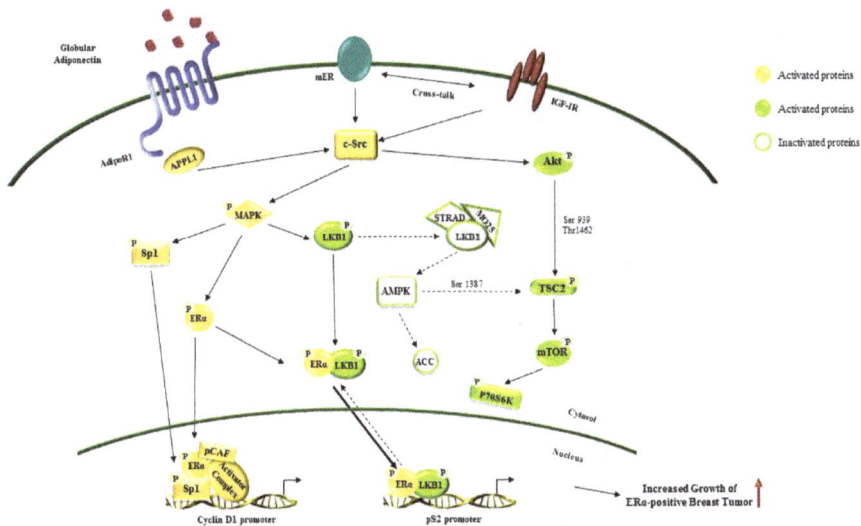

Figure 3. Effects of adiponectin in estrogen receptor alpha (ERα)-positive breast cancer growth. Globular adiponectin binds its receptor AdipoR1 on breast cancer cell surface. Adiponectin/AdipoR1 cross-talk with ERα and insulin growth factor 1 receptor (IGF1R) activating several downstream pathways involved in sustaining breast cancer cell growth and progression. The red ↑ Indicates increased growth of ERα-positive breast cancer. Dotted arrows show signaling inhibition. Solid arrows marks signaling activation. The arrows from cytosol to nucleus and vice versa indicate protein translocation. Solid arrows show a greater localization of the proteins in the nucleus. Dotted arrows mark a cytosolic localization.

6. Potential Therapeutic of Adiponectin

A balanced and healthy diet may control all the factors that have been described to sustain obesity-related disease (i.e., IGF-1, insulin, leptin) [159]. Thus, a healthy lifestyle and personal behavior should be considered as the most important prevention in this pathological condition. Indeed, the reduction of calories in diet, physical exercise and moderating consumption alcohol prevents obesity and cancer development [128]. It has been reported that vigorous aerobic exercise leads to a peak of adiponectin circulating level [160,161]. Furthermore, understanding all molecular mechanisms through which adiponectin influences tumorigenesis might provide new potential therapeutic targets. In this concern, pharmacological increase of serum adiponectin levels, up-regulation of adiponectin receptors expression, or synthesis of adiponectin receptor agonists may also be considered a promising therapeutic approach. Due to the higher frequency of breast cancer among female malignancies, most of the therapeutic strategies, aimed to ameliorate adiponectin's response, have been proposed in breast tumor models. Interestingly, Otvos et al. developed a new adiponectin-based short peptide (H-DAsn-Ile-Pro-Nva-Leu-Tyr-DSer-Phe-Ala-DSer-NH2) named ADP 355, which could be suitable for treatment in cancer. ADP 355 showed high affinity with AdipoR1, and through the regulation of the canonical adiponectin-regulated pathways (i.e., AMPK, Akt, STAT3, and ERK1/2), reduced breast tumor growth both in in vitro and in vivo studies [162,163]. Even though, ADP 355 showed promising efficacy in several malignancies, it is particularly important to design a therapeutic strategy that also impacts leptin signaling in order to functionally and physiologically re-equilibrate the adiponectin/leptin ratio [162]. AdipoRon is an oral AdipoR1/R2 agonist that successfully reestablished adiponectin functions, mainly activating AMPK and PPAR-α pathways, in obesity-related type 2 diabetes [164]. BHD1028, BHD43, and BHD44 are three other peptides designed to fully mimic adiponectin actions. In particular, Kim et al. found that BHD1028 was the peptide that showed the highest affinity with AdipoR1 and the main activation of AMPK already at low-level concentration, more than ADP 355. In addition, the PEGylation of BHD1028 improved its stability and solubility indicating this peptide as a promising candidate for anti-diabetes and metabolic disorders [165]. PPARγ agonists, such as thiazolidinediones, rosiglitazone and pioglitazone also augment the circulating level of adiponectin through directly enhancing adiponectin gene and protein expression in a dose-dependent manner [53,166,167]. Nevertheless, the use of these drugs is still limited for their potential side effects. Another pharmacological agent that presents a tangible benefit in breast cancer treatment is the anti-diabetic drug metformin. It can prevent breast cancer cell growth through the stimulation of AMPK, inhibition of mTOR signaling, and reduction of the HER2 protein [168]. In addition, metformin reduced estrogen circulating levels via AMPK signaling, blocking aromatase promoter activity [169]. Thus, metformin appears to partially mimic adiponectin signal in the treatment of obesity-related breast cancer [56,57].

Recent findings demonstrated that adiponectin differently regulated the LKB1/AMPK/mTOR signaling in breast cancer cells. In ERα-negative cells, adiponectin phosphorylated AMPK and blocked mTOR activation, thus inhibiting breast tumor growth [139]. On the other hand, in MCF-7 cells adiponectin induced MAPK phosphorylation, which in turn transactivated ERα and activated mTOR, promoting breast tumor growth [139]. On the basis of these evidences, in a breast cancer setting it is becoming important to discriminate ERα-positive and ERα-negative tumors to specifically assess the best therapeutic approaches designed to impact adiponectin functions [64].

7. Conclusions

Obesity is a serious health condition and a well-recognized risk factor for many diseases, such as type 2 diabetes, cardiovascular diseases, hypertension, and cancer [6,7]. Obese female breast cancer patients are more likely to have a worse prognosis [170] and recent meta-analyses also estimated an approximately 30% increased risk of disease recurrence or death in obese versus normal weight women [171,172]. Several hypotheses have been proposed to unravel the direct link between obesity and cancer including hyperinsulinemia, estrogen signalling, inflammation and adipokine expression [173,174]. Indeed, bioactive molecules secreted from adipose tissue raised a wide spark interest in this field and among them adiponectin seems to play a potential role in influencing tumor development and progression. The effects of adiponectin, the most abundant secreted adipokine, have been largely studied in obesity-associated female-specific tumors. Although in cervical, ovarian, and endometrial cancers adiponectin exerts anti-proliferative actions, in breast cancer a new and contradictory function of this adipokine is emerging. Thus, therapeutic strategies aiming to regulate adiponectin concentrations and AdipoR1/2 activation are considered an encouraging tool in the management of obesity-related cancer, such as cervical, ovarian, endometrial, while a lot of controversial issues still remain in adiponectin treatment of breast cancer.

Author Contributions: L.G., G.D.N prepared the manuscript, collected data, wrote, edited, and prepared figures. S.C., L.M., S.A., prepared, revised, and provided critical consideration for the manuscript, design, and editing. All authors reviewed and approved the final version of the manuscript.

Funding: This work was supported by the Associazione Italiana Ricerca sul Cancro (AIRC; IG-18602 and IG-21414) and the Progetti di Ricerca di Interesse Nazionale-Ministero Istruzione Università e Ricerca (Grant 2015B7M39T_001).

Conflicts of Interest: The authors declare no conflict of interest.

Abbreviations

WHO	World Health Organization
BMI	Body Mass Index
IGF-1	Insulin-like Growth Factor-1
fAd	full-length Adiponectin
LMW	Low Molecular Weight
MMW	Middle Molecular Weight
HMW	High Molecular Weight
gAd	globular Adiponectin
TNFα	Tumor Necrosis Factor α
PPAR-γ	Peroxisome Proliferator-Activated Receptor gamma
AdipoR1	Adiponectin receptor 1
AdipoR2	Adiponectin receptor2
LKB1	Liver Kinase B 1
AMPK	AMP-activated protein Kinase
Akt	Protein Kinase B
mTOR	mammalian Target of Rapamycin
S6K	ribosomal protein S6 Kinase
TSC2	Tuberous Sclerosis Complex 2
ERK1/2	Extracellular signal-Regulated Kinases
PI3K	Phosphatidylinositol 3-Kinases
cJNK	c-Jun N-terminal kinase
STAT3	Signal Transducer and Activator of Transcription
NF-kB	Nuclear Factor k B
E2	Estradiol
ERα	Estrogen Receptor alpha
IGF1R	Insulin Growth Factor 1 Receptor
PR	Progesterone Receptor
TGF-β1	Transforming growth factor beta 1
SMAD2	Small Mother Against Decapentaplegic 2

References

1. Risk, N. Factor Collaboration (NCD-RisC). Trends in adult body-mass index in 200 countries from 1975 to 2014: A pooled analysis of 1698 population-based measurement studies with 19.2 million participants. *Lancet* **2016**, *387*, 1377–1396.

2. Hubert, H.B.; Feinleib, M.; McNamara, P.M.; Castelli, W.P. Obesity as an independent risk factor for cardiovascular disease: A 26-year follow-up of participants in the Framingham Heart Study. *Circulation* **1983**, *67*, 968–977. [CrossRef]

3. Mokdad, A.H.; Ford, E.S.; Bowman, B.A.; Dietz, W.H.; Vinicor, F.; Bales, V.S.; Marks, J.S. Prevalence of obesity, diabetes, and obesity-related health risk factors, 2001. *JAMA* **2003**, *289*, 76–79. [CrossRef]

4. Ogden, C.L.; Carroll, M.D.; Curtin, L.R.; McDowell, M.A.; Tabak, C.J.; Flegal, K.M. Prevalence of overweight and obesity in the United States, 1999-2004. *JAMA* **2006**, *295*, 1549–1555. [CrossRef]

5. Renehan, A.G.; Roberts, D.L.; Dive, C. Obesity and cancer: Pathophysiological and biological mechanisms. *Arch. Physiol. Biochem.* **2008**, *114*, 71–83. [CrossRef] [PubMed]

6. Renehan, A.G.; Tyson, M.; Egger, M.; Heller, R.F.; Zwahlen, M. Body-mass index and incidence of cancer: A systematic review and meta-analysis of prospective observational studies. *Lancet* **2008**, *371*, 569–578. [CrossRef]

7. Calle, E.E.; Rodriguez, C.; Walker-Thurmond, K.; Thun, M.J. Overweight, obesity, and mortality from cancer in a prospectively studied cohort of US adults. *Engl. J. Med.* **2003**, *348*, 1625–1638. [CrossRef]

8. Larsson, S.C.; Wolk, A. Obesity and colon and rectal cancer risk: A meta-analysis of prospective studies. *Am. J. Clin. Nutr.* **2007**, *86*, 556–565. [CrossRef]

9. Hsing, A.W.; Sakoda, L.C.; Chua, S.C., Jr. Obesity, metabolic syndrome, and prostate cancer. *Am. J. Clin. Nutr.* **2007**, *86*, 843S–857S. [CrossRef]

10. Basen-Engquist, K.; Chang, M. Obesity and cancer risk: Recent review and evidence. *Curr. Oncol. Rep.* **2011**, *13*, 71–76. [CrossRef]

11. Goodwin, P.J.; Stambolic, V. Impact of the obesity epidemic on cancer. *Annu. Rev. Med.* **2015**, *66*, 281–296. [CrossRef] [PubMed]

12. Park, J.; Morley, T.S.; Kim, M.; Clegg, D.J.; Scherer, P.E. Obesity and cancer—Mechanisms underlying tumour progression and recurrence. *Nat. Rev. Endocrinol.* **2014**, *10*, 455. [CrossRef] [PubMed]

13. Van Kruijsdijk, R.C.; Van Der Wall, E.; Visseren, F.L. Obesity and cancer: The role of dysfunctional adipose tissue. *Cancer Epidemiol. Prev. Biomark.* **2009**, *18*, 2569–2578. [CrossRef] [PubMed]

14. Gallagher, E.J.; LeRoith, D.; Karnieli, E. The metabolic syndrome—From insulin resistance to obesity and diabetes. *Endocrinol. Metab. Clin. North Am.* **2008**, *37*, 559–579. [CrossRef] [PubMed]

15. Weyer, C.; Funahashi, T.; Tanaka, S.; Hotta, K.; Matsuzawa, Y.; Pratley, R.E.; Tataranni, P.A. Hypoadiponectinemia in obesity and type 2 diabetes: Close association with insulin resistance and hyperinsulinemia. *J. Clin. Endocrinol. Metab.* **2001**, *86*, 1930–1935. [CrossRef]

16. Ouchi, N.; Kobayashi, H.; Kihara, S.; Kumada, M.; Sato, K.; Inoue, T.; Funahashi, T.; Walsh, K. Adiponectin stimulates angiogenesis by promoting cross-talk between AMP-activated protein kinase and Akt signaling in endothelial cells. *J. Biol. Chem.* **2004**, *279*, 1304–1309. [CrossRef]

17. Arita, Y.; Kihara, S.; Ouchi, N.; Takahashi, M.; Maeda, K.; Miyagawa, J.-i.; Hotta, K.; Shimomura, I.; Nakamura, T.; Miyaoka, K. Paradoxical decrease of an adipose-specific protein, adiponectin, in obesity. *Biochem. Biophys. Res. Commun.* **1999**, *257*, 79–83. [CrossRef]

18. Hu, E.; Liang, P.; Spiegelman, B.M. AdipoQ is a novel adipose-specific gene dysregulated in obesity. *J. Biol. Chem.* **1996**, *271*, 10697–10703. [CrossRef]

19. Barb, D.; Williams, C.J.; Neuwirth, A.K.; Mantzoros, C.S. Adiponectin in relation to malignancies: A review of existing basic research and clinical evidence. *Am. J. Clin. Nutr.* **2007**, *86*, 858S–866S. [CrossRef]

20. Tilg, H.; Moschen, A.R. Adipocytokines: Mediators linking adipose tissue, inflammation and immunity. *Nat. Rev. Immunol.* **2006**, *6*, 772. [CrossRef]

21. Dalamaga, M.; Diakopoulos, K.N.; Mantzoros, C.S. The role of adiponectin in cancer: A review of current evidence. *Endocr. Rev.* **2012**, *33*, 547–594. [CrossRef]

22. Chandran, M.; Phillips, S.A.; Ciaraldi, T.; Henry, R.R. Adiponectin: More than just another fat cell hormone? *Diabetes Care* **2003**, *26*, 2442–2450. [CrossRef]

23. Mantzoros, C.; Petridou, E.; Dessypris, N.; Chavelas, C.; Dalamaga, M.; Alexe, D.M.; Papadiamantis, Y.; Markopoulos, C.; Spanos, E.; Chrousos, G. Adiponectin and breast cancer risk. *J. Clin. Endocrinol. Metab.* **2004**, *89*, 1102–1107. [CrossRef]

24. Petridou, E.; Mantzoros, C.; Dessypris, N.; Koukoulomatis, P.; Addy, C.; Voulgaris, Z.; Chrousos, G.; Trichopoulos, D. Plasma adiponectin concentrations in relation to endometrial cancer: A case-control study in Greece. *J. Clin. Endocrinol. Metab.* **2003**, *88*, 993–997. [CrossRef]

25. Hotta, K.; Funahashi, T.; Arita, Y.; Takahashi, M.; Matsuda, M.; Okamoto, Y.; Iwahashi, H.; Kuriyama, H.; Ouchi, N.; Maeda, K. Plasma concentrations of a novel, adipose-specific protein, adiponectin, in type 2 diabetic patients. *Arterioscler. Thromb. Vasc. Biol.* **2000**, *20*, 1595–1599. [CrossRef]

26. Di Zazzo, E.; Polito, R.; Bartollino, S.; Nigro, E.; Porcile, C.; Bianco, A.; Daniele, A.; Moncharmont, B. Adiponectin as Link Factor between Adipose Tissue and Cancer. *Int. J. Mol. Sci.* **2019**, *20*, 839. [CrossRef]

27. Ziemke, F.; Mantzoros, C.S. Adiponectin in insulin resistance: Lessons from translational research. *Am. J. Clin. Nutr.* **2009**, *91*, 258S–261S. [CrossRef]

28. Brochu-Gaudreau, K.; Rehfeldt, C.; Blouin, R.; Bordignon, V.; Murphy, B.D.; Palin, M.-F. Adiponectin action from head to toe. *Endocrine* **2010**, *37*, 11–32. [CrossRef]

29. Lee, C.; Woo, Y.; Wang, Y.; Yeung, C.; Xu, A.; Lam, K. Obesity, adipokines and cancer: An update. *Clin. Endocrinol.* **2015**, *83*, 147–156. [CrossRef]

30. Maeda, K.; Okubo, K.; Shimomura, I.; Funahashi, T.; Matsuzawa, Y.; Matsubara, K. cDNA cloning and expression of a novel adipose specific collagen-like factor, apM1 (AdiPoseMost abundant Gene transcript 1). *Biochem. Biophys. Res. Commun.* **1996**, *221*, 286–289. [CrossRef]

31. Fujimoto, N.; Matsuo, N.; Sumiyoshi, H.; Yamaguchi, K.; Saikawa, T.; Yoshimatsu, H.; Yoshioka, H. Adiponectin is expressed in the brown adipose tissue and surrounding immature tissues in mouse embryos. *Biochim. Biophys. Acta* **2005**, *1731*, 1–12. [CrossRef]

32. Chen, J.; Tan, B.; Karteris, E.; Zervou, S.; Digby, J.; Hillhouse, E.; Vatish, M.; Randeva, H. Secretion of adiponectin by human placenta: Differential modulation of adiponectin and its receptors by cytokines. *Diabetologia* **2006**, *49*, 1292. [CrossRef]

33. Fayad, R.; Pini, M.; Sennello, J.A.; Cabay, R.J.; Chan, L.; Xu, A.; Fantuzzi, G. Adiponectin deficiency protects mice from chemically induced colonic inflammation. *Gastroenterology* **2007**, *132*, 601–614. [CrossRef]

34. Delaigle, A.l.M.; Jonas, J.-C.; Bauche, I.B.; Cornu, O.; Brichard, S.M. Induction of adiponectin in skeletal muscle by inflammatory cytokines: In vivo and in vitro studies. *Endocrinology* **2004**, *145*, 5589–5597. [CrossRef]

35. Katsiougiannis, S.; Kapsogeorgou, E.K.; Manoussakis, M.N.; Skopouli, F.N. Salivary gland epithelial cells: A new source of the immunoregulatory hormone adiponectin. *Arthritis Rheum.* **2006**, *54*, 2295–2299. [CrossRef]

36. Kaser, S.; Moschen, A.; Cayon, A.; Kaser, A.; Crespo, J.; Pons-Romero, F.; Ebenbichler, C.; Patsch, J.; Tilg, H. Adiponectin and its receptors in non-alcoholic steatohepatitis. *Gut* **2005**, *54*, 117–121. [CrossRef]

37. Nishida, M.; Funahashi, T.; Shimomura, I. Pathophysiological significance of adiponectin. *Med Mol. Morphol.* **2007**, *40*, 55–67. [CrossRef]

38. Kadowaki, T.; Yamauchi, T. Adiponectin and adiponectin receptors. *Endocr. Rev.* **2005**, *26*, 439–451. [CrossRef]

39. Wong, G.W.; Wang, J.; Hug, C.; Tsao, T.-S.; Lodish, H.F. A family of Acrp30/adiponectin structural and functional paralogs. *Proc. Natl. Acad. Sci. USA* **2004**, *101*, 10302–10307. [CrossRef]

40. Wong, G.W.; Krawczyk, S.A.; Kitidis-Mitrokostas, C.; Revett, T.; Gimeno, R.; Lodish, H.F. Molecular, biochemical and functional characterizations of C1q/TNF family members: Adipose-tissue-selective expression patterns, regulation by PPAR-γ agonist, cysteine-mediated oligomerizations, combinatorial associations and metabolic functions. *Biochem. J.* **2008**, *416*, 161–177. [CrossRef]

41. Hada, Y.; Yamauchi, T.; Waki, H.; Tsuchida, A.; Hara, K.; Yago, H.; Miyazaki, O.; Ebinuma, H.; Kadowaki, T. Selective purification and characterization of adiponectin multimer species from human plasma. *Biochem. Biophys. Res. Commun.* **2007**, *356*, 487–493. [CrossRef]

42. Tsao, T.-S.; Tomas, E.; Murrey, H.E.; Hug, C.; Lee, D.H.; Ruderman, N.B.; Heuser, J.E.; Lodish, H.F. Role of disulfide bonds in Acrp30/adiponectin structure and signaling specificity: Different oligomers activate different signal transduction pathways. *J. Biol. Chem.* **2003**, *278*, 50810–50817. [CrossRef]

43. Wang, Y.; Xu, A.; Knight, C.; Xu, L.Y.; Cooper, G.J. Hydroxylation and glycosylation of the four conserved lysine residues in the collagenous domain of adiponectin potential role in the modulation of its insulin-sensitizing activity. *J. Biol. Chem.* **2002**, *277*, 19521–19529. [CrossRef]

44. Waki, H.; Yamauchi, T.; Kamon, J.; Ito, Y.; Uchida, S.; Kita, S.; Hara, K.; Hada, Y.; Vasseur, F.; Froguel, P. Impaired multimerization of human adiponectin mutants associated with diabetes: Molecular structure and multimer formation of adiponectin. *J. Biol. Chem.* **2003**, *278*, 40352–40363. [CrossRef]

45. Pajvani, U.B.; Du, X.; Combs, T.P.; Berg, A.H.; Rajala, M.W.; Schulthess, T.; Engel, J.; Brownlee, M.; Scherer, P.E. Structure-function studies of the adipocyte-secreted hormone Acrp30/adiponectin implications for metabolic regulation and bioactivity. *J. Biol. Chem.* **2003**, *278*, 9073–9085. [CrossRef]

46. Fruebis, J.; Tsao, T.-S.; Javorschi, S.; Ebbets-Reed, D.; Erickson, M.R.S.; Yen, F.T.; Bihain, B.E.; Lodish, H.F. Proteolytic cleavage product of 30-kDa adipocyte complement-related protein increases fatty acid oxidation in muscle and causes weight loss in mice. *Proc. Natl. Acad. Sci. USA* **2001**, *98*, 2005–2010. [CrossRef]

47. Waki, H.; Yamauchi, T.; Kamon, J.; Kita, S.; Ito, Y.; Hada, Y.; Uchida, S.; Tsuchida, A.; Takekawa, S.; Kadowaki, T. Generation of globular fragment of adiponectin by leukocyte elastase secreted by monocytic cell line THP-1. *Endocrinology* **2005**, *146*, 790–796. [CrossRef]

48. Goldstein, B.J.; Scalia, R. Adiponectin: A novel adipokine linking adipocytes and vascular function. *J. Clin. Endocrinol. Metab.* **2004**, *89*, 2563–2568. [CrossRef]

49. Kadowaki, T.; Yamauchi, T.; Kubota, N.; Hara, K.; Ueki, K.; Tobe, K. Adiponectin and adiponectin receptors in insulin resistance, diabetes, and the metabolic syndrome. *J. Clin. Investig.* **2006**, *116*, 1784–1792. [CrossRef]

50. Nishizawa, H.; Shimomura, I.; Kishida, K.; Maeda, N.; Kuriyama, H.; Nagaretani, H.; Matsuda, M.; Kondo, H.; Furuyama, N.; Kihara, S. Androgens decrease plasma adiponectin, an insulin-sensitizing adipocyte-derived protein. *Diabetes* **2002**, *51*, 2734–2741. [CrossRef]

51. Cnop, M.; Havel, P.; Utzschneider, K.; Carr, D.; Sinha, M.; Boyko, E.; Retzlaff, B.; Knopp, R.; Brunzell, J.; Kahn, S.E. Relationship of adiponectin to body fat distribution, insulin sensitivity and plasma lipoproteins: Evidence for independent roles of age and sex. *Diabetologia* **2003**, *46*, 459–469. [CrossRef]

52. Swarbrick, M.M.; Havel, P.J. Physiological, pharmacological, and nutritional regulation of circulating adiponectin concentrations in humans. *Metab. Syndr. Relat. Disord.* **2008**, *6*, 87–102. [CrossRef]

53. Combs, T.P.; Wagner, J.A.; Berger, J.; Doebber, T.; Wang, W.-J.; Zhang, B.B.; Tanen, M.; Berg, A.H.; O'rahilly, S.; Savage, D.B. Induction of adipocyte complement-related protein of 30 kilodaltons by PPARγ agonists: A potential mechanism of insulin sensitization. *Endocrinology* **2002**, *143*, 998–1007. [CrossRef]

54. Maeda, N.; Takahashi, M.; Funahashi, T.; Kihara, S.; Nishizawa, H.; Kishida, K.; Nagaretani, H.; Matsuda, M.; Komuro, R.; Ouchi, N. PPARγ ligands increase expression and plasma concentrations of adiponectin, an adipose-derived protein. *Diabetes* **2001**, *50*, 2094–2099. [CrossRef]

55. Joseph, G.Y.; Javorschi, S.; Hevener, A.L.; Kruszynska, Y.T.; Norman, R.A.; Sinha, M.; Olefsky, J.M. The effect of thiazolidinediones on plasma adiponectin levels in normal, obese, and type 2 diabetic subjects. *Diabetes* **2002**, *51*, 2968–2974.

56. Surmacz, E. Leptin and adiponectin: Emerging therapeutic targets in breast cancer. *J. Mammary Gland Biol. Neoplasia* **2013**, *18*, 321–332. [CrossRef]

57. Khan, S.; Shukla, S.; Sinha, S.; Meeran, S.M. Role of adipokines and cytokines in obesity-associated breast cancer: Therapeutic targets. *Cytokine Growth Factor Rev.* **2013**, *24*, 503–513. [CrossRef]

58. Takahashi, M.; Arita, Y.; Yamagata, K.; Matsukawa, Y.; Okutomi, K.; Horie, M.; Shimomura, I.; Hotta, K.; Kuriyama, H.; Kihara, S. Genomic structure and mutations in adipose-specific gene, adiponectin. *Int. J. Obes.* **2000**, *24*, 861. [CrossRef]

59. Kaklamani, V.G.; Sadim, M.; Hsi, A.; Offit, K.; Oddoux, C.; Ostrer, H.; Ahsan, H.; Pasche, B.; Mantzoros, C. Variants of the adiponectin and adiponectin receptor 1 genes and breast cancer risk. *Cancer Res.* **2008**, *68*, 3178–3184. [CrossRef]

60. Simpson, F.; Whitehead, J.P. Adiponectin—It's all about the modifications. *Int. J. Biochem. Cell Biol.* **2010**, *42*, 785–788. [CrossRef]

61. Trujillo, M.; Hanif, W.; Barnett, A.; McTernan, P.; Scherer, P.; Kumar, S. Serum high molecular weight complex of adiponectin correlates better with glucose tolerance than total serum adiponectin in Indo-Asian males. *Diabetologia* **2005**, *48*, 1084–1087.

62. Trujillo, M.; Scherer, P. Adiponectin–journey from an adipocyte secretory protein to biomarker of the metabolic syndrome. *J. Intern. Med.* **2005**, *257*, 167–175. [CrossRef]

63. Yamauchi, T.; Kamon, J.; Ito, Y.; Tsuchida, A.; Yokomizo, T.; Kita, S.; Sugiyama, T.; Miyagishi, M.; Hara, K.; Tsunoda, M. Cloning of adiponectin receptors that mediate antidiabetic metabolic effects. *Nature* **2003**, *423*, 762. [CrossRef]

64. Panno, M.L.; Naimo, G.D.; Spina, E.; Andò, S.; Mauro, L. Different molecular signaling sustaining adiponectin action in breast cancer. *Curr. Opin. Pharmacol.* **2016**, *31*, 1–7. [CrossRef]

65. Hug, C.; Wang, J.; Ahmad, N.S.; Bogan, J.S.; Tsao, T.-S.; Lodish, H.F. T-cadherin is a receptor for hexameric and high-molecular-weight forms of Acrp30/adiponectin. *Proc. Natl. Acad. Sci. USA* **2004**, *101*, 10308–10313. [CrossRef]

66. Asada, K.; Yoshiji, H.; Noguchi, R.; Ikenaka, Y.; Kitade, M.; Kaji, K.; Yoshii, J.; Yanase, K.; Namisaki, T.; Yamazaki, M. Crosstalk between high-molecular-weight adiponectin and T-cadherin during liver fibrosis development in rats. *Int. J. Mol. Med.* **2007**, *20*, 725–729.

67. Chan, D.W.; Lee, J.M.; Chan, P.C.; Ng, I.O. Genetic and epigenetic inactivation of T-cadherin in human hepatocellular carcinoma cells. *Int. J. Cancer* **2008**, *123*, 1043–1052. [CrossRef]

68. Lee, M.-H.; Klein, R.L.; El-Shewy, H.M.; Luttrell, D.K.; Luttrell, L.M. The adiponectin receptors AdipoR1 and AdipoR2 activate ERK1/2 through a Src/Ras-dependent pathway and stimulate cell growth. *Biochemistry* **2008**, *47*, 11682–11692. [CrossRef]

69. Hebbard, L.W.; Garlatti, M.; Young, L.J.; Cardiff, R.D.; Oshima, R.G.; Ranscht, B. T-cadherin supports angiogenesis and adiponectin association with the vasculature in a mouse mammary tumor model. *Cancer Res.* **2008**, *68*, 1407–1416. [CrossRef]

70. Berg, A.H.; Combs, T.P.; Scherer, P.E. ACRP30/adiponectin: An adipokine regulating glucose and lipid metabolism. *Trends Endocrinol. Metab.* **2002**, *13*, 84–89. [CrossRef]

71. Nagaraju, G.P.; Rajitha, B.; Aliya, S.; Kotipatruni, R.P.; Madanraj, A.S.; Hammond, A.; Park, D.; Chigurupati, S.; Alam, A.; Pattnaik, S. The role of adiponectin in obesity-associated female-specific carcinogenesis. *Cytokine Growth Factor Rev.* **2016**, *31*, 37–48. [CrossRef]

72. Kharroubi, I.; Rasschaert, J.; Eizirik, D.L.; Cnop, M. Expression of adiponectin receptors in pancreatic β cells. *Biochem. Biophys. Res. Commun.* **2003**, *312*, 1118–1122. [CrossRef]

73. Igata, M.; Motoshima, H.; Tsuruzoe, K.; Kojima, K.; Matsumura, T.; Kondo, T.; Taguchi, T.; Nakamaru, K.; Yano, M.; Kukidome, D. Adenosine monophosphate-activated protein kinase suppresses vascular smooth muscle cell proliferation through the inhibition of cell cycle progression. *Circ. Res.* **2005**, *97*, 837–844. [CrossRef]

74. Wilcox, G. Insulin and insulin resistance. *Clin. Biochem. Rev.* **2005**, *26*, 19.

75. Iwabu, M.; Yamauchi, T.; Okada-Iwabu, M.; Sato, K.; Nakagawa, T.; Funata, M.; Yamaguchi, M.; Namiki, S.; Nakayama, R.; Tabata, M. Adiponectin and AdipoR1 regulate PGC-1α and mitochondria by Ca^{2+} and AMPK/SIRT1. *Nature* **2010**, *464*, 1313. [CrossRef]

76. Miyazaki, T.; Bub, J.D.; Uzuki, M.; Iwamoto, Y. Adiponectin activates c-Jun NH2-terminal kinase and inhibits signal transducer and activator of transcription 3. *Biochem. Biophys. Res. Commun.* **2005**, *333*, 79–87. [CrossRef]

77. Pearson, G.; Robinson, F.; Beers Gibson, T.; Xu, B.-E.; Karandikar, M.; Berman, K.; Cobb, M.H. Mitogen-activated protein (MAP) kinase pathways: Regulation and physiological functions. *Endocr. Rev.* **2001**, *22*, 153–183. [CrossRef]

78. Inoki, K.; Zhu, T.; Guan, K.-L. TSC2 mediates cellular energy response to control cell growth and survival. *Cell* **2003**, *115*, 577–590. [CrossRef]

79. Dieudonne, M.-N.; Bussiere, M.; Dos Santos, E.; Leneveu, M.-C.; Giudicelli, Y.; Pecquery, R. Adiponectin mediates antiproliferative and apoptotic responses in human MCF7 breast cancer cells. *Biochem. Biophys. Res. Commun.* **2006**, *345*, 271–279. [CrossRef]

80. Ouchi, N.; Kihara, S.; Arita, Y.; Okamoto, Y.; Maeda, K.; Kuriyama, H.; Hotta, K.; Nishida, M.; Takahashi, M.; Muraguchi, M. Adiponectin, an adipocyte-derived plasma protein, inhibits endothelial NF-κB signaling through a cAMP-dependent pathway. *Circulation* **2000**, *102*, 1296–1301. [CrossRef]

81. Wang, Y.; Lam, J.B.; Lam, K.S.; Liu, J.; Lam, M.C.; Hoo, R.L.; Wu, D.; Cooper, G.J.; Xu, A. Adiponectin modulates the glycogen synthase kinase-3β/β-catenin signaling pathway and attenuates mammary tumorigenesis of MDA-MB-231 cells in nude mice. *Cancer Res.* **2006**, *66*, 11462–11470. [CrossRef]

82. Matafome, P.; Santos-Silva, D.; Sena, C.; Seica, R. Common mechanisms of dysfunctional adipose tissue and obesity-related cancers. *Diabetes Metab. Res. Rev.* **2013**, *29*, 285–295. [CrossRef]

83. Choi, J.; Cha, Y.J.; Koo, J.S. Adipocyte biology in breast cancer: From silent bystander to active facilitator. *Prog. Lipid Res.* **2017**. [CrossRef]

84. Bray, F.; Ferlay, J.; Soerjomataram, I.; Siegel, R.L.; Torre, L.A.; Jemal, A. Global cancer statistics 2018: GLOBOCAN estimates of incidence and mortality worldwide for 36 cancers in 185 countries. *CA Cancer J. Clin.* **2018**, *68*, 394–424. [CrossRef]

85. Crosbie, E.J.; Einstein, M.H.; Franceschi, S.; Kitchener, H.C. Human papillomavirus and cervical cancer. *Lancet* **2013**, *382*, 889–899. [CrossRef]

86. Benedetto, C.; Salvagno, F.; Canuto, E.M.; Gennarelli, G. Obesity and female malignancies. *Best Pract. Res. Clin. Obstet. Gynaecol.* **2015**, *29*, 528–540. [CrossRef]

87. Gu, W.; Chen, C.; Zhao, K.-N. Obesity-associated endometrial and cervical cancers. *Front. Biosci. (Elite Ed.)* **2013**, *5*, 109–118. [CrossRef]

88. Jee, S.H.; Yun, J.E.; Park, E.J.; Cho, E.R.; Park, I.S.; Sull, J.W.; Ohrr, H.; Samet, J.M. Body mass index and cancer risk in Korean men and women. *Int. J. Cancer* **2008**, *123*, 1892–1896. [CrossRef]

89. Kemp, T.J.; Hildesheim, A.; García-Piñeres, A.; Williams, M.C.; Shearer, G.M.; Rodriguez, A.C.; Schiffman, M.; Burk, R.; Freer, E.; Bonilla, J. Elevated systemic levels of inflammatory cytokines in older women with persistent cervical human papillomavirus infection. *Cancer Epidemiol. Prev. Biomark.* **2010**, *19*, 1954–1959. [CrossRef]

90. Ulmer, H.; Bjørge, T.; Concin, H.; Lukanova, A.; Manjer, J.; Hallmans, G.; Borena, W.; Häggström, C.; Engeland, A.; Almquist, M. Metabolic risk factors and cervical cancer in the metabolic syndrome and cancer project (Me–Can). *Gynecol. Oncol.* **2012**, *125*, 330–335. [CrossRef]

91. Lacey, J.V., Jr.; Swanson, C.A.; Brinton, L.A.; Altekruse, S.F.; Barnes, W.A.; Gravitt, P.E.; Greenberg, M.D.; Hadjimichael, O.C.; McGowan, L.; Mortel, R. Obesity as a potential risk factor for adenocarcinomas and squamous cell carcinomas of the uterine cervix. *Cancer* **2003**, *98*, 814–821. [CrossRef]

92. Maruthur, N.M.; Bolen, S.D.; Brancati, F.L.; Clark, J.M. The association of obesity and cervical cancer screening: A systematic review and meta-analysis. *Obesity* **2009**, *17*, 375–381. [CrossRef]

93. Xie, L.; Wang, Y.; Wang, S.; Wu, N.; Chen, Y.; Yan, J. Adiponectin induces growth inhibition and apoptosis in cervical cancer HeLa cells. *Biologia* **2011**, *66*, 712–720. [CrossRef]

94. Otsuka, I.; Kameda, S.; Hoshi, K. Early detection of ovarian and fallopian tube cancer by examination of cytological samples from the endometrial cavity. *Br. J. Cancer* **2013**, *109*, 603. [CrossRef]

95. Romero, I.; Bast, R.C., Jr. Minireview: Human ovarian cancer: Biology, current management, and paths to personalizing therapy. *Endocrinology* **2012**, *153*, 1593–1602. [CrossRef]

96. Nagle, C.; Dixon, S.; Jensen, A.; Kjaer, S.; Modugno, F.; Fereday, S.; Hung, J.; Johnatty, S.; Fasching, P.; Beckmann, M. Obesity and survival among women with ovarian cancer: Results from the Ovarian Cancer Association Consortium. *Br. J. Cancer* **2015**, *113*, 817. [CrossRef]

97. Olsen, C.M.; Green, A.C.; Whiteman, D.C.; Sadeghi, S.; Kolahdooz, F.; Webb, P.M. Obesity and the risk of epithelial ovarian cancer: A systematic review and meta-analysis. *Eur. J. Cancer* **2007**, *43*, 690–709. [CrossRef]

98. Leitzmann, M.F.; Koebnick, C.; Danforth, K.N.; Brinton, L.A.; Moore, S.C.; Hollenbeck, A.R.; Schatzkin, A.; Lacey, J.V., Jr. Body mass index and risk of ovarian cancer. *Cancer* **2009**, *115*, 812–822. [CrossRef]

99. Cancer, C.G.o.E.S.o.O. Ovarian cancer and oral contraceptives: Collaborative reanalysis of data from 45 epidemiological studies including 23 257 women with ovarian cancer and 87 303 controls. *Lancet* **2008**, *371*, 303–314.

100. Bhaskaran, K.; Douglas, I.; Forbes, H.; dos-Santos-Silva, I.; Leon, D.A.; Smeeth, L. Body-mass index and risk of 22 specific cancers: A population-based cohort study of 5·24 million UK adults. *Lancet* **2014**, *384*, 755–765. [CrossRef]

101. Ose, J.; Fortner, R.T.; Rinaldi, S.; Schock, H.; Overvad, K.; Tjonneland, A.; Hansen, L.; Dossus, L.; Fournier, A.; Baglietto, L. Endogenous androgens and risk of epithelial invasive ovarian cancer by tumor characteristics in the European Prospective Investigation into Cancer and Nutrition. *Int. J. Cancer* **2015**, *136*, 399–410. [CrossRef]

102. Uddin, S.; Bu, R.; Ahmed, M.; Abubaker, J.; Al-Dayel, F.; Bavi, P.; Al-Kuraya, K.S. Overexpression of leptin receptor predicts an unfavorable outcome in Middle Eastern ovarian cancer. *Mol. Cancer* **2009**, *8*, 74. [CrossRef]

103. Chen, C.; Chang, Y.-C.; Lan, M.S.; Breslin, M. Leptin stimulates ovarian cancer cell growth and inhibits apoptosis by increasing cyclin D1 and Mcl-1 expression via the activation of the MEK/ERK1/2 and PI3K/Akt signaling pathways. Corrigendum in/10.3892/ijo. 2016.3564. *Int. J. Oncol.* **2013**, *42*, 1113–1119. [CrossRef]

104. Aune, G.; Stunes, A.K.; Lian, A.-M.; Reseland, J.E.; Tingulstad, S.; Torp, S.H.; Syversen, U. Circulating interleukin-8 and plasminogen activator inhibitor-1 are increased in women with ovarian carcinoma. *Results Immunol.* **2012**, *2*, 190–195. [CrossRef]

105. Otokozawa, S.; Tanaka, R.; Akasaka, H.; Ito, E.; Asakura, S.; Ohnishi, H.; Saito, S.; Miura, T.; Saito, T.; Mori, M. Associations of serum isoflavone, adiponectin and insulin levels with risk for epithelial ovarian cancer: Results of a case-control study. *Asian Pac. J. Cancer Prev.* **2015**, *16*, 4987–4991. [CrossRef]

106. Jin, J.H.; Kim, H.-J.; Kim, C.Y.; Kim, Y.H.; Ju, W.; Kim, S.C. Association of plasma adiponectin and leptin levels with the development and progression of ovarian cancer. *Obstet. Gynecol. Sci.* **2016**, *59*, 279–285. [CrossRef]

107. Wu, M.-M.; Chen, H.-C.; Chen, C.-L.; You, S.-L.; Cheng, W.-F.; Chen, C.-A.; Lee, T.-C.; Chen, C.-J. A prospective study of gynecological cancer risk in relation to adiposity factors: Cumulative incidence and association with plasma adipokine levels. *PLoS ONE* **2014**, *9*, e104630. [CrossRef]

108. Diaz, E.S.; Karlan, B.Y.; Li, A.J. Obesity-associated adipokines correlate with survival in epithelial ovarian cancer. *Gynecol. Oncol.* **2013**, *129*, 353–357. [CrossRef]

109. Hoffmann, M.; Gogola, J.; Ptak, A. Adiponectin Reverses the Proliferative Effects of Estradiol and IGF-1 in Human Epithelial Ovarian Cancer Cells by Downregulating the Expression of Their Receptors. *Horm. Cancer* **2018**, *9*, 166–174. [CrossRef]

110. Li, X.; Yu, Z.; Fang, L.; Liu, F.; Jiang, K. Expression of adiponectin receptor-1 and prognosis of epithelial ovarian cancer patients. *Med Sci. Monit.* **2017**, *23*, 1514. [CrossRef]

111. Dupont, J.; Reverchon, M.; Cloix, L.; Froment, P.; Ramé, C. Involvement of adipokines, AMPK, PI3K and the PPAR signaling pathways in ovarian follicle development and cancer. *Int. J. Dev. Biol.* **2013**, *56*, 959–967. [CrossRef]

112. Huijgens, A.; Mertens, H. Factors predicting recurrent endometrial cancer. *Facts Views Vis. ObGyn* **2013**, *5*, 179.

113. Arem, H.; Irwin, M. Obesity and endometrial cancer survival: A systematic review. *Int. J. Obes.* **2013**, *37*, 634. [CrossRef]

114. Gunter, M.J.; Hoover, D.R.; Yu, H.; Wassertheil-Smoller, S.; Manson, J.E.; Li, J.; Harris, T.G.; Rohan, T.E.; Xue, X.; Ho, G.Y. A prospective evaluation of insulin and insulin-like growth factor-I as risk factors for endometrial cancer. *Cancer Epidemiol. Prev. Biomark.* **2008**, *17*, 921–929. [CrossRef]

115. Berstein, L.; Kvatchevskaya, J.; Poroshina, T.; Kovalenko, I.; Tsyrlina, E.; Zimarina, T.; Ourmantcheeva, A.; Ashrafian, L.; Thijssen, J. Insulin resistance, its consequences for the clinical course of the disease, and possibilities of correction in endometrial cancer. *J. Cancer Res. Clin. Oncol.* **2004**, *130*, 687–693. [CrossRef]

116. Cust, A.E.; Kaaks, R.; Friedenreich, C.; Bonnet, F.; Laville, M.; Lukanova, A.; Rinaldi, S.; Dossus, L.; Slimani, N.; Lundin, E. Plasma adiponectin levels and endometrial cancer risk in pre-and postmenopausal women. *J. Clin. Endocrinol. Metab.* **2007**, *92*, 255–263. [CrossRef]

117. Ashizawa, N.; Yahata, T.; Quan, J.; Adachi, S.; Yoshihara, K.; Tanaka, K. Serum leptin–adiponectin ratio and endometrial cancer risk in postmenopausal female subjects. *Gynecol. Oncol.* **2010**, *119*, 65–69. [CrossRef]

118. Gong, T.T.; Wu, Q.J.; Wang, Y.L.; Ma, X.X. Circulating adiponectin, leptin and adiponectin–leptin ratio and endometrial cancer risk: Evidence from a meta-analysis of epidemiologic studies. *Int. J. Cancer* **2015**, *137*, 1967–1978. [CrossRef]

119. Li, Z.J.; Yang, X.L.; Yao, Y.; Han, W.Q.; Li, B. Circulating adiponectin levels and risk of endometrial cancer: Systematic review and meta-analysis. *Exp. Ther. Med.* **2016**, *11*, 2305–2313. [CrossRef]

120. Lin, T.; Zhao, X.; Kong, W.-m. Association between adiponectin levels and endometrial carcinoma risk: Evidence from a dose–response meta-analysis. *BMJ Open* **2015**, *5*, e008541. [CrossRef]

121. Zeng, F.; Shi, J.; Long, Y.; Tian, H.; Li, X.; Zhao, A.Z.; Li, R.F.; Chen, T. Adiponectin and endometrial cancer: A systematic review and meta-analysis. *Cell. Physiol. Biochem.* **2015**, *36*, 1670–1678. [CrossRef]

122. Moon, H.-S.; Chamberland, J.P.; Aronis, K.; Tseleni-Balafouta, S.; Mantzoros, C.S. Direct role of adiponectin and adiponectin receptors in endometrial cancer: In vitro and ex vivo studies in humans. *Mol. Cancer Ther.* **2011**, *10*, 2234–2243. [CrossRef]

123. Cong, L.; Gasser, J.; Zhao, J.; Yang, B.; Li, F.; Zhao, A.Z. Human adiponectin inhibits cell growth and induces apoptosis in human endometrial carcinoma cells, HEC-1-A and RL95-2. *Endocr. Relat. Cancer* **2007**, *14*, 713–720. [CrossRef]

124. Harvie, M.; Hooper, L.; Howell, A. Central obesity and breast cancer risk: A systematic review. *Obes. Rev.* **2003**, *4*, 157–173. [CrossRef]

125. Lahmann, P.H.; Hoffmann, K.; Allen, N.; Van Gils, C.H.; Khaw, K.T.; Tehard, B.; Berrino, F.; Tjønneland, A.; Bigaard, J.; Olsen, A. Body size and breast cancer risk: Findings from the European Prospective Investigation into Cancer And Nutrition (EPIC). *Int. J. Cancer* **2004**, *111*, 762–771. [CrossRef]

126. Michels, K.B.; Terry, K.L.; Willett, W.C. Longitudinal study on the role of body size in premenopausal breast cancer. *Arch. Intern. Med.* **2006**, *166*, 2395–2402. [CrossRef]

127. Barone, I.; Catalano, S.; Gelsomino, L.; Marsico, S.; Giordano, C.; Panza, S.; Bonofiglio, D.; Bossi, G.; Covington, K.R.; Fuqua, S.A. Leptin mediates tumor–stromal interactions that promote the invasive growth of breast cancer cells. *Cancer Res.* **2012**, *72*, 1416–1427. [CrossRef]

128. Katira, A.; Tan, P.H. Evolving role of adiponectin in cancer-controversies and update. *Cancer Biol. Med.* **2016**, *13*, 101. [CrossRef]

129. Miyoshi, Y.; Funahashi, T.; Kihara, S.; Taguchi, T.; Tamaki, Y.; Matsuzawa, Y.; Noguchi, S. Association of serum adiponectin levels with breast cancer risk. *Clin. Cancer Res.* **2003**, *9*, 5699–5704.

130. Tworoger, S.S.; Eliassen, A.H.; Kelesidis, T.; Colditz, G.A.; Willett, W.C.; Mantzoros, C.S.; Hankinson, S.E. Plasma adiponectin concentrations and risk of incident breast cancer. *J. Clin. Endocrinol. Metab.* **2007**, *92*, 1510–1516. [CrossRef]

131. Oh, S.W.; Park, C.-Y.; Lee, E.S.; Yoon, Y.S.; Lee, E.S.; Park, S.S.; Kim, Y.; Sung, N.J.; Yun, Y.H.; Lee, K.S. Adipokines, insulin resistance, metabolic syndrome, and breast cancer recurrence: A cohort study. *Breast Cancer Res.* **2011**, *13*, R34. [CrossRef] [PubMed]

132. Macis, D.; Guerrieri-Gonzaga, A.; Gandini, S. Circulating adiponectin and breast cancer risk: A systematic review and meta-analysis. *Int. J. Epidemiol.* **2014**, *43*, 1226–1236. [CrossRef]

133. Tan, P.H.; Tyrrell, H.E.; Gao, L.; Xu, D.; Quan, J.; Gill, D.; Rai, L.; Ding, Y.; Plant, G.; Chen, Y. Adiponectin receptor signaling on dendritic cells blunts antitumor immunity. *Cancer Res.* **2014**, *74*, 5711–5722. [CrossRef]

134. Kang, J.H.; Lee, Y.Y.; Yu, B.Y.; Yang, B.-S.; Cho, K.-H.; Yoon, D.K.; Roh, Y.K. Adiponectin induces growth arrest and apoptosis of MDA-MB-231 breast cancer cell. *Arch. Pharmacal Res.* **2005**, *28*, 1263–1269. [CrossRef]

135. Dos Santos, E.; Benaitreau, D.; Dieudonne, M.-N.; Leneveu, M.-C.; Serazin, V.; Giudicelli, Y.; Pecquery, R. Adiponectin mediates an antiproliferative response in human MDA-MB 231 breast cancer cells. *Oncol. Rep.* **2008**, *20*, 971–977.

136. Grossmann, M.; Nkhata, K.; Mizuno, N.; Ray, A.; Cleary, M. Effects of adiponectin on breast cancer cell growth and signaling. *Br. J. Cancer* **2008**, *98*, 370. [CrossRef]

137. Nakayama, S.; Miyoshi, Y.; Ishihara, H.; Noguchi, S. Growth-inhibitory effect of adiponectin via adiponectin receptor 1 on human breast cancer cells through inhibition of S-phase entry without inducing apoptosis. *Breast Cancer Res. Treat.* **2008**, *112*, 405–410. [CrossRef] [PubMed]

138. Andò, S.; Gelsomino, L.; Panza, S.; Giordano, C.; Bonofiglio, D.; Barone, I.; Catalano, S. Obesity, Leptin and Breast Cancer: Epidemiological Evidence and Proposed Mechanisms. *Cancers* **2019**, *11*, 62. [CrossRef]

139. Mauro, L.; Naimo, G.D.; Gelsomino, L.; Malivindi, R.; Bruno, L.; Pellegrino, M.; Tarallo, R.; Memoli, D.; Weisz, A.; Panno, M.L. Uncoupling effects of estrogen receptor α on LKB1/AMPK interaction upon adiponectin exposure in breast cancer. *FASEB J.* **2018**, *32*, 4343–4355. [CrossRef]

140. Mauro, L.; Pellegrino, M.; De Amicis, F.; Ricchio, E.; Giordano, F.; Rizza, P.; Catalano, S.; Bonofiglio, D.; Sisci, D.; Panno, M.L. Evidences that estrogen receptor α interferes with adiponectin effects on breast cancer cell growth. *Cell Cycle* **2014**, *13*, 553–564. [CrossRef]

141. Mauro, L.; Pellegrino, M.; Giordano, F.; Ricchio, E.; Rizza, P.; De Amicis, F.; Catalano, S.; Bonofiglio, D.; Panno, M.L.; Andò, S. Estrogen receptor-α drives adiponectin effects on cyclin D1 expression in breast cancer cells. *FASEB J.* **2015**, *29*, 2150–2160. [CrossRef]

142. Pfeiler, G.H.; Buechler, C.; Neumeier, M.; Schäffler, A.; Schmitz, G.; Ortmann, O.; Treeck, O. Adiponectin effects on human breast cancer cells are dependent on 17-β estradiol. *Oncol. Rep.* **2008**, *19*, 787–793. [CrossRef]

143. Lam, J.B.; Chow, K.H.; Xu, A.; Lam, K.S.; Liu, J.; Wong, N.-S.; Moon, R.T.; Shepherd, P.R.; Cooper, G.J.; Wang, Y. Adiponectin haploinsufficiency promotes mammary tumor development in MMTV-PyVT mice by modulation of phosphatase and tensin homolog activities. *PLoS ONE* **2009**, *4*, e4968. [CrossRef]

144. Kim, K.-y.; Baek, A.; Hwang, J.-E.; Choi, Y.A.; Jeong, J.; Lee, M.-S.; Cho, D.H.; Lim, J.-S.; Kim, K.I.; Yang, Y. Adiponectin-activated AMPK stimulates dephosphorylation of AKT through protein phosphatase 2A activation. *Cancer Res.* **2009**, *69*, 4018–4026. [CrossRef] [PubMed]

145. Liu, J.; Lam, J.B.; Chow, K.H.; Xu, A.; Lam, K.S.; Moon, R.T.; Wang, Y. Adiponectin stimulates Wnt inhibitory factor-1 expression through epigenetic regulations involving the transcription factor specificity protein 1. *Carcinogenesis* **2008**, *29*, 2195–2202. [CrossRef]

146. Taliaferro-Smith, L.; Nagalingam, A.; Knight, B.B.; Oberlick, E.; Saxena, N.K.; Sharma, D. Integral role of PTP1B in adiponectin-mediated inhibition of oncogenic actions of leptin in breast carcinogenesis. *Neoplasia (New York, NY)* **2013**, *15*, 23. [CrossRef]

147. Denzel, M.S.; Hebbard, L.W.; Shostak, G.; Shapiro, L.; Cardiff, R.D.; Ranscht, B. Adiponectin deficiency limits tumor vascularization in the MMTV-PyV-mT mouse model of mammary cancer. *Clin. Cancer Res.* **2009**, *15*, 3256–3264. [CrossRef]

148. Landskroner-Eiger, S.; Qian, B.; Muise, E.S.; Nawrocki, A.R.; Berger, J.P.; Fine, E.J.; Koba, W.; Deng, Y.; Pollard, J.W.; Scherer, P.E. Proangiogenic contribution of adiponectin toward mammary tumor growth in vivo. *Clin. Cancer Res.* **2009**, *15*, 3265–3276. [CrossRef] [PubMed]

149. Ward, P.S.; Thompson, C.B. Metabolic reprogramming: A cancer hallmark even warburg did not anticipate. *Cancer Cell* **2012**, *21*, 297–308. [CrossRef]

150. Luo, Z.; Zang, M.; Guo, W. AMPK as a metabolic tumor suppressor: Control of metabolism and cell growth. *Future Oncol.* **2010**, *6*, 457–470. [CrossRef]

151. Mihaylova, M.M.; Shaw, R.J. The AMPK signalling pathway coordinates cell growth, autophagy and metabolism. *Nature Cell Biol.* **2011**, *13*, 1016. [CrossRef]

152. Shackelford, D.B.; Shaw, R.J. The LKB1–AMPK pathway: Metabolism and growth control in tumour suppression. *Nature Rev. Cancer* **2009**, *9*, 563. [CrossRef]

153. Zhang, Y.; Yu, M.; Tian, W. Physiological and pathological impact of exosomes of adipose tissue. *Cell Prolif.* **2016**, *49*, 3–13. [CrossRef]

154. Guo, W.; Gao, Y.; Li, N.; Shao, F.; Wang, C.; Wang, P.; Yang, Z.; Li, R.; He, J. Exosomes: New players in cancer. *Oncol. Rep.* **2017**, *38*, 665–675. [CrossRef]

155. Lin, R.; Wang, S.; Zhao, R.C. Exosomes from human adipose-derived mesenchymal stem cells promote migration through Wnt signaling pathway in a breast cancer cell model. *Mol. Cell. Biochem.* **2013**, *383*, 13–20. [CrossRef]

156. Gernapudi, R.; Yao, Y.; Zhang, Y.; Wolfson, B.; Roy, S.; Duru, N.; Eades, G.; Yang, P.; Zhou, Q. Targeting exosomes from preadipocytes inhibits preadipocyte to cancer stem cell signaling in early-stage breast cancer. *Breast Cancer Res. Treat.* **2015**, *150*, 685–695. [CrossRef]

157. Philley, J.V.; Kannan, A.; Griffith, D.E.; Devine, M.S.; Benwill, J.L.; Wallace, R.J., Jr.; Brown-Elliott, B.A.; Thakkar, F.; Taskar, V.; Fox, J.G. Exosome secretome and mediated signaling in breast cancer patients with nontuberculous mycobacterial disease. *Oncotarget* **2017**, *8*, 18070. [CrossRef]

158. Obata, Y.; Kita, S.; Koyama, Y.; Fukuda, S.; Takeda, H.; Takahashi, M.; Fujishima, Y.; Nagao, H.; Masuda, S.; Tanaka, Y. Adiponectin/T-cadherin system enhances exosome biogenesis and decreases cellular ceramides by exosomal release. *JCI Insight* **2018**, *3*. [CrossRef]

159. Kang, D.-W.; Lee, J.; Suh, S.-H.; Ligibel, J.; Courneya, K.S.; Jeon, J.Y. Effects of exercise on insulin, IGF axis, adipocytokines, and inflammatory markers in breast cancer survivors: A systematic review and meta-analysis. *Cancer Epidemiol. Prev. Biomark.* **2017**, *26*, 355–365. [CrossRef]

160. Kriketos, A.D.; Gan, S.K.; Poynten, A.M.; Furler, S.M.; Chisholm, D.J.; Campbell, L.V. Exercise increases adiponectin levels and insulin sensitivity in humans. *Diabetes Care* **2004**, *27*, 629–630. [CrossRef]

161. Saunders, T.J.; Palombella, A.; McGuire, K.A.; Janiszewski, P.M.; Després, J.-P.; Ross, R. Acute exercise increases adiponectin levels in abdominally obese men. *J. Nutr. Metab.* **2012**, *2012*. [CrossRef]

162. Otvos, L., Jr.; Kovalszky, I.; Olah, J.; Coroniti, R.; Knappe, D.; Nollmann, F.I.; Hoffmann, R.; Wade, J.D.; Lovas, S.; Surmacz, E. Optimization of adiponectin-derived peptides for inhibition of cancer cell growth and signaling. *Pept. Sci.* **2015**, *104*, 156–166. [CrossRef]

163. Otvos, L.; Haspinger, E.; La Russa, F.; Maspero, F.; Graziano, P.; Kovalszky, I.; Lovas, S.; Nama, K.; Hoffmann, R.; Knappe, D. Design and development of a peptide-based adiponectin receptor agonist for cancer treatment. *BMC Biotechnol.* **2011**, *11*, 90. [CrossRef]

164. Okada-Iwabu, M.; Yamauchi, T.; Iwabu, M.; Honma, T.; Hamagami, K.-i.; Matsuda, K.; Yamaguchi, M.; Tanabe, H.; Kimura-Someya, T.; Shirouzu, M. A small-molecule AdipoR agonist for type 2 diabetes and short life in obesity. *Nature* **2013**, *503*, 493. [CrossRef]

165. Kim, S.; Lee, Y.; Kim, J.W.; Son, Y.-J.; Ma, M.J.; Um, J.-H.; Kim, N.D.; Min, S.H.; Kim, D.I.; Kim, B.B. Discovery of a novel potent peptide agonist to adiponectin receptor 1. *PLoS ONE* **2018**, *13*, e0199256. [CrossRef]

166. Wei, S.; Yang, J.; Lee, S.-L.; Kulp, S.K.; Chen, C.-S. PPARγ-independent antitumor effects of thiazolidinediones. *Cancer Lett.* **2009**, *276*, 119–124. [CrossRef]

167. Yamauchi, T.; Kamon, J.; Waki, H.; Terauchi, Y.; Kubota, N.; Hara, K.; Mori, Y.; Ide, T.; Murakami, K.; Tsuboyama-Kasaoka, N. The fat-derived hormone adiponectin reverses insulin resistance associated with both lipoatrophy and obesity. *Nature Med.* **2001**, *7*, 941. [CrossRef]

168. Dowling, R.J.; Zakikhani, M.; Fantus, I.G.; Pollak, M.; Sonenberg, N. Metformin inhibits mammalian target of rapamycin–dependent translation initiation in breast cancer cells. *Cancer Res.* **2007**, *67*, 10804–10812. [CrossRef]

169. Brown, K.A.; Simpson, E.R. Obesity and breast cancer: Mechanisms and therapeutic implications. *Front. Biosci. (Elite Ed.)* **2012**, *4*, 2515–2524. [CrossRef]

170. Renehan, A.G.; Soerjomataram, I.; Tyson, M.; Egger, M.; Zwahlen, M.; Coebergh, J.W.; Buchan, I. Incident cancer burden attributable to excess body mass index in 30 European countries. *Int. J. Cancer* **2010**, *126*, 692–702. [CrossRef]

171. Protani, M.; Coory, M.; Martin, J.H. Effect of obesity on survival of women with breast cancer: Systematic review and meta-analysis. *Breast Cancer Res. Treat.* **2010**, *123*, 627–635. [CrossRef] [PubMed]

172. Chan, D.; Vieira, A.; Aune, D.; Bandera, E.; Greenwood, D.; McTiernan, A.; Navarro Rosenblatt, D.; Thune, I.; Vieira, R.; Norat, T. Body mass index and survival in women with breast cancer—Systematic literature review and meta-analysis of 82 follow-up studies. *Ann. Oncol.* **2014**, *25*, 1901–1914. [CrossRef] [PubMed]

173. Taubes, G. *Unraveling the Obesity-Cancer Connection*; American Association for the Advancement of Science: Washington, DC, USA, 2012.

174. Tahergorabi, Z.; Khazaei, M.; Moodi, M.; Chamani, E. From obesity to cancer: A review on proposed mechanisms. *Cell Biochem. Funct.* **2016**, *34*, 533–545. [CrossRef] [PubMed]

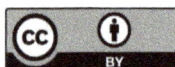

International Journal of
Molecular Sciences

MDPI

Review

Mechanisms of Adiponectin Action in Fertility: An Overview from Gametogenesis to Gestation in Humans and Animal Models in Normal and Pathological Conditions

Alix Barbe [1,2,3,†], Alice Bongrani [1,2,3,†], Namya Mellouk [1,2,3], Anthony Estienne [1,2,3], Patrycja Kurowska [4], Jérémy Grandhaye [1,2,3], Yaelle Elfassy [5,6,7], Rachel Levy [5,6,7], Agnieszka Rak [2], Pascal Froment [1,2,3] and Joëlle Dupont [1,2,3,*]

[1] INRA UMR85 Physiologie de la Reproduction et des Comportements, F-37380 Nouzilly, France; alix.barbe@inra.fr (A.B.); alice.bongrani@inra.fr (A.B.); namya.mellouk@inra.fr (N.M.); anthony.estienne@inra.fr (A.E.); jeremy.grandhaye@inra.fr (J.G.); pascal.froment@inra.fr (P.F.)
[2] CNRS UMR7247 Physiologie de la Reproduction et des Comportements, F-37380 Nouzilly, France; agnieszka.rak@uj.edu.pl
[3] Université François Rabelais de Tours, F-37041 Tours, France
[4] Department of Physiology and Toxicology of Reproduction, Institute of Zoology and Biomedical Research, Jagiellonian University, 31-007 Krakow, Poland; patrycja.kurowska@doctoral.uj.edu.pl
[5] Assistance Publique des Hôpitaux de Paris, Hôpital Tenon, Service de Biologie de la Reproduction, F-75020 Paris, France; yaelle.elfassy@hotmail.fr (Y.E.); rachel.levy@orange.fr (R.L.)
[6] Université Pierre et Marie Curie Paris 6, F-75005 Paris, France
[7] INSERM UMRS_938, Centre de Recherche Saint-Antoine, F-75571 Paris, France
* Correspondence: Joelle.dupont@inra.fr; Tel.: 33-2-4742-7789; Fax: 33-2-4742-7743
† These authors contributed equally to this work.

Received: 28 February 2019; Accepted: 22 March 2019; Published: 27 March 2019

Abstract: Adiponectin is the most abundant plasma adipokine. It mainly derives from white adipose tissue and plays a key role in the control of energy metabolism thanks to its insulin-sensitising, anti-inflammatory, and antiatherogenic properties. In vitro and in vivo evidence shows that adiponectin could also be one of the hormones controlling the interaction between energy balance and fertility in several species, including humans. Indeed, its two receptors—AdipoR1 and AdipoR2—are expressed in hypothalamic–pituitary–gonadal axis and their activation regulates Kiss, GnRH and gonadotropin expression and/or secretion. In male gonads, adiponectin modulates several functions of both somatic and germ cells, such as steroidogenesis, proliferation, apoptosis, and oxidative stress. In females, it controls steroidogenesis of ovarian granulosa and theca cells, oocyte maturation, and embryo development. Adiponectin receptors were also found in placental and endometrial cells, suggesting that this adipokine might play a crucial role in embryo implantation, trophoblast invasion and foetal growth. The aim of this review is to characterise adiponectin expression and its mechanism of action in male and female reproductive tract. Further, since features of metabolic syndrome are associated with some reproductive diseases, such as polycystic ovary syndrome, gestational diabetes mellitus, preeclampsia, endometriosis, foetal growth restriction and ovarian and endometrial cancers, evidence regarding the emerging role of adiponectin in these disorders is also discussed.

Keywords: fertility; adipose tissue; reproductive tract; adipokines; cell signaling

1. Introduction

It is well known that white adipose tissue is no longer the main storage compartment of triglycerides but it is a real endocrine organ releasing a number of biologically active proteins, also known as adipokines [1]. Adipokines are considered as main regulators of the whole body energy homeostasis. One of these adipokines, named adiponectin, is recognised to play a major role in regulation of the insulin sensitivity and the pathogenesis of the metabolic syndrome. In recent years, its role in the modulation of reproductive functions has become increasingly important. There has therefore been a spate of research investigating its role in the hypothalamic–pituitary–gonadal axis but also in placenta and uterus. In this review, we will discuss the structure of adiponectin and its physiological role in the male and female reproductive tract, with a predominant emphasis on its role in several human reproductive diseases including polycystic ovary syndrome, gestational diabetes mellitus, foetal growth restriction, ovarian and endometrial cancer, endometriosis and preeclampsia.

2. Structure and Mechanism of Adiponectin Action

2.1. Structure of Adiponectin Gene and Proteins

2.1.1. Adiponectin Gene

Adiponectin, also known as ACRP30 (adipocyte complement-related protein of 30 kDa), GBP28 (Gelatin-binding protein 28), ADIPOQ (Adiponectin, C1Q And Collagen Domain Containing) and apM1 (Adipose most abundant gene transcript 1), has been discovered as a factor produced by the white adipose tissue almost simultaneously by four different teams using different approaches. The term "adiponectin" appears in 1999 following the alignment of nucleotide sequences of these four factors [2]. In human, apM1 is a 16 kb gene consisting of three exons and two introns (Figure 1), showing sequence homologies with the genes encoding collagen VIII, collagen X and the C1q factor of complement [3]. Several regulatory regions of apM1 gene expression have been identified in one region promoter of the gene surrounding exon 1. Unlike many genes, the promoter of apM1 does not include a TATA sequence, but contains several elements of response to many transcriptional factors [4], as described in Figure 1. So, the transcriptional activity of the adiponectin gene can be regulated by many mechanisms.

2.1.2. Adiponectin Protein

The full length of human adiponectin (244 amino acids, 30 kDa) consists of four domains: an amino-terminal signal peptide made up of 18 amino acids, a species specific hypervariable domain of 23 amino acids, a 66-amino acid collagen-like domain consisting of 22 repeats of the motif (Glycine-X-Y) where X and Y are variable amino acids, and a 137-amino acid carboxy-terminal globular domain [5] (Figure 2). It represents the long form of adiponectin. However, it exists also a short form of adiponectin resulting from the cleavage made by an elastase secreted by monocytes and neutrophils. Several proteolytic sites have been described located within the variable sequence and the collagen domain. The short form of adiponectin preserves its globular domain integrity and can exert its effects by binding to its receptor [6] (Figure 2). In contrast to humans, mouse adiponectin is a 247-amino acid protein [7].

Adiponectin is secreted from adipocytes into the bloodstream as three oligomeric complexes including trimer (67 kDa), hexamer (complex of two trimers, 130 kDa) and a high molecular weight (300 kDa) [8] Figure 2. Adiponectin as a monomer is undetectable in native conditions. Polymerisation is therefore an essential mechanism in regulating the biological activity of the protein [9] Thus, adiponectin forms trimers (low molecular weight form or LMW) following the establishment of hydrophobic bonds between the globular domains and noncovalent interactions within α-helices of the collagenous domains [10]. The short form of the protein does not polymerise further [11]. In contrast, in its long form adiponectin trimers form hexamers (intermediate or medium molecular weight form or MMW) and much more complex structures composed of 18 or more monomers (high molecular weight form or HMW) [12,13]. This polymerisation of adiponectin requires post-translational modifications. Indeed, the formation of hexamers is achieved by the establishment of disulphide bridges between two cysteines located in the variable region of adiponectin. Experimental evidence suggests that different forms of adiponectin fractions exhibit different biological activities. For example, non-HMW adiponectin (i.e., complexes with lower molecular weight) shows stronger anti-inflammatory actions, whereas the HMW form, whose active form constitutes nearly 70% of circulating adiponectin in healthy people, may be related to insulin sensitivity [14,15].

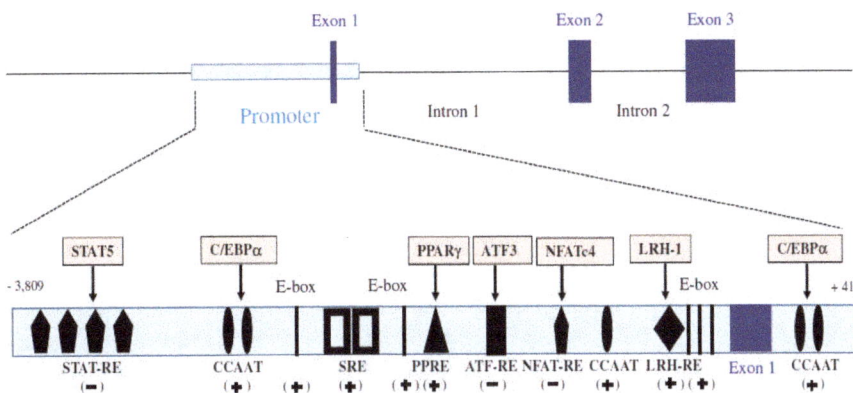

Figure 1. Structure of adiponectin gene and its promoter region. Binding sites (cis-elements) are STAT-RE: Signal Transducers and Activators of Transcription Response Element; CCAAT: CCAAT box is a distinct pattern of nucleotides with GGCCAATCT consensus sequence; SRE: Serum Response Element; PPRE: Peroxisome Proliferator Response Element; ATF-RE: Activating Transcription Factor-Response Element; LRH-RE: Liver Receptor Homolog 1 Response Element; E-box: Enhancer-box; NFAT-RE: Nuclear Factor of Activated T cells Response Element. Transcription factors (trans-elements) are STAT5: Signal transducer and activator of transcription 5; C.EBPα: CCAAT/enhancer-binding protein alpha; PPAR: Peroxisome Proliferator-activated Receptor gamma; ATF3: Activating Transcription Factor 3; NFATc4: Nuclear Factor of Activated T cells 4; LRH-1: Liver Receptor Homolog-1. The stimulatory (+) and inhibitory (−) roles of each transcription factor in the adiponectin gene expression are shown below the binding sites.

Adiponectin is considered as the adipokine most widely present in the bloodstream. It circulates at relatively high levels (3 to 30 μg/mL) representing thus 0.01% of the total plasma proteins [16] in different species like human, pigs, dairy cows, rats, chicken and turkeys [17–23]. In human, MMW and HMW forms represent 90% of the protein in the circulation and the LMW form represents only 10% [24]. The globular form remains extremely minor [12]. In cows, it is well known that the plasma concentration of adiponectin reaches its minimum before calving and its maximum during early lactation [25–29]. Unlike rodents and humans, the main circulating form is HMW in cows [26], while trimeric forms and globular forms are not detected [28,30]. In various species, the plasma adiponectin level is likely related to reproductive pathologies (polycystic ovary syndrome, gestational diabetes mellitus, preeclampsia, endometriosis, foetal growth restriction and ovarian and endometrial cancer) that are detailed below (Section 9 of this review). Expression of the adiponectin in the body is closely related to many physiological and physiopathological processes.

Adiponectin plasma concentrations are correlated with the adipose tissue level. They are also regulated by the nutritional status. Indeed, they are increased during fasting and decreased after refeeding in rodents and sheep [31,32]. Moreover, they are higher in females compared to males in humans and rodents [21]. Adiponectin levels are lower in women under certain conditions. Indeed, Cnop et al. (2003) showed that adiponectin levels in the postmenopausal women are higher than in the premenopausal women [33], while data from Nishizawa et al. (2002) found no significant differences [21]. In mice, plasma adiponectin levels are 4-fold higher in mature female than in immature female [34]. In obese compared to control patients, adiponectin concentrations in adipose tissue and in the circulation have consistently been found to be abnormally low [35], suggesting that adiponectin is strongly associated with obesity and is a potentially important hormone in the link between obesity and women's pathology.

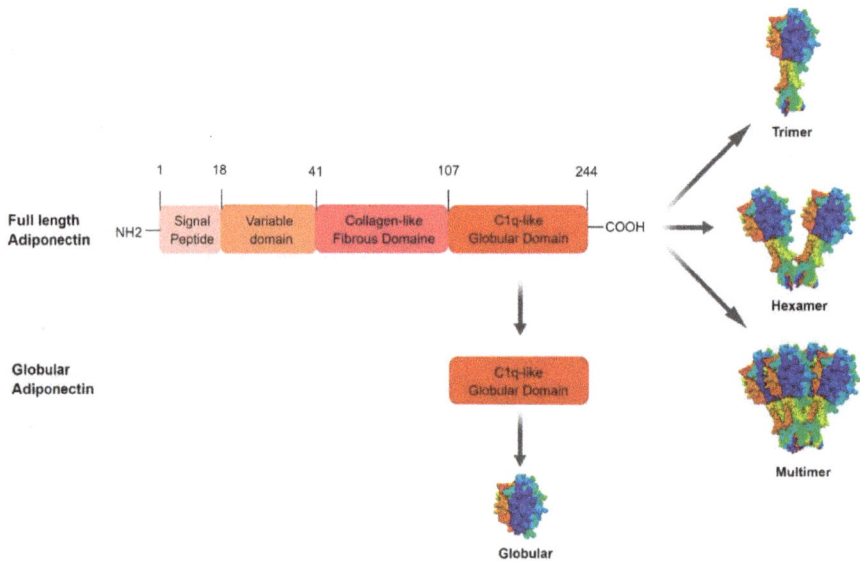

Figure 2. Structure and specific forms of human adiponectin (trimer, hexamer, multimer and globular).

2.1.3. Regulation of Adiponectin Expression

Adiponectin expression can be regulated by various factors and physiological processes. As shown in Figure 1, human adiponectin gene contains binding sites for many transcription factors including PPAR (peroxisome proliferator-activated receptor gamma [36] and its coactivator PPARγ, coactivator 1α (PGC1α) [37], C/EBPα (CCAAT/enhancer-binding protein alpha) [38], LRH-1 (liver receptor homolog-1) [36], FoxO1 (forkhead box O1) [39], SREBP-1c (sterol-regulatory element-binding protein 1c) [40], ATF3 (Activating Transcription Factor 3) [41], NFATc4 (nuclear factor of activated T cells 4) [41], Id3 (inhibitor of differentiation 3) [42], STAT5 (Signal transducer and activator of transcription 5) [43] and the clock helix–loop–helix transcription factors CLOCK and BMAL1 [44]. The activation and the repression of these transcription factors are finely regulated by endogenous and exogenous signals inducing the activation of many signalling pathways in the secretory cell. Once released in the bloodstream, adiponectin exerts its physiological effects by binding to specific membrane receptors.

2.2. Adiponectin Receptors and Adiponectin Signalling Pathways

2.2.1. AdipoR1 and AdipoR2

Adiponectin acts mainly through two seven-transmembrane domain receptors—AdipoR1 and AdipoR2—that differ from other G protein-coupled receptors. Indeed, their topology is opposite of that of the G protein-coupled receptors; their C-terminal end is located extracellularly whereas the N-terminal end is located intracellularly (Figure 3). AdipoR1 and AdipoR2 have a zinc binding motif that appears to be essential for signal transduction in the intracellular compartment [45]. They are structurally conserved (67% amino acid identity) [22]. AdipoR1 is expressed in all tissues and the highest expression is in skeletal muscles, while AdipoR2 is expressed mainly in the white adipose tissue and liver. These receptors have differing affinities for specific forms of adiponectin. AdipoR1 is a high-affinity receptor for the globular adiponectin form, and acts as a low-affinity receptor for the long form of adiponectin in skeletal muscle. In contrast, AdipoR2 is an intermediate-affinity receptor for both globular and full length adiponectin form in the liver [19,22,46].

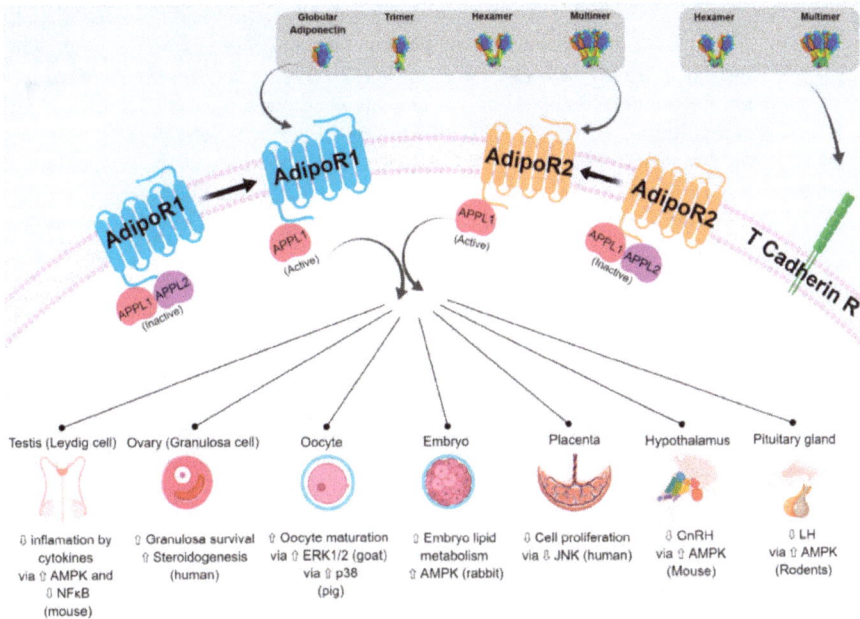

Figure 3. Adiponectin receptors and some examples of biological effects of adiponectin in reproductive tissues or cells. Adiponectin interacts with adiponectin receptors (mainly AdipoR1 and AdipoR2) to activate or inhibit a number of signalling pathways. T Cadherin receptor (T Cadherin R) binds the hexameric and high molecular weight isoforms of adiponectin but it has no intracellular domain. AdipoR1- and R2-dependent signalling is mediated through APPL 1 and APPL2. In the absence of adiponectin signal, APPL2 can bind to the N-terminal domain of the adiponectin receptors or it can form an APPL1/APPL2 heterodimer which prevents the APPL1/adiponectin receptors binding. On the other hand, the binding of adiponectin to its receptors favours the dissociation of this heterodimer. In peripheral tissues, adiponectin receptors have differing affinities for specific forms of adiponectin. In the reproductive tissues the affinities for specific forms of adiponectin is unknown. However, in these tissues, adiponectin regulates different biological effects through various signalling pathways. ⇧ Increase/stimulation. ⇩ Decrease/inhibition.

2.2.2. The Other Adiponectin Receptors

The T-cadherin receptor protein has been identified as a receptor for the MMW and HMW forms of adiponectin [47]. This membrane receptor does not have an intracellular domain. Thus, T-cadherin could regulate the bioavailability of adiponectin, rather than exerting its own effects [22]. Indeed, mice deficient in T-cadherin have increased circulating adiponectin levels, especially of the HMW form [48]. Some data also suggest that there are other AdipoR isoforms still unknown to date. AdipoR-independent effects of adiponectin have been observed in hypothalamic cells expressing the AdipoR1 and AdipoR2 receptors. Similarly, macrophages whose expression of AdipoR1, AdipoR2 and T-cadherin have been invalidated by interfering RNA still show biological effects of adiponectin [49].

2.2.3. APPL1 and APPL2

Adiponectin induces activation of many signalling pathways. However, adiponectin receptors do not appear to exhibit kinase or phosphorylation domains. Indeed the targeted mutagenesis of tyrosine residues of these receptors does not induce disruption of adiponectin signalling [50]. Thus, the activation of the transduction pathways following the binding of adiponectin to its receptor involves intermediate molecules binding to adiponectin receptors in response to their conformational change. The protein APPL1 (Adaptor protein, phosphotyrosine interacting with PH (Pleckstrin Homology) domain and leucine zipper 1) has thus been identified as an adapter protein capable of binding to the intracellular domains of AdipoR1 and AdipoR2 receptors [50] (Figure 3). The binding of the APPL1 protein to adiponectin receptors is regulated by a second adapter protein, the APPL2 protein (Figure 3). In the absence of adiponectin signal, APPL2 can bind to the N-terminal domain of the adiponectin receptors or it can form an APPL1/APPL2 heterodimer which prevents the APPL1/adiponectin receptors binding [22]. On the other hand, the binding of adiponectin to its receptors favours the dissociation of this heterodimer. Thus the APPL proteins regulate the adiponectin signal according to the Yin and Yang model proposed by Wang et al. [49,51].

2.2.4. Signalling Pathways Regulated by Adiponectin

Upon binding to its receptors, adiponectin activates different signalling pathways in various cell types: mitogen-activated protein kinase (MAPK), such as p38 and extracellular signal-regulated kinases 1/2 (ERK1/2); serine/threonine protein kinase (Akt); and AMP-activated protein kinase (AMPK). It is also able to phosphorylate the transcription factor, peroxisome proliferator-activated receptor alpha (PPARα). Thus, adiponectin regulates through these signalling pathways different functions in the organism [19,22]. Figure 3 shows some examples of cell signalling pathways regulated in reproductive tissues or cells.

3. Expression, Regulation and Effect of Adiponectin and Adiponectin Receptors in the Hypothalamic–Pituitary Axis

The hypothalamic–pituitary–gonadal (HPG) axis plays a critical role in regulating reproductive function. Gonadotropin-releasing hormone (GnRH), which is secreted by the hypothalamus, acts on pituitary gonadotrophs to stimulate luteinising hormone (LH) and follicle-stimulating hormone (FSH) synthesis and secretion, ultimately affecting the animal's fertility. Adiponectin and its AdipoR1 and AdipoR2 receptors are expressed in the human hypothalamus and pituitary [52,53]. Adiponectin appears to play an important role in regulating the activity of hypothalamic–pituitary axis, because its deficiency disrupts FSH and LH secretion as well as LH surge [54]. Adiponectin mutation also causes significant reduction in GnRH immunoreactive neurons, which helps explain the disrupted estrous cyclicity and ovarian functions [54].

3.1. Adiponectin and Hypothalamus: A Role in the Fertility Regulation?

Adiponectin receptors expression in the hypothalamus has been observed in many species, including humans, rodents and pigs [52,55,56]. Adiponectin is also present in the human, mice and rat cerebrospinal fluid (CSF), suggesting an autocrine or paracrine action of this adipokine on the hypothalamic–pituitary axis [52,57,58]. In the CSF, the adiponectin trimer is the predominate form [57]. In addition, studies in mice show that peripheral intravenous application of adiponectin leads to a concurrent rise in CSF adiponectin [59]. Therefore, adiponectin does cross the blood–brain barrier, although concentrations in the CSF are approximately 1000-fold lower than that in serum [57]. Cerebrospinal fluid concentrations of adiponectin are increased during fasting and decreased after refeeding in rodent and sheep [31,32].

In the hypothalamus, GnRH neurons are key components of the reproductive axis, controlling the synthesis and release of gonadotropins. In vitro studies have notably described an inhibitory effect of adiponectin on the secretion of GnRH by hypothalamic cells through activation of AMPK [60]. Indeed, in GT1-7 cells (subset strains of GT1 cell lines) adiponectin inhibits GnRH secretion but also suppresses *KISS1* mRNA transcription [61,62]. Kisspeptins are hypothalamic neuropeptides discovered in the

2000s. The binding of kisspeptins to their KISS1-R receptors appears to be the mechanism that triggers puberty by inducing secretion of GnRH.

Thus, adiponectin appears to decrease the secretion of GnRH via the reduction of the signal emitted by kisspeptins. A more recent study showed that AdipoR2 was expressed in mouse GnRH neurons and adiponectin rapidly decreased GnRH neuronal activity in a subpopulation of GnRH neurons via a PKCζ/LKB1/AMPK signalling cascade [63].

3.2. Adiponectin and Pituitary: A Role in the Fertility Regulation?

Adiponectin and its receptors were also described in the pituitary of various species including human, mouse, rat, chicken and pig [53,64–66]. In human, adiponectin was present mainly in growth hormone (GH)-, follicle-stimulating hormone (FSH)-, luteinising hormone (LH)- and thyroid-stimulating hormone (TSH)-producing cells, whereas adiponectin receptors were located in the gonadotrophs, somatotrophs and thyrotrophs, but not in corticotrophs or lactotrophs. [53]. In cultured rat and mouse pituitary cells, adiponectin inhibited basal and GnRH-induced LH secretion [64,67]. Furthermore, it decreased the expression of the gene encoding the GnRH receptor (GnRH-R) [64]. In the porcine primary pituitary cells, adiponectin increased basal FSH release [66]. In this latter study, adiponectin also modulated GnRH and insulin-induced LH and FSH secretion dependently on the stage of the oestrous cycle. At the opposite, Sarmento-Cabral A et al., 2017 showed recently that adiponectin did not affect LH and FSH release by primary pituitary cell cultures from two normal nonhuman-primate species [68].

The presence of adiponectin receptors in the GnRH neurons and pituitary cells, and its influence on the GnRH, LH and FSH release suggests an important role of adiponectin at the hypothalamic–pituitary axis in the control of fertility in both male and female. Both LH and FSH ultimately control gonadal function. In female, ovarian follicles are stimulated by FSH to grow and mature; LH stimulates ovulation and corpus luteum formation. In men, FSH initiates, and in conjunction with high intratesticular testosterone, sustains spermatogenesis, whereas LH controls androgen synthesis by the testicular Leydig cells. As described below, adiponectin system is expressed and regulates gonadal functions.

4. Expression, Regulation and Effect of Adiponectin in Gonads

4.1. Expression, Regulation and Effect of Adiponectin System in Ovary

The involvement of adiponectin in ovary of multiple species has already been well reviewed by our and other groups [69,70]. Here we briefly summarise the major published works with an emphasis on differences between human, rodents and agronomic species.

4.1.1. Plasma and Follicular Fluids Profiles

Adiponectin is detected in follicular fluids (FF). Adiponectin levels are higher in FF than in plasma in women [71], and the opposite is observed in cows [30]. In human, FF adiponectin concentrations are positively correlated with the serum values [71–73]. In addition to the differences in adiponectin concentrations, adiponectin isoform distribution varies between the serum and FF compartments in women. Indeed, the HMW fraction is significantly higher in serum than in FF [72]. Moreover, adiponectin levels are lower in FF from women with repeated implantation failures [74]. Taken together, all these data suggest that ovarian cells could produce adiponectin and FF adiponectin could be involved in the success of the techniques of medical assistance to procreation.

4.1.2. Expression in Ovarian Cells

In granulosa cells, adiponectin expression is low and almost undetectable in humans, rodents and chickens [17,69]. However, adiponectin is strongly produced by human theca cells and even more so during follicular maturation. In contrast, the expression of AdipoR1 and AdipoR2 is greater in granulosa cells than in theca cells of hens [17]. In addition, adiponectin, AdipoR1 and AdipoR2 are present in the corpus luteum of mammalian species (human, rat, cow and sows) [69]. In avian species, the expression of adiponectin in granulosa cells is positively correlated with the weight of F3 preovulatory follicle and is upregulated in ovarian tissues during the laying period compared with the prelaying period [75,76].

4.1.3. Regulation by Physiologic Status

As adiponectin system was simultaneously involved in metabolism and reproduction, modulation of the body energy status may regulate their expression in ovarian tissues. The expression pattern of adiponectin and its receptors increases in bovine granulosa cell during follicular development and the opposite was observed in bovine theca cells [77]. In human, stable levels of plasma adiponectin have been observed during the phases of the physiological menstrual cycle [78], whereas Galván and coworkers have shown lower plasma adiponectin levels in the luteal than in the follicular and the mid-cycle phase [79]. So, the plasma adiponectin profile is contradictory during the menstrual cycle in women. In pig, both gene and protein expression of adiponectin are enhanced during the luteal phase of the cycle [20]. More recently, we demonstrated that the plasma adiponectin concentration is higher in cows fed high energy diets than cows fed low energy diets presenting reproductive defects [29]. In sheep, feeding restriction increases circulating level of adiponectin and the expression level of both AdipoR1 and AdipoR2 in ovary [32]. On the other hand, the expression of AdipoR1 and AdipoR2 is decreased in theca cells of hens fed with fish oil supplementation, while the expression of AdipoR2 is increased in restricted hens [76]. Thus, adiponectin system is modulated by the energy status in various species.

4.1.4. Regulation by Hormones

Hormones may regulate the production and action of adiponectin at different levels: adiponectin secretion, adiponectin receptor expression and cellular responses. In humans, LH treatment increases the level of adiponectin FF as well as in theca and granulosa cells [20,69,80,81]. In addition, FSH and hCG (a substitute for LH) treatment contribute to activate LH receptors and consequently upregulate by more than 2-fold the expression of AdipoR2 (but not AdipoR1) in human granulosa cells [69]. Conversely, an hCG injection increases the expression of adiponectin and AdipoR1 (but not AdipoR2) genes in rat ovaries [17,69]. Furthermore, the expression of AdipoR2 is increased by LH and reduced by IGF1 in bovine theca cells [69,82].

4.1.5. Effect on Steroidogenesis

Adiponectin can modulate and mediate the actions of hormones production by ovarian cells. In mammals, numerous studies have shown beneficial effects of adiponectin on various physiological functions. The work published by our team has clearly demonstrated an effect of adiponectin on the steroidogenesis of ovarian cells trough variability across species. In human granulosa cells, adiponectin enhances the secretion of progesterone and oestradiol in the presence of FSH or IGF-1 [71,83]. Furthermore, depletion of adiponectin gene in mice disturbs steroidogenesis, follicular development and reduces fertility [54]. In cattle, adiponectin inhibits insulin-induced steroidogenesis in granulosa and theca cells [82,84]. In hens, adiponectin increases IGF-1-induced progesterone production by granulosa cells from F2 and F3/4 follicles and decreases LH or FSH-induced production by granulosa cells from F3/4 follicles [17].

Adiponectin also inhibits synthesis androgens including androstenedione in the murine ovary [85], as described in Section 9.1.1. In women with polycystic ovary syndrome, characterised by hyperandrogenism, circulating levels of adiponectin are decreased [86]. Adiponectin and its receptors are also present in the male reproductive tract.

4.2. Expression, Regulation and Effect of Adiponectin System in Testis

4.2.1. Blood Plasma and Seminal Fluid Profiles

Seminal fluid (SF) is the male body fluid related to reproduction. It contains adiponectin at concentrations approximately 66- and 180-fold lower than serum in men and bulls, respectively [30,87]. In addition, a positive correlation between the adiponectin concentrations in both SF and blood plasma was observed suggesting that adiponectin is transferred from the blood to testis tissue, particularly via gaps in the blood–testis barrier.

4.2.2. Expression in Testicular Cells

Adiponectin and adiponectin receptors are expressed in human testes and more precisely in the Leydig cells. Adiponectin receptors are also present in the spermatozoa [88–90]. AdipoR2 null mice demonstrated atrophic seminiferous tubules with aspermia (lack of semen) and enlarged brains, but displayed normal testosterone levels; whether these testicular defects reflect central or peripheral responses to the loss of AdipoR2 signalling remains unknown [91]. Expression of adiponectin and its receptors (AdipoR1 and AdipoR2) declines significantly in the testis of old mice [92].

Thus, an adequate concentration of adiponectin and its receptors may be required for normal testicular functions and adiponectin treatment could be a promising antiageing therapy promoting normal reproductive activities in the testis of aging mice.

4.2.3. Regulation by Physiologic Status

In chicken, the expression of AdipoR1 and AdipoR2 mRNA is modified during the puberty; the expression of these two mRNA is increased in adulthood compared to prepubertal animals [93]. This suggests that the sexual maturation induces an upregulation of testicular adiponectin receptors genes expressions. AdipoR2 protein expression is also increased in Leydig cells during the puberty in rats [89,94] and mouse making the cells more sensitive to circulating adiponectin. Moreover, in the mouse, it has been shown that the serum concentration of adiponectin is also increased during this period [24,95].

4.2.4. Regulation by Hormones

Several studies have shown a link between the steroid secretion and adiponectin. For example, an ablation of gonads in adult male mice led to an increase of circulating adiponectin [95,96]. However, when an injection of testosterone was performed on the same animals, the levels of circulating adiponectin were restored [96]. In men with hypogonadism, high concentrations of serum adiponectin were reduced by androgen supplementation [97]. A study in the rat has shown a relationship between testosterone and adiponectin. In this study, a developmental exposure to isoflavones has increased serum adiponectin levels and decreased serum testosterone levels [94]. The testis extract from the pig, enhanced adiponectin secretion in adipocyte through the peroxisome proliferator-activated receptor signalling pathway [98]. Taken together, these studies suggest that a reciprocal relationship and a possible regulation exist between gonadal steroid hormones and adipose tissue-derived factors.

4.2.5. Effect on Steroidogenesis, Lactate Production and Cytokine-Mediated Cytotoxicity

Adiponectin regulates both spermatogenesis and steroidogenesis in adult testis via its two receptors, AdipoR1 and AdipoR2 [89,99]. Indeed, in vitro experiments showed that adiponectin acted directly in Leydig cells to decrease androgen secretion, which was associated with inhibition of the StAR protein in Leydig cells [94].

Following adiponectin binding, AdipoR1 and AdipoR2 activate downstream targets such as AMPK, PPAR-α, and MAPK [19]. In the testis, AMPK and PPAR-α signalling pathways have been shown to be functional and involved in the regulation of steroidogenesis [100]. Therefore, adiponectin could interact through these signalling pathways to alter testosterone production.

However, adiponectin did not modulate anti-Mullerian hormone (AMH) transcript levels [101]. Another important role of adiponectin is to maintain insulin sensitivity by stimulating glucose uptake in the testes [99]. Indeed, intratesticular glucose level was shown to be associated with testicular functions like testosterone production [102]. Furthermore, adiponectin administration ameliorates testicular mass and functions in aged mice by enhanced expression of insulin receptor, antioxidative enzyme activity, testosterone synthesis and glucose and lactate uptake by enhanced expression of transporters GLUT8 (glucose transporter) and MCT2 & MCT4 (lactate transporters) [92].

As potent anti-inflammatory mediators, adiponectin has been demonstrated to protect Leydig cells against cytokine-mediated cytotoxicity, acting as a testicular defence mechanism to attenuate the negative impact of proinflammatory molecules, particularly those released by macrophages (e.g., interleukin 1 (IL-1), tumour necrosis factor alpha (TNF-α) and interferon gamma (IFN-γ)) on steroidogenesis [103].

Thus, while adiponectin signalling appears to be present in male gonadal tissue, the extent to which this signalling contributes to normal testicular function and fertility potential need to be clarified.

5. Expression, Regulation and Effect of Adiponectin System in Gametogenesis (Oocyte and Spermatozoa)

5.1. Oocyte

The expression of adiponectin (gene and protein) was found in the oocytes of rats [17] and cows [77,84], whereas that of AdipoR1 and AdipoR2 has been shown in oocytes of cows [84], pigs [104], goats [105] and rats [17]. Several studies have shown that adiponectin supplementation during in vitro maturation (IVM) of human, mouse, goat and swine oocytes exerts positive effects on meiotic progression and initial embryonic development [104,106,107] (Figure 4A). In goat oocytes, adiponectin has a positive effect on the meiotic maturation through the classical MAPK pathway [105]. In contrast, no significant effects of adiponectin were observed on bovine IVM, cleavage and blastocyst formation rates [84] (Figure 4A). These results indicate that species differences may exist with regard to the specific oocyte response to adiponectin. In human, a decrease in DNA methylation levels in the promoter of adiponectin has been described in response to glucose IVM exposed to 10 mM glucose as compared to controls [108].

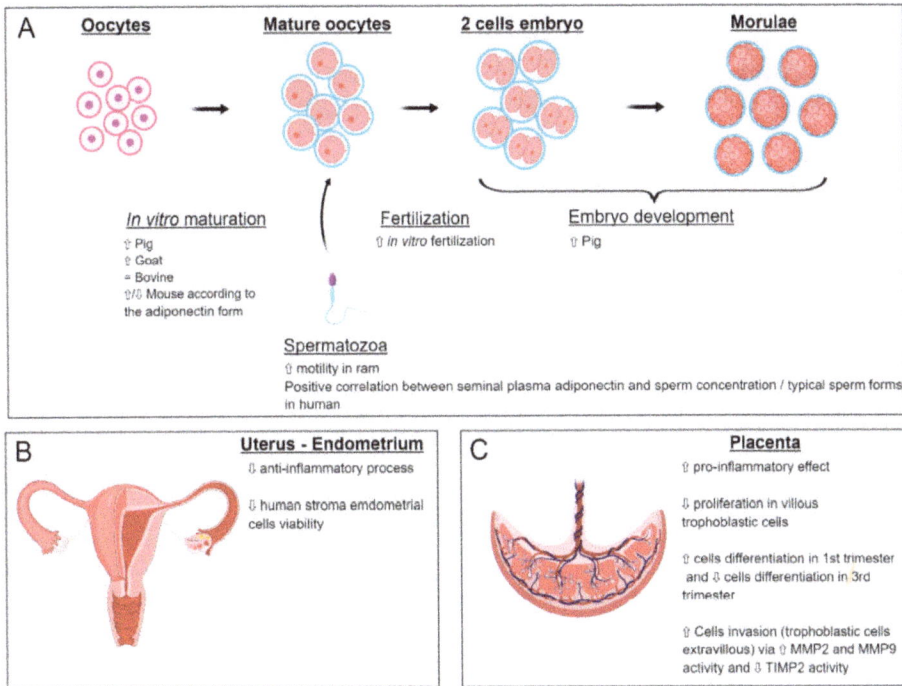

Figure 4. Effects of adiponectin on in vitro maturation and embryo development (**A**), uterus (**B**) and placenta (**C**). ⇧ Increase/stimulation. ⇩ Decrease/inhibition. = no effect.

5.2. Spermatozoa

5.2.1. Localisation of Adiponectin and Its Receptor

The presence of adiponectin receptors on spermatozoa has been reported by Kawwass et al. 2015 [70]. In bulls, adiponectin is abundantly found on flagellum whereas AdipoR1 can be observed particularly on the equatorial and acrosome regions, and AdipoR2 on the sperm head region and on equatorial line [109].

5.2.2. Role of Adiponectin on Sperm Motility and Capacitation

In bull, plasma adiponectin concentration and spermatozoa mRNA abundances for AdipoR1 and AdipoR2 are positively related to sire conception rate [109]. In ram, an association between adiponectin and its receptors and sperm motility parameters has been reported [110] (Figure 4A). In human, adiponectin levels in seminal plasma have been shown to be positively correlated with sperm concentration, sperm count and percentage of typical sperm forms [87] (Figure 4A). After capacitation, the levels of adiponectin and its receptors are lowered, suggesting a direct role on sperm motility [87].

6. Expression, Regulation and Effect of Adiponectin System in Embryo Development and Implantation: The Evolution of the Adiponectin System during Pregnancy

6.1. Adiponectin System during Embryo Development

Adiponectin and its receptors are expressed in embryos at different stages of development, in different species of mammals, chickens and fishes [111,112].

Kim et al. (2011) demonstrated, in mouse, the expression of adiponectin mRNA in 2-cell and 8-cell embryos [113]. The receptors were detected at all stages of the preimplantation embryo, although levels were lowest at the blastocyst stage. AdipoR1 mRNA level was raised in 8- to 16-cell embryos. In morulas and blastocysts, the level of adipoR1 mRNA was significantly higher than in oocytes. AdipoR2 mRNA level was lower in 4-cell embryos and 8- to 16-cells embryos than in oocytes, and significantly increased in morulas and blastocysts [114]. By in situ hybridisation, adiponectin mRNA was detected in the mouse embryo at day 7 and day 8. In bovine embryo, AdipoR1 was clearly expressed but AdipoR2 and adiponectin were weakly present and undetectable, respectively [84].

The effects of adiponectin on in vitro oocyte maturation and early embryo development were assessed in different species (Figure 4A). In bovine, when culture medium of embryos was supplemented with recombinant adiponectin, any effect of adiponectin was observed in the 48 h-cleavage and day 8 blastocyst rates [84]. In mouse, when 4-cell embryos were cultured in vitro and supplemented with 10 µg/mL of different isoforms of adiponectin, most of the embryos in all groups reached the blastocyst stage; however, the full-length and the trimeric isoforms had opposite effects on the embryo distribution. With the full-length isoform, the proportion of embryos with lower cell numbers decreased while the proportion of embryos with high cell numbers increased. Opposite results were observed with the trimeric isoform [114]. In pig, when oocytes were matured in vitro in medium alone, and then cultured for 7 days with adiponectin, development to the blastocyst stage was significantly improved compared to the control group (medium alone). These results provide evidence that adiponectin has positive effects in both oocyte maturation and embryo culture in this species [104] (Figure 4A). Furthermore, a recent study shows that in pig embryos, the methylation level of AdipoR2 increased in response to female nutritional restriction [115], suggesting that the nutritional status of the mother can affect the adiponectin system in the offspring.

Mammalian preimplantation embryos contain lipid droplets [116] that serve as an energy source. They influence cell–cell interactions, cell proliferation and intracellular transport mechanisms [117]. However, excess lipid accumulation above the normal level is linked with impaired embryo quality due to cellular dysfunction and/or cell death caused by increased lipid peroxidation and mitochondrial dysfunction. In rabbit, adiponectin regulates embryonic lipid metabolism by AMPK signalling [118].

6.2. Evolution of Serum Adiponectin during Pregnancy

After several controversies, it is now well established that adiponectin is not a placental hormone [119,120]. Maternal adiponectinemia is constant throughout pregnancy and results mainly from adipocyte production. However, a decrease in circulating adiponectin levels is observed after delivery [121]. This suggests that placental factors contribute to increased adiponectinemia early in pregnancy and persist until parturition. It has also been shown that the HMW form of adiponectin is present in the bloodstream of the pregnant woman compared to the nonpregnant woman [122].

7. Expression, Regulation and Effect of Adiponectin System in Endometrium, Placenta and Relation between the Foetus and Mother

7.1. Expression and Effects of Adiponectin on Uterine Functions

The role of adiponectin in the endometrium is relatively unknown. The AdipoR1, AdipoR2 and adiponectin receptors themselves are present in this tissue [123,124]. A variation in AdipoR1 and AdipoR2 protein expression was measured during the menstrual cycle. Specifically, this expression is maximal in the middle of the secretory phase of the cycle, corresponding to the period of uterine receptivity to the embryo [123]. This study therefore suggests an important role of the adiponectin signal during human embryonic implantation. This hypothesis has been reinforced by a study showing that the endometrium of women with repeated implantation failures underexpresses AdipoR1 and AdipoR2 compared to fertile endometrium [124]. Adiponectin would also exert an anti-inflammatory effect in the endometrium by inhibiting the production of proinflammatory cytokines such as IL-6, IL-8 and MCP-1 (monocyte chemotactic protein-1) [123]. Finally, adiponectin decreases cell viability of human endometrial cells [125] (Figure 4B).

7.2. Expression and Effects of Adiponectin on the Placenta

Adiponectin appears to exert an endocrine action (via adipose tissue) or paracrine (via the endometrium) in the placenta. Thus, it regulates many placental processes:

- Inflammatory Response:

Interestingly, while its anti-inflammatory role has been described in many organs, including the endometrium, it appears that adiponectin exerts a proinflammatory effect in the third trimester placenta. Adiponectin induces the production of CD24 and Siglec-10 inflammatory molecules and interleukins IL-8 and IL-1β by trophoblasts derived from term placenta [126]. These proinflammatory effects were also observed during the in vitro culture of placental explants of the third trimester, in the presence of adiponectin. The authors observed an increase in the secretion of interleukins IL-6 and IL-1β and TNF-α via the NF-κB pathway [127]. These factors may be necessary to trigger the immunotolerance phenomenon in the mother (Figure 4C).

- Cell Proliferation

Adiponectin exerts its "classic" role of antiproliferative hormone in villous trophoblastic cells in the first trimester [128]. These results are also observed in the placenta at term, where adiponectin reduces the number of cells entering into mitosis by control of the MAPK pathway [129] (Figure 4C).

- Cell Differentiation

Adiponectin stimulates the biochemical (secretion of hCG and leptin secretion) and morphological (increased expression of syncytin-2 and decreased expression of E-cadherin) differentiation of first-trimester villous trophoblasts early (obtained before the arrival of the blood in the intervillous chamber) [120]. On the other hand, it inhibits the biochemical differentiation of villous trophoblastic cells from "late" first-trimester placentas and third-trimester placentas [119,130]. However, it has no effect on morphological differentiation in the term placenta [130] (Figure 4C).

- Cellular Invasion

Adiponectin increases the invasive abilities of trophoblastic cells by stimulating the activity of metalloproteases MMP-2 and MMP-9—two major enzymes of the invasion process—which digest the extracellular matrix of the endometrium. These enzymes thus promote the migration of trophoblastic cells within the deciduous. At the same time, adiponectin decreases the expression of the metalloprotease inhibitor, TIMP-2 [119] (Figure 4C).

7.3. Relation between Foetus and Mother

Recurrent spontaneous abortion (RSA) is associated with abnormal maternal tolerance to the semiallogenic foetus. A recent study shows that recombinant adiponectin therapy improves pregnancy outcome in a murine model of abortion by expanding the Treg cell population and function and decreasing the Th17 cell population and function via a p38MAPK-STAT5 pathway. This therapy reduced the abortion rate in abortion-prone model. Recombinant adiponectin administration induced the expression of AdipoR1 and AdipoR2 mRNA at the maternofetal interface [131].

Throughout the entire first trimester of pregnancy, foetal growth is sustained by endometrial secretions, i.e., histiotrophic nutrition. Endometrial stromal cells (EnSCs) accumulate and secrete a variety of nutritive molecules which are absorbed by trophoblastic cells and transmitted to the foetus. Glycogen appears to have a critical role in the early stages of foetal development, since infertile women have low endometrial glycogen levels. Duval et al., 2018 showed that adiponectin exerts a dual role at the foetal–maternal interface by promoting glycogen synthesis in the endometrium and conversely reducing trophoblastic glycogen uptake [132].

8. Foetus Growth

It has been observed in a mouse model that the injection of adiponectin into the mother induces a reduction in the foetal growth of young mice [133]. In humans, a negative correlation between maternal adiponectinemia and infant weight has also been observed [134]. This effect of adiponectin on foetal growth may be related to the effects of this adipokine on the expression of nutrient transporters in the placenta. Indeed, adiponectin inhibits the expression of amino acid transporters (SNAT) in the human placenta at term [135]. In the same way in the pregnant rat, adiponectin reduces the expression of the GLUT3 glucose transporter and that of lipoprotein lipase transporting fatty acids in the placenta [136]. Similar results were observed in the mouse. Indeed, chronic administration of adiponectin during pregnancy reduces placental transport of amino acids in this species [133]. Thus, by inhibiting the transport of nutrients, adiponectin appears to negatively regulate foetal growth.

It has been suggested that the hyper-growth pattern of the foetus when there is maternal obesity may be due to the relatively lesser maternal concentrations of total and HMW adiponectin. This endocrine and physiological paradigm may result in increased insulin and mammalian target of rapamycin complex 1 (mTORC1) placental signalling, as well as an upregulation of transplacental glucose and sodium-coupled neutral amino acid transporters (GLUT and SNAT) [133,137,138]. Furthermore, nutrients available for foetal growth are greater when there is maternal hypoadiponectinemia and insulin resistance [139,140].

In pregnancies where there are not symptomatic problems, increased maternal adiponectin regulates foetal growth [135]. As pregnancy progresses, the physiologic decrease in adiponectin concentrations, as well as insulin sensitivity, result in increased amounts of nutrients from the maternal to foetal circulation, increasing foetal growth [133,135,138]. With maternal obesity or gestational diabetes, total and HMW concentrations of adiponectin, however, are relatively less, even before pregnancy as compared to when the obesity condition does not exist [140]. Hypoadiponectinemia exacerbates the loss of insulin sensitivity and the increases in nutrient partitioning from the maternal to foetal circulation, resulting in larger foetuses and macrosomic babies [140–142]. The body weight of foetuses from adiponectin $(-/-)$ dams was significantly greater than that of wild type dams at both embryonic day (E)14.5 and (E)18.5. In addition to nutrient supply, maternal adiponectin inhibits foetal growth by increasing IGFBP-1 expression in trophoblast cells [143].

9. Adiponectin and Reproductive Diseases:

Diseases associated with abnormal adiponectin levels are polycycstic ovary syndrome, ovarian and endometrial cancer, endometriosis, gestational diseases, preeclampsia and foetal growth restriction, all of which are associated with subfertility.

9.1. Ovarian Pathologies

9.1.1. Polycystic Ovary Syndrome (PCOS)

Polycystic ovary syndrome (PCOS) is a very common endocrinopathy affecting 6 to 13% of women of reproductive age and one of the leading causes of female poor fertility [144]. Since Rotterdam Consensus Conference in 2003, its diagnosis requires the presence of at least two of the following features; oligo-/anovulation, hyperandrogenism and polycystic ovaries on ultrasound (corresponding to a follicle number per ovary ≥ 20 and/or an ovarian volume ≥ 10 mL in either ovary) [145]. PCOS is frequently associated with insulin resistance (IR), abdominal obesity [146] and an increased risk of developing type 2 diabetes since as many as 10% of women with PCOS develop diabetes by the age of 40 years [147]. Hyperandrogenism is the other main feature of the syndrome with elevated circulating androgen levels observed in 60 to 80% of PCOS patients [148]. Development of hyperandrogenism happens in part because high insulin levels and free insulin growth factor (IGF) stimulate androgens production by ovarian theca cells [149]. Furthermore, an increase in abdominal adipose tissue, stimulated by compensatory hyperinsulinemia, creates an imbalance in sex steroids with decreased sex hormone binding globulin (SHBG) levels and increased free androgens levels [149]. Although IR and hyperandrogenaemia are the essential abnormalities of the syndrome, mounting evidence supports that also genetic factors play a key role in PCOS pathogenesis [150].

The implication of adiponectin in energy metabolism as an insulin-sensitising, antiatherogenic and anti-inflammatory molecule is largely admitted. Notably, obesity and insulin-resistant states have been associated with reduced plasma adiponectin concentrations [146]. In women with PCOS, adiponectin signalling in adipose tissue seems to be impaired with decreased expression of AdipoR1 and AdipoR2, suggesting that adiponectin dysregulation may be one of the possible mechanisms responsible for lessening insulin-sensitivity [147] (Figure 6). As accumulating evidence supports a direct role of this adipokine in female reproductive tissues, altered adiponectin levels could thus be causally involved in both the reproductive and metabolic disturbances associated with PCOS (Figure 5A,B).

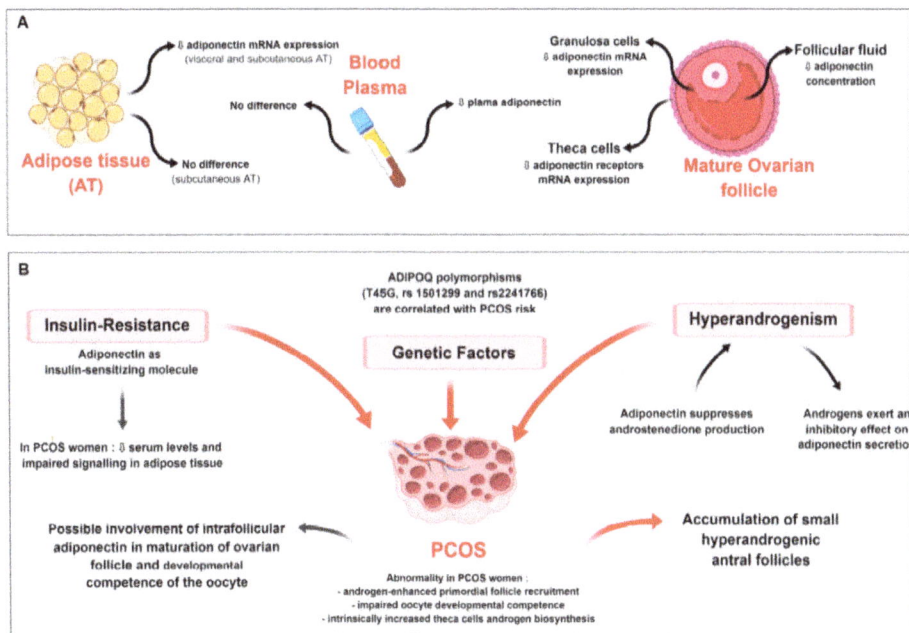

Figure 5. (**A**) Adiponectin system in ovary (granulosa and theca cells and follicular fluid), plasma and adipose tissue (AT) in polycystic ovary syndrome (PCOS) patient as compared to control. (**B**) Description of PCOS syndrome and possible involvement of adiponectin in this syndrome. ⇣ Decrease/inhibition.

According to two meta-analyses [146,151], after controlling for BMI-related effects, serum adiponectin concentrations in PCOS women are lower than in non-PCOS controls. Notably, HMW adiponectin appears to be selectively reduced in women with PCOS independently of IR severity [152] (Figure 5). Nevertheless, other studies found no difference in adiponectin plasma levels between PCOS patients and controls [153–156]. Similarly, data concerning adiponectin expression in adipose tissue are controversial. Carmina et al. demonstrated that adiponectin mRNA levels were reduced in visceral and subcutaneous (SC) adipose tissue of PCOS patients compared to controls [101], while no changes of adiponectin expression in SC fat were found by Lecke et al. and Svendsen et al. [155,156] (Figure 5A).

Regarding the reproductive tissues, adiponectin concentration in follicular fluid (FF) is decreased in PCOS women [157–159]. In PCOS and control groups, a strong positive correlation was observed between HMW adiponectin concentrations in serum and FF samples [158]. Intrafollicular HMW adiponectin levels were 2 times lower than in plasma, suggesting a combined effect endocrine factors, including insulin and gonadotropins, rather than passive diffusion result [157]. Compared to normal ovaries, in PCOS a lower proportion of theca cells expresses adiponectin receptors [147] and granulosa cells show decreased expression of adiponectin, APPL1 [160], AdipoR1 and AdipoR2, possibly affecting follicular development and selection of a dominant follicle [158].

The downregulation of adiponectin expression in PCOS women may contribute to their characteristically lower insulin sensitivity [101] and even contribute to the hyperandrogenic environment (Figure 5B). Indeed, adiponectin suppresses production of androstenedione and key enzymes of the androgen synthesis pathway in mice ovaries [85] and cultured human theca cells [147]. Further, in granulosa cells, it increases the expression of the enzymes involved in oestradiol and progesterone synthesis [17], enhancing aromatase activity and limiting androgens production by theca cells. On the other hand, the inhibitory effect of testosterone on adiponectin synthesis has been suggested by the sexual dimorphism observed in humans, with adiponectin concentrations significantly higher in women than in men [21], and confirmed in castrated rats [161]. Similarly, in hypogonadal men, elevated adiponectin levels are reduced to rates similar to healthy individuals by a testosterone replacement therapy [97]. In vitro, androgens suppress adiponectin expression by decreasing its secretion [21], but treatment of adipose tissue with testosterone and oestradiol increases the expression of AdipoR1 and AdipoR2 [162]. According to this observation, in women with PCOS, possibly as the result of high levels of androgens, adiponectin receptors are upregulated in both subcutaneous and visceral fats, this may be a compensatory mechanism to achieve some insulin sensitivity [162] (Figure 5B).

The existence of a potentially causal relationship between adiponectin and PCOS is strengthened by genomic studies. At first, a single nucleotide polymorphism of human adiponectin precursor gene (ADIPOQ)—T45G—has been investigated in relation to PCOS, and a statistically definable correlation between the occurrence of this gene form and the ovarian disorder was found [163]. More recently, others two functional ADIPOQ polymorphisms—rs1501299 and rs2241766—were reported to be significantly correlated with PCOS risk in Caucasian women [150]. Specifically, the ADIPOQ rs2241766 TT genotype [164] and the G allele of rs1501299 [165] were associated with a significantly increased risk of developing PCOS. As previous studies have found that the presumably "protective" T allele of rs1501299 was accompanied by higher adiponectin expression, this observation further supports the hypothesis that decreased adiponectin levels are associated with PCOS [165].

Finally, data from clinical investigations in PCOS women confirm adiponectin relevant role in the physiopathology of this syndrome. Thus, Mohammadi et al. demonstrated that 8-week omega-3 fatty acid supplementation in overweight and obese PCOS patients significantly increased the mean baseline levels of adiponectin and concomitantly decreased IR [166]. This effect of omega-3 fatty acids on adiponectin has been recently confirmed by Yang et al. They also reported a significant decrease in total cholesterol, triglycerides and LDL-cholesterol, resulting in a global beneficial effect on cardiometabolic risk factors characteristic of PCOS women [167]. Further, using a dehydroepiandrosterone (DHEA)-treated PCOS mouse model, Singh et al. showed that exogenous adiponectin treatment enhanced the ovarian expression of insulin receptors and decreased theca androgen synthesis [168], which was accompanied by restored ovulation and normalised circulating androgens and glucose levels [169]. Thus, systemic adiponectin treatment could be even a promising therapeutic aid for PCOS management.

9.1.2. Ovarian Cancers

Ovarian cancer is the most lethal gynaecologic malignancy among women, with an estimated 150,000 annual deaths [170]. However, due to the unspecific and inconspicuous symptoms in the early stage of ovarian cancer, there are no effective and accurate detection methods for this disease [171]. There are many types of ovarian cancer that originate from different ovarian cell types [172], including mucinous ovarian cancer, epithelial ovarian cancer, germ cell cancer, stromal cell cancer (which forms from the cells that secrete female hormones), ovarian endometrioid adenocarcinoma, clear cell carcinoma, squamous cell carcinoma and serous carcinoma [173]. Epithelial ovarian cancer, the most common ovarian malignancy, originates in the epithelial cells on the surface of the ovary and accounts for 85–89% of ovarian cancers. Germ cell cancer accounts for only 5% of ovarian cancers and originates from the cells of any one ovary. This rare cancer affects mainly adolescent girls and young women. Two other rare cancers that account for 7% of all ovarian cancers are interstitial and endocrine ovarian tumours.

Literature data have found that lower adiponectin levels are associated with higher incidence of various human cancers, such as ovarian, endometrial and breast cancers [174,175]. The inhibitory effect of adiponectin on the proliferation of several types of cancer cells has also been reported [176,177]. Brakenhielm et al. (2004) found that adiponectin inhibits primary tumour growth and is linked to decreased angiogenesis [177]. These findings suggest that adiponectin may be the link between obesity and increased cancer risk in women. The expression of AdipoR1 and AdipoR2 has been reported in a human granulosa tumour KGN cell line [83] and in various epithelial ovarian cancer cell lines. Their expression in these cell lines was lower than in the granulosa tumour cell line (COV434) [178]. Li et al. (2017) illustrated that epithelial ovarian cancer patients with AdipoR1-positive expression survived longer than those with AdipoR1-negative expression [179]. The last study of Hoffmann et al. (2018) indicated that adiponectin decreased epithelial ovarian cancer cell proliferation, and that this effect was independent of apoptosis [178]. Nagaraju et al. (2016) proposed that adiponectin action on ovarian cancer can be induced through activation of AMPK/PKA pathway and PPARγ regulation [180].

9.2. Uterine/Endometrial Diseases

9.2.1. Endometriosis and Endometrial Cancer

Endometriosis corresponds to ectopic implantation and a high invasiveness of the endometrial tissue. Some studies have indicated that serum adiponectin level decreases in women with endometriosis [181] and endometrial cancer [182]. Also, adiponectin level in peritoneal fluid of endometriosis patients decreased dramatically in advanced endometriosis [183]. Takemura et al. (2006) compared adiponectin concentrations in serum and peritoneal fluid in women with and without endometriosis [123]. They reported that adiponectin concentrations were lower in women with endometriosis than in those without endometriosis. However, Pandey et al. (2010) observed similar adiponectin levels in women with pelvic endometriosis compared to women without endometriosis [184]. Similar results were reported by Choi et al. (2013), who did not find any difference in the expression of adiponectin or AdipoR in normal endometrium and ovarian endometrioma [185]. Adiponectin inhibit endometrial stromal cell proliferation in dose and time dependant manner, and cause cell death, suggest as antiendometriosis agent [125].

So, adiponectin could be a beneficial factor to limit the endometriosis. However, further studies are necessary to better understand its effects in this gynaecologic disease.

9.2.2. Endometrial Cancer

Endometrial (uterine) cancer starts in the layer of cells that form the lining (endometrium) of the uterus. Over 80% of endometrial cancers are adenocarcinomas (endometrioid). Endometrial cancer is most commonly found in women 55 years and older and rarely occurs in women below 45 years of age [180]. Women with high leptin levels, lower circulating levels of adiponectin in serum due to obesity, hyperinsulinaemia, and high leptin/adiponectin ratio have the highest risk of developing endometrial cancer [186]. Several study documented that adiponectin and obesity act independently in promoting endometrial cancer [187,188]. High circulating levels of adiponectin are related to a reduced risk of developing endometrial cancer, independent of the other risk factors such as insulin resistance and hypothyroidism that cause obesity [189]. The effect of adiponectin and obesity, synergistically, was associated with a 6-fold increase in the risk of developing endometrial cancer. Study of Hyun-Seuk Moon et al. documented that the adiponectin receptors expression is similar in normal and cancerous tissues, but AdipoR1 was higher than that AdipoR2 in the human endometrial cancer cell lines KLE and RL95-2 [190]. Moon et al. hypothesised that adiponectin mediates activation of the AMPK pathway by LKB1 (an adapter molecule with growth-suppressing effects on tumour cells) [190]. Adiponectin-mediated AMPK activation inhibits cell proliferation, colony formation, and adhesion and invasion properties of endometrial cancer cells [191], and inhibits angiogenesis and the neovascularisation process in mouse [177]. Decreased expression of cyclin D1 and E2, different pro-growth regulators of cell cycle, and the signalling proteins ERK1/2 and Akt are all associated with PTEN (phosphatase tensin homolog, tumour suppressor gene) activity and LKB1-mediated adiponectin signalling in inhibiting endometrial carcinogenesis. These results suggest that additional studies are needed to determine the significance of adiponectin and adiponectin receptors as prognostic markers and therapeutic targets in endometrial cancer [180].

9.3. Gestational Pathologies

9.3.1. Gestational Diabetes Mellitus (Figure 6)

Gestational diabetes mellitus (GDM) is defined as "diabetes first diagnosed in the second or third trimester of pregnancy that was not clearly overt diabetes prior to gestation" [192]. According to last International Diabetes Federation estimation, it affects approximately 14% of pregnancies worldwide, representing ←18 million births annually [193]. During pregnancy, GDM can result in serious complications for both mother and child, including preeclampsia, preterm birth, stillbirth, macrosomia and hypoglycaemia in the newborns. Moreover, although it usually resolves following delivery, in the long-term, women with a past history of GDM and babies born of GDM pregnancies are at increased risk of obesity, type 2 diabetes mellitus (T2DM) and cardiovascular diseases [193].

In healthy pregnancy, insulin sensitivity (IS) increases during early gestation to promote glucose uptake into adipose stores in preparation for the energy demands of later pregnancy. As pregnancy progresses, however, IS lessens under the effect of several local and placental hormones. As result, glycaemia is slightly elevated and glucose is readily transported across the placenta to fuel foetal growth. This physiological state of insulin resistance (IR) also promotes endogenous hepatic glucose production and lipolysis in adipose tissue, resulting in a further increase in blood glucose and free fatty acid (FFA) concentrations [193]. Pregnant women compensate for these changes through hypertrophy and hyperplasia of pancreatic β cells, as well as increased glucose-stimulated insulin secretion [194]. Failure of this compensatory response gives raise to maternal hyperglycaemia or GDM [195]. Thus, GDM is usually the result of β cell dysfunction on a background of chronic IR during pregnancy. In most cases, both β cell impairment and tissue IR exist prior to pregnancy and can progress, representing the basis for increased risk of T2DM in post-pregnancy [193]. Indeed, GDM is often considered as a prediabetic state [196].

Human pregnancy is a physiological condition characterised by decreased circulating adiponectin [197]. In late pregnancy adiponectin mRNA levels in white adipose tissue were 2.5-fold lower compared to pre pregnancy assessments, most likely suggesting reduced adiponectin production, possibly due to gestation-related adipose tissue accumulation in abdominal compartment [197]. Interestingly, lowering in total adiponectin is reflected primarily at the level of HMW adiponectin complexes resulting in decreased HMW/LMW ratio, further suggesting that HMW adiponectin is the active form of the protein [197,198]. Pregnancy-mediated adiponectin changes seem related to impairment of peripheral IS to glucose, but not to lipid metabolism as, contrary to what happens in nonpregnant women [198], in late pregnancy plasma adiponectin concentrations were independent of FFA levels under conditions of hyperinsulinemia [197].

Interestingly, during pregnancy, adiponectin is expressed and circulates in maternal and foetal compartments separately [199]. It can be found in foetal circulation at the 24th week of gestation at the earliest [200] and its levels increase in parallel with gestational age [201]. Compared to maternal plasma, umbilical vein serum adiponectin concentration was found 3-fold higher [202]. As no correlation between adiponectin levels in the maternal and foetal circulation was shown, and since there is no transplacental crossing of molecules larger than 500 Da, it is likely that different mechanisms are implicated in adiponectin production and regulation in the foetus and the mother. Notably, adiponectin may have an important role in foetal carbohydrate metabolism, especially in the presence of GDM [200].

These findings even suggest that human placenta might be an independent source of adiponectin [203]. Indeed, although the results were controversial [119], there are evidences that adiponectin and its receptors are present in rat and human placenta [136,163] and that human placenta is able to secrete adiponectin in an in vitro model [203]. Interestingly, Chen et al. demonstrated also that, compared to normal placenta, GDM placenta has significantly lower adiponectin gene expression but increased AdipoR1 levels [203].

Hypoadiponectinemia has been widely observed in women with GDM [200,204–206]. In particular, compared to pregnant control women, plasma adiponectin concentration in patients with GDM markedly decreased in the 3rd trimester of pregnancy, but significantly raised up 24 h postpartum [200], strongly supporting a straight correlation between hypoadiponectinemia and pregnancy- related IR. Several authors have also linked hypoadiponectinemia to the low-grade inflammatory condition typical of pregnancy further exacerbated by GDM [197,203,204], derived from white adipose tissue and placenta increased production of IL-6 and TNF-α [207]. Indeed, TNF-α is known to inhibit adiponectin synthesis ([208] and a significant negative correlation was found between this proinflammatory cytokine and adipose tissue mRNA/plasma adiponectin levels [209]. Thus, the upregulation of proinflammatory cytokines may represent an important functional link between hypoadiponectinemia and IR in GDM [197].

A recent meta-analysis showed that circulating adiponectin levels during the first or early second trimester of pregnancy were significantly lower in women who late developed GDM [210]. This result was confirmed by Illiodromiti et al., suggesting that prepregnancy and early pregnancy assessment of plasma adiponectin may improve the detection of women at high risk of developing GDM [211]. These findings also confirm that the decline in maternal adiponectin levels precedes clinical diagnosis of GDM [212], implying that women with GDM are most likely metabolically different before gestation [213]. Remarkably, the association between adiponectin levels and subsequent risk of GDM appears to be independent of adiposity in early pregnancy [212–214], suggesting that other pathways may be involved.

The potential role of adiponectin in pathophysiology of GDM is further supported by recent genomic studies. Indeed, the G allele of ADIPOQ gene rs266729 polymorphism is associated with an increased risk of GDM, independently of age, BMI before pregnancy and past pregnancies [215,216]. Further, the association between the G allele of rs2241766 polymorphism and GDM was independently found in a Chinese population [217], an Iranian population [218] and a Malaysian population [219]. Interestingly, the G allele of rs266729 polymorphism is associated with lower adiponectin levels and is considered a risk factor for developing T2DM [215]. Similarly, in the cohort of Han et al., women with TG or GG phenotypes presented significantly lower plasma adiponectin concentrations than TT homozygotes women [217].

Results from animal investigations strongly suggest that hypoadiponectinemia may even underlie GDM. In particular, Qiao et al. demonstrated that pregnant mice with adiponectin deficiency (Adipoq$^{-/-}$) spontaneously developed the main characteristics of GDM, as glucose intolerance, hyperlipidaemia and foetal overgrowth [199]. Interestingly, compared to wild type, in Adipoq$^{-/-}$ dams, despite higher blood glucose concentrations, plasma insulin levels were significantly lower as the result of decreased β cell mass. Remarkably, adiponectin reconstitution during late pregnancy restored maternal metabolism, β cell mass and foetal body weight [199]. Thus, adiponectin is most likely involved in controlling maternal metabolic adaptation to pregnancy and hypoadiponectinemia may play a causal role in the development of GDM [199]. Particularly, adiponectin may represent a factor in the expansion of β cell mass that is believed to be necessary for the maintenance of glucose homeostasis in pregnancy [195]. Indeed, adiponectin is known to enhance β cell proliferation [220] and a strong association between blood adiponectin concentration in late pregnancy and β cell function has been repeatedly found [221,222]. Moreover, ante-partum hypoadiponectinemia seem to predict postpartum IR, β cell dysfunction and fasting glycaemia, providing a means of stratifying women with GDM with respect to their future risk of T2DM [206].

In summary, adiponectin may be associated with GDM development through impaired insulin sensitivity, decreased β cell mass and attenuated anti-inflammatory capacity, thus representing a potential target for treatment or prevention of GDM [195] (Figure 6).

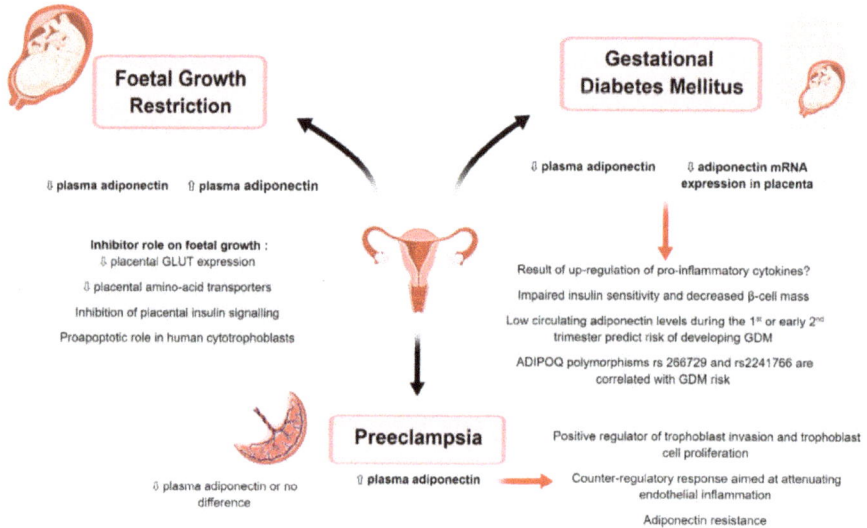

Figure 6. Plasma adiponectin in foetal growth restriction, preeclampsia and gestational diabetes mellitus (GDM) as compared to control patients ⇧ Increase/stimulation. ⇩ Decrease/inhibition.

9.3.2. Preeclampsia (Figure 6)

Preeclampsia (PE) is a severe pregnancy complication affecting 4.6% of pregnant women worldwide [223]. It is at the second or third place in the world ranking of maternal morbidity and mortality causes [224]. It is defined as the association of arterial hypertension appearing from the 20th week of gestation onward and one of the following conditions: proteinuria, maternal organs dysfunction (renal insufficiency, hepatic impairment, neurological complication or haematological disorder like thrombocytopenia or haemolysis) and uteroplacental dysfunction including foetal growth restriction [224]. The pathophysiology of PE has not yet been fully elucidated. However, the two main characteristics of the syndrome appear to be an abnormal placentation and an exaggerated maternal inflammatory response [224]. Indeed, initial incomplete trophoblast invasion and abnormal uterine spiral artery remodelling would be followed by the release into maternal circulation of placental factors, such as inflammatory cytokines and reactive oxygen species, able to trigger a broad intravascular inflammatory response resulting in endothelial dysfunction [225]. As clinical manifestations of PE regress after delivery, it is likely that placental trophoblast cells function may play a central role in its pathogenesis [226]. Like GDM, PE shares risk factors with metabolic syndrome including IR, subclinical inflammation and obesity [227], and women with a history of hypertensive pregnancy disorders present 1.4–3 times higher risk of future cardiovascular diseases compared to women with normotensive pregnancies [228]. Notably, IR was suggested to be part of the pathophysiology that links obesity and PE and would explain the increased rate of this syndrome in obese pregnant women [225].

Strong evidence supports the association between PE and hypoadiponectinemia during the first trimester of pregnancy [163]. In late pregnancy however a paradoxical significant increase in circulating adiponectin has been repeatedly found [201,229–233]. Indeed, this result is highly controversial, with some studies reporting hypoadiponectinemia [234–236] and others finding no significant difference in serum adiponectin levels during pregnancy compared to normal pregnant women [237,238]. Likewise, Haugen et al. failed to demonstrate significant differences in adipose tissue adiponectin mRNA expression in PE patients compared to healthy controls [231]. Reasons for these conflicting results include PE definition, ethnic background of patients, BMI, renal function and smoking [227]. Moreover, Takemura et al. showed that adiponectin changes between PE patients and normal pregnant women were limited to HMW isoform, since no significant difference was found in low- or medium-molecular weight isoforms [234].

Similarly, studies that evaluated the potential prediction of PE by adiponectin measurement in early pregnancy showed conflicting results [227]. Analyses of the relationship between circulating adiponectin and BMI in PE were also inconsistent. Plasma adiponectin levels decreased in women with severe PE and BMI > 25 kg/m^2, whereas they increased in normal weight PE patients [233]. Likewise, Eleuterio et al. showed a negative correlation between serum adiponectin concentration and BMI in normal pregnant women but not in PE patients [232].

The association of genetic variations of the single-nucleotide polymorphism (SNP) type in the adiponectin gene (ADIPOQ) with IR, metabolic syndrome, GDM, T2DM and hypertension has been widely reported [239]. Interestingly, PE was found to be associated with one of the same polymorphisms, 276G>T, that correlates with ovarian disorders [163]. Notably, the TT genotype seems to be related with protection against the development of PE [240]. A significant association was also found between PE and the CT genotype of the −11377C>G polymorphism [239], suggesting that adiponectin may be involved in PE development.

Regarding the pathophysiological role of adiponectin in PE, it has been hypothesised that increased adiponectin concentrations could be part of a physiological feedback mechanism aimed at improving IS and mitigating endothelial dysfunction and cardiovascular risk associated with this syndrome [231]. Actually, adiponectin might attenuate the excessive inflammatory response in the vascular wall through inhibition of NF-κB signalling, decreased CRP (C-reactive protein) and increased nitric oxide generation [227] via endothelial nitric oxide synthase activation and superoxide inhibition in endothelial cells [241]. Further, some reports proposed adiponectin as a positive regulator in the process of trophoblast invasion by modulation of MMP/TIMP balance [232]. In particular, adiponectin showed the ability to increase MMP2 and MMP9 activity in human extra villous trophoblast cells via a reduction of TIMP2 expression [119]. Interestingly, Eleuterio et al. found a negative correlation between circulating adiponectin and MMP2 and TIMP2 in PE patients, suggesting that hyperadiponectinaemia may contribute to the systemic endothelial dysfunction characterising PE [232]. The role of adiponectin in proliferation of trophoblast cells and invasive mechanisms was also demonstrated in rat placenta, where adiponectin and ADIPOR2 expression has been repeatedly reported [136,163]. Intriguingly, some authors have also suggested that adiponectin upregulation in PE patients might represent the result of an adiponectin resistance state, as already described in different animal models [227].

In summary, until now data about the relationships between adiponectin and PE are poor. Nevertheless, its insulin-sensitising and anti-inflammatory activities and its ability in modulating trophoblast cells proliferation and trophoblast invasion led us to speculate that this adipokine might play a role in PE pathogenesis (Figure 6).

9.3.3. Foetal Growth Restriction (Figure 6)

Foetal Growth Restriction (FGR) is a common complication of pregnancy affecting 3 to 9% of pregnancies in the developed world and up to 25% of pregnancies in low-middle income countries [242]. Traditionally, an estimated foetal weight less than the 10th percentile for the population at a given gestational age is highly suggestive of FGR. The main feature of this pathological condition is a placental failure to adequately supply oxygen and nutrients to the developing foetus, thus resulting in a stunted foetal growth [243] This phenomenon, named placental insufficiency, is idiopathic in up to 60% of cases and it is due to a physiological deficiency in uterine spiral arteries remodelling, resulting in restricted uteroplacental perfusion [244]. Placentas from FGR foetuses are then small and show vascular defects that seem to be associated with excessive apoptosis and impaired trophoblast invasion [245]. Moreover, the altered expression of glucose, amino acids and fatty acids carriers in placental syncytiotrophoblast contributes to reduced nutrients transport from mother to foetus [245–247]. Indeed, nutrient supply, a key determinant of foetal growth, depends mainly on placental nutrient transport rather than maternal nutrient levels [133]. In the foetus, hypoxia derived from placental insufficiency results in the so-called brain sparing, that is, the preferential blood flow redistribution to vital organs like brain, myocardium and adrenal glands. Prolonged foetal hypoxia reduces foetal weight and has an adverse impact on foetal organ development and vascular remodelling, resulting in increased rates of neonatal mortality and morbidity [243]. FGR is the greatest risk factor for stillbirth [248] and FGR newborns more likely present transient neonatal morbidities including hypothermia, altered glucose metabolism, polycythaemia, jaundice and sepsis [249]. Interestingly, Small-for-Gestational-Age (SGA) is also a likely risk factor for the development of metabolic complications in later life, such as obesity, high blood pressure, glucose metabolism disorders and adipose tissue dysfunction [250].

Data concerning the relationship between adiponectin concentration in maternal circulation and FGR are controversial. Some studies showed increased serum adiponectin levels [251,252], whereas others reported a negative correlation between circulating adiponectin and FGR [253,254]. Interestingly, mothers who gave birth to Large-for-Gestational-Age (LGA) children had lower plasma adiponectin levels, and hypoadiponectinemia was accompanied by a decrease in mRNA levels of adiponectin receptor AdipoR2 [255]. It is even noteworthy that, according to a very recent meta-analysis [250], blood adiponectin concentration at birth is significantly lower in SGA newborns than in healthy controls.F

Compared to adults, adiponectin concentration in human foetal circulation and umbilical cord blood is 2 to 3 times higher, suggesting that adiponectin may be involved in foetal growth. This hypothesis was confirmed by four independent studies which demonstrated that adiponectin downregulates placental nutrient transport functions. In particular, adiponectin inhibited glucose transporter GLUT1 and GLUT2 expression in human villous cytotrophoblasts [256] and downregulated GLUT3 mRNA expression in placentas of rats exposed to a chronic adiponectin treatment during pregnancy [136]. Besides, in vivo experiments showed that adiponectin chronic infusion in pregnant mice was associated with downregulation of placental amino acid transporters via inhibition of mTOR signalling and resulted in a 19% foetal weight drop [133]. The same result was found in human villous cytotrophoblasts [256]. Using a mouse model of obesity in pregnancy, Aye et al. further confirmed that maternal adiponectin supplementation prevents foetal overgrowth caused by maternal obesity by the inhibition of placental insulin and mTORC1 signalling resulting in normalisation of placental nutrient transport [138]. Surprisingly, in human villous cytotrophoblasts, adiponectin seems also to inhibit mitochondrial biogenesis and to play a proapoptotic role via caspase activity, suggesting a causative role of this adipokine in foetal growth regulation [256].

Hence, adiponectin seems to function as an endocrine link between maternal adipose tissue and foetal growth by regulating placental functions [138]. This may further explain the strong association between maternal BMI and birth weight. Indeed, based on these postulates, low adiponectin levels characterising women with obesity and GDM would remove the inhibition of this adipokine on placental insulin signalling and amino acid transport, thereby promoting increased foetal growth [133] (Figure 6).

10. Conclusions

Adiponectin and its receptors are largely expressed in the central and peripheral reproductive tissues in both male and female in different species. In mice, adiponectin deficiency leads to female subfertility associated to central and ovarian dysfunctions. These data suggest that adiponectin is essential for normal mouse reproduction. However, the role of the local versus systemic adiponectin in the fertility is still unclear. Moreover, the involvement of the different forms of adiponectin in reproductive tract remains also to be investigated. Interestingly, plasma and/or tissue expression of adiponectin might be associated to various reproductive diseases like PCOS syndrome, gestational diabetes, preeclampsia and uterine growth restriction. Studies on animal models and human data

Int. J. Mol. Sci. **2019**, *20*, 1526

suggest that adiponectin could be a potential target for treatment or prevention of these pathologies. Finally, all the data suggest that additional studies are needed to determine the significance of adiponectin and adiponectin receptors as prognostic markers and therapeutic targets in different ovarian or endometrial cancers.

Author Contributions: All authors read and approved the final manuscript.

Funding: This research was funded by INRA, Val de Loire Region (France), grant APR IR-2016 "PREVADI" and grant Agence de Biomedecine "Obésité et qualité des spermatozoïdes humains: importance des adipocytokines". A. Barbe and A. Bongrani were funded by Val de Loire Region (France).

Acknowledgments: The authors thank to BIORENDER for the figures.

Conflicts of Interest: The authors declare no conflicts of interest.

Abbreviations

STAT	Signal Transducers and Activators of Transcription
CCAAT	*CCAAT* box is a distinct pattern of nucleotides with GGCCAATCT consensus sequence
SRE	Serum Response Element
PPRE	Peroxisome Proliferator Response Element
AP-1	Activator Protein 1
LRH-RE	Liver Receptor Homolog 1 Response Element
LMW	Low Molecular Weight
MMW	Medium Molecular Weight
HMW	High Molecular Weight
PCOS	Polycystic Ovary Syndrome
CSF	CerebroSpinal Fluid
HPG	Hypothalamic–Pituitary–Gonadal axis
AMH	Anti-Mullerian Hormone
MMP	Matrix MetalloProteinases
TIMP	Tissue Inhibitors of MetalloProteinases
PE	PreEclempsia
IGFBP-1	Insulin-like Growth Factor Binding Protein 1
hCG	human Chorionic Gonadotropin
FF	Follicular Fluid
TNF	Tumour Necrosis Factor
IFN	InterFeroN
PKA	Protein Kinase A
SF	Seminal Fluid
IVM	In Vitro Maturation
IGF-1	Insulin like Growth Factor 1
IR	Insulin Resistance
IS	Insulin Sensitivity
FFA	Free Fatty Acid
BMI	Body Mass Index
StAR	Steroid Acute Regulatory protein
T2DM	Type 2 Diabetes Mellitus
DHEA	DeHydroEpiAndrosterone
PTEN	Phosphatase and TENsin homolog
LKB1	Liver Kinase B1
NFkB	Transcription factor Nuclear Factor-kappa B
IL8/1	InterLeukin 8/1
ERK1/2	Extracellular signal-Regulated Kinases 1 & 2
MAPK	Mitogen-Activated Protein Kinases
PPAR	Peroxisome Proliferator-Activated Receptor
AMPK	AMP-activated Protein Kinase

APPL1/2　Adaptor Protein, Phosphotyrosine interacting with PH domain and Leucine zipper 1/2
BMAL1　Brain and Muscle Arnt-Like protein-1
CLOCK　Circadian Locomoter Output Cycles protein Kaput
Siglec10　Sialic acid binding ig like lectin 10
SNAT　Sodium-coupled Neutral Amino acid Transporters
mTORC1　Mammalian Target Of Rapamycin Complex 1 or mechanistic target of rapamycin complex 1
GLUT　GLUcose Transporter
MCT2/4　MonoCarboxylate Transporter (lactate transporter)

References

1. Trayhurn, P.; Beattie, J.H. Physiological role of adipose tissue: White adipose tissue as an endocrine and secretory organ. *Proc. Nutr. Soc.* **2001**, *60*, 329–339. [CrossRef] [PubMed]
2. Arita, Y.; Kihara, S.; Ouchi, N.; Takahashi, M.; Maeda, K.; Miyagawa, J.; Hotta, K.; Shimomura, I.; Nakamura, T.; Miyaoka, K.; et al. Paradoxical decrease of an adipose-specific protein, adiponectin, in obesity. *Biochem. Biophys. Res. Commun.* **1999**, *257*, 79–83. [CrossRef]
3. Takahashi, M.; Arita, Y.; Yamagata, K.; Matsukawa, Y.; Okutomi, K.; Horie, M.; Shimomura, I.; Hotta, K.; Kuriyama, H.; Kihara, S.; et al. Genomic structure and mutations in adipose-specific gene, adiponectin. *Int. J. Obes. Relat. Metab. Disord.* **2000**, *24*, 861–868. [CrossRef] [PubMed]
4. Liu, M.; Liu, F. Transcriptional and post-translational regulation of adiponectin. *Biochem. J.* **2009**, *425*, 41–52. [CrossRef] [PubMed]
5. Nishida, M.; Funahashi, T.; Shimomura, I. Pathophysiological significance of adiponectin. *Med. Mol. Morphol.* **2007**, *40*, 55–67. [CrossRef]
6. Waki, H.; Yamauchi, T.; Kamon, J.; Kita, S.; Ito, Y.; Hada, Y.; Uchida, S.; Tsuchida, A.; Takekawa, S.; Kadowaki, T. Generation of globular fragment of adiponectin by leukocyte elastase secreted by monocytic cell line THP-1. *Endocrinology* **2005**, *146*, 790–796. [CrossRef]
7. Scherer, P.E.; Williams, S.; Fogliano, M.; Baldini, G.; Lodish, H.F. A novel serum protein similar to C1q, produced exclusively in adipocytes. *J. Biol. Chem.* **1995**, *270*, 26746–26749. [CrossRef]
8. Hada, Y.; Yamauchi, T.; Waki, H.; Tsuchida, A.; Hara, K.; Yago, H.; Miyazaki, O.; Ebinuma, H.; Kadowaki, T. Selective purification and characterization of adiponectin multimer species from human plasma. *Biochem. Biophys. Res. Commun.* **2007**, *356*, 487–493. [CrossRef]
9. Wang, Y.; Lam, K.S.; Yau, M.H.; Xu, A. Post-translational modifications of adiponectin: Mechanisms and functional implications. *Biochem. J.* **2008**, *409*, 623–633. [CrossRef] [PubMed]
10. Shapiro, L.; Scherer, P.E. The crystal structure of a complement-1q family protein suggests an evolutionary link to tumor necrosis factor. *Curr. Biol.* **1998**, *8*, 335–338. [CrossRef]
11. Wang, Y.; Lam, K.S.; Chan, L.; Chan, K.W.; Lam, J.B.; Lam, M.C.; Hoo, R.C.; Mak, W.W.; Cooper, G.J.; Xu, A. Post-translational modifications of the four conserved lysine residues within the collagenous domain of adiponectin are required for the formation of its high molecular weight oligomeric complex. *J. Biol. Chem.* **2006**, *281*, 16391–16400. [CrossRef] [PubMed]
12. Waki, H.; Yamauchi, T.; Kamon, J.; Ito, Y.; Uchida, S.; Kita, S.; Hara, K.; Hada, Y.; Vasseur, F.; Froguel, P.; et al. Impaired multimerization of human adiponectin mutants associated with diabetes. Molecular structure and multimer formation of adiponectin. *J. Biol. Chem.* **2003**, *278*, 40352–40363. [CrossRef]
13. Wedellova, Z.; Kovacova, Z.; Tencerova, M.; Vedral, T.; Rossmeislova, L.; Siklova-Vitkova, M.; Stich, V.; Polak, J. The Impact of Full-Length, Trimeric and Globular Adiponectin on Lipolysis in Subcutaneous and Visceral Adipocytes of Obese and Non-Obese Women. *PLoS ONE* **2013**, *8*, e66783. [CrossRef]
14. Nakano, Y.; Tajima, S.; Yoshimi, A.; Akiyama, H.; Tsushima, M.; Tanioka, T.; Negoro, T.; Tomita, M.; Tobe, T. A novel enzyme-linked immunosorbent assay specific for high-molecular-weight adiponectin. *J. Lipid Res.* **2006**, *47*, 1572–1582. [CrossRef]
15. Tishinsky, J.M.; Robinson, L.E.; Dyck, D.J. Insulin-sensitizing properties of adiponectin. *Biochimie* **2012**, *94*, 2131–2136. [CrossRef]
16. Swarbrick, M.M.; Havel, P.J. Physiological, pharmacological, and nutritional regulation of circulating adiponectin concentrations in humans. *Metab. Syndr. Relat. Disord.* **2008**, *6*, 87–102. [CrossRef]

17. Chabrolle, C.; Tosca, L.; Dupont, J. Regulation of adiponectin and its receptors in rat ovary by human chorionic gonadotrophin treatment and potential involvement of adiponectin in granulosa cell steroidogenesis. *Reproduction* **2007**, *133*, 719–731. [CrossRef]

18. Diot, M.; Reverchon, M.; Rame, C.; Froment, P.; Brillard, J.P.; Briere, S.; Leveque, G.; Guillaume, D.; Dupont, J. Expression of adiponectin, chemerin and visfatin in plasma and different tissues during a laying season in turkeys. *Reprod. Biol. Endocrinol.* **2015**, *13*, 81. [CrossRef] [PubMed]

19. Kadowaki, T.; Yamauchi, T. Adiponectin and adiponectin receptors. *Endocr. Rev.* **2005**, *26*, 439–451. [CrossRef] [PubMed]

20. Maleszka, A.; Smolinska, N.; Nitkiewicz, A.; Kiezun, M.; Chojnowska, K.; Dobrzyn, K.; Szwaczek, H.; Kaminski, T. Adiponectin Expression in the Porcine Ovary during the Oestrous Cycle and Its Effect on Ovarian Steroidogenesis. *Int. J. Endocrinol.* **2014**, *2014*, 957076. [CrossRef] [PubMed]

21. Nishizawa, H.; Shimomura, I.; Kishida, K.; Maeda, N.; Kuriyama, H.; Nagaretani, H.; Matsuda, M.; Kondo, H.; Furuyama, N.; Kihara, S.; et al. Androgens decrease plasma adiponectin, an insulin-sensitising adipocyte-derived protein. *Diabetes* **2002**, *51*, 2734–2741. [CrossRef] [PubMed]

22. Yamauchi, T.; Iwabu, M.; Okada-Iwabu, M.; Kadowaki, T. Adiponectin receptors: A review of their structure, function and how they work. *Best Pract. Res. Clin. Endocrinol. Metab.* **2014**, *28*, 15–23. [CrossRef] [PubMed]

23. Hendricks, G.L., 3rd; Hadley, J.A.; Krzysik-Walker, S.M.; Prabhu, K.S.; Vasilatos-Younken, R.; Ramachandran, R. Unique profile of chicken adiponectin, a predominantly heavy molecular weight multimer, and relationship to visceral adiposity. *Endocrinology* **2009**, *150*, 3092–3100. [CrossRef]

24. Combs, T.P.; Marliss, E.B. Adiponectin signaling in the liver. *Rev. Endocr. Metab. Disord.* **2014**, *15*, 137–147. [CrossRef]

25. Singh, S.P.; Haussler, S.; Gross, J.J.; Schwarz, F.J.; Bruckmaier, R.M.; Sauerwein, H. Short communication: Circulating and milk adiponectin change differently during energy deficiency at different stages of lactation in dairy cows. *J. Dairy Sci.* **2014**, *97*, 1535–1542. [CrossRef]

26. Giesy, S.L.; Yoon, B.; Currie, W.B.; Kim, J.W.; Boisclair, Y.R. Adiponectin deficit during the precarious glucose economy of early lactation in dairy cows. *Endocrinology* **2012**, *153*, 5834–5844. [CrossRef]

27. Ohtani, Y.; Takahashi, T.; Sato, K.; Ardiyanti, A.; Song, S.H.; Sato, R.; Onda, K.; Wada, Y.; Obara, Y.; Suzuki, K.; et al. Changes in circulating adiponectin and metabolic hormone concentrations during periparturient and lactation periods in Holstein dairy cows. *Anim. Sci. J.* **2012**, *83*, 788–795. [CrossRef] [PubMed]

28. Mielenz, M.; Mielenz, B.; Singh, S.P.; Kopp, C.; Heinz, J.; Haussler, S.; Sauerwein, H. Development, validation, and pilot application of a semiquantitative Western blot analysis and an ELISA for bovine adiponectin. *Domest. Anim. Endocrinol.* **2013**, *44*, 121–130. [CrossRef]

29. Mellouk, N.; Rame, C.; Touze, J.L.; Briant, E.; Ma, L.; Guillaume, D.; Lomet, D.; Caraty, A.; Ntallaris, T.; Humblot, P.; et al. Involvement of plasma adipokines in metabolic and reproductive parameters in Holstein dairy cows fed with diets with differing energy levels. *J. Dairy Sci.* **2017**, *100*, 8518–8533. [CrossRef]

30. Heinz, J.F.; Singh, S.P.; Janowitz, U.; Hoelker, M.; Tesfaye, D.; Schellander, K.; Sauerwein, H. Characterization of adiponectin concentrations and molecular weight forms in serum, seminal plasma, and ovarian follicular fluid from cattle. *Theriogenology* **2015**, *83*, 326–333. [CrossRef] [PubMed]

31. Kubota, N.; Yano, W.; Kubota, T.; Yamauchi, T.; Itoh, S.; Kumagai, H.; Kozono, H.; Takamoto, I.; Okamoto, S.; Shiuchi, T.; et al. Adiponectin stimulates AMP-activated protein kinase in the hypothalamus and increases food intake. *Cell Metab.* **2007**, *6*, 55–68. [CrossRef] [PubMed]

32. Wang, R.; Kuang, M.; Nie, H.; Bai, W.; Sun, L.; Wang, F.; Mao, D.; Wang, Z. Impact of Food Restriction on the Expression of the Adiponectin System and Genes in the Hypothalamic-Pituitary-Ovarian Axis of Pre-Pubertal Ewes. *Reprod. Domest. Anim.* **2016**, *51*, 657–664. [CrossRef]

33. Cnop, M.; Havel, P.J.; Utzschneider, K.M.; Carr, D.B.; Sinha, M.K.; Boyko, E.J.; Retzlaff, B.M.; Knopp, R.H.; Brunzell, J.D.; Kahn, S.E. Relationship of adiponectin to body fat distribution, insulin sensitivity and plasma lipoproteins: Evidence for independent roles of age and sex. *Diabetologia* **2003**, *46*, 459–469. [CrossRef]

34. Combs, T.P.; Berg, A.H.; Rajala, M.W.; Klebanov, S.; Iyengar, P.; Jimenez-Chillaron, J.C.; Patti, M.E.; Klein, S.L.; Weinstein, R.S.; Scherer, P.E. Sexual differentiation, pregnancy, calorie restriction, and aging affect the adipocyte-specific secretory protein adiponectin. *Diabetes* **2003**, *52*, 268–276. [CrossRef] [PubMed]

35. Ouchi, N.; Kihara, S.; Funahashi, T.; Matsuzawa, Y.; Walsh, K. Obesity, adiponectin and vascular inflammatory disease. *Curr. Opin. Lipidol.* **2003**, *14*, 561–566. [CrossRef] [PubMed]

36. Iwaki, M.; Matsuda, M.; Maeda, N.; Funahashi, T.; Matsuzawa, Y.; Makishima, M.; Shimomura, I. Induction of adiponectin, a fat-derived antidiabetic and antiatherogenic factor, by nuclear receptors. *Diabetes* **2003**, *52*, 1655–1663. [CrossRef]

37. Berg, A.H.; Combs, T.P.; Scherer, P.E. ACRP30/adiponectin: An adipokine regulating glucose and lipid metabolism. *Trends Endocrinol. Metab.* **2002**, *13*, 84–89. [CrossRef]

38. Qiao, L.; Maclean, P.S.; Schaack, J.; Orlicky, D.J.; Darimont, C.; Pagliassotti, M.; Friedman, J.E.; Shao, J. C/EBPalpha regulates human adiponectin gene transcription through an intronic enhancer. *Diabetes* **2005**, *54*, 1744–1754. [CrossRef]

39. Qiao, L.; Shao, J. SIRT1 regulates adiponectin gene expression through Foxo1-C/enhancer-binding protein alpha transcriptional complex. *J. Biol. Chem.* **2006**, *281*, 39915–39924. [CrossRef]

40. Seo, J.B.; Moon, H.M.; Noh, M.J.; Lee, Y.S.; Jeong, H.W.; Yoo, E.J.; Kim, W.S.; Park, J.; Youn, B.S.; Kim, J.W.; et al. Adipocyte determination- and differentiation-dependent factor 1/sterol regulatory element-binding protein 1c regulates mouse adiponectin expression. *J. Biol. Chem.* **2004**, *279*, 22108–22117. [CrossRef]

41. Kim, H.B.; Kong, M.; Kim, T.M.; Suh, Y.H.; Kim, W.H.; Lim, J.H.; Song, J.H.; Jung, M.H. NFATc4 and ATF3 negatively regulate adiponectin gene expression in 3T3-L1 adipocytes. *Diabetes* **2006**, *55*, 1342–1352. [CrossRef] [PubMed]

42. Doran, A.C.; Meller, N.; Cutchins, A.; Deliri, H.; Slayton, R.P.; Oldham, S.N.; Kim, J.B.; Keller, S.R.; McNamara, C.A. The helix-loop-helix factors Id3 and E47 are novel regulators of adiponectin. *Circ. Res.* **2008**, *103*, 624–634. [CrossRef]

43. White, U.A.; Maier, J.; Zhao, P.; Richard, A.J.; Stephens, J.M. The modulation of adiponectin by STAT5-activating hormones. *Am. J. Physiol. Endocrinol. Metab.* **2016**, *310*, E129–E136. [CrossRef]

44. Barnea, M.; Chapnik, N.; Genzer, Y.; Froy, O. The circadian clock machinery controls adiponectin expression. *Mol. Cell. Endocrinol.* **2015**, *399*, 284–287. [CrossRef] [PubMed]

45. Tanabe, H.; Fujii, Y.; Okada-Iwabu, M.; Iwabu, M.; Nakamura, Y.; Hosaka, T.; Motoyama, K.; Ikeda, M.; Wakiyama, M.; Terada, T.; et al. Crystal structures of the human adiponectin receptors. *Nature* **2015**, *520*, 312–316. [CrossRef]

46. Kadowaki, T.; Yamauchi, T.; Kubota, N.; Hara, K.; Ueki, K.; Tobe, K. Adiponectin and adiponectin receptors in insulin resistance, diabetes, and the metabolic syndrome. *J. Clin. Investig.* **2006**, *116*, 1784–1792. [CrossRef]

47. Hug, C.; Wang, J.; Ahmad, N.S.; Bogan, J.S.; Tsao, T.S.; Lodish, H.F. T-cadherin is a receptor for hexameric and high-molecular-weight forms of Acrp30/adiponectin. *Proc. Natl. Acad. Sci. USA* **2004**, *101*, 10308–10313. [CrossRef] [PubMed]

48. Denzel, M.S.; Scimia, M.C.; Zumstein, P.M.; Walsh, K.; Ruiz-Lozano, P.; Ranscht, B. T-cadherin is critical for adiponectin-mediated cardioprotection in mice. *J. Clin. Investig.* **2010**, *120*, 4342–4352. [CrossRef]

49. Ruan, H.; Dong, L.Q. Adiponectin signaling and function in insulin target tissues. *J. Mol. Cell Biol.* **2016**, *8*, 101–109. [CrossRef] [PubMed]

50. Mao, X.; Kikani, C.K.; Riojas, R.A.; Langlais, P.; Wang, L.; Ramos, F.J.; Fang, Q.; Christ-Roberts, C.Y.; Hong, J.Y.; Kim, R.Y.; et al. APPL1 binds to adiponectin receptors and mediates adiponectin signalling and function. *Nat. Cell Biol.* **2006**, *8*, 516–523. [CrossRef] [PubMed]

51. Wang, C.; Xin, X.; Xiang, R.; Ramos, F.J.; Liu, M.; Lee, H.J.; Chen, H.; Mao, X.; Kikani, C.K.; Liu, F.; et al. Yin-Yang regulation of adiponectin signaling by APPL isoforms in muscle cells. *J. Biol. Chem.* **2009**, *284*, 31608–31615. [CrossRef] [PubMed]

52. Kos, K.; Harte, A.L.; da Silva, N.F.; Tonchev, A.; Chaldakov, G.; James, S.; Snead, D.R.; Hoggart, B.; O'Hare, J.P.; McTernan, P.G.; et al. Adiponectin and resistin in human cerebrospinal fluid and expression of adiponectin receptors in the human hypothalamus. *J. Clin. Endocrinol. Metab.* **2007**, *92*, 1129–1136. [CrossRef] [PubMed]

53. Psilopanagioti, A.; Papadaki, H.; Kranioti, E.F.; Alexandrides, T.K.; Varakis, J.N. Expression of adiponectin and adiponectin receptors in human pituitary gland and brain. *Neuroendocrinology* **2009**, *89*, 38–47. [CrossRef] [PubMed]

54. Cheng, L.; Shi, H.; Jin, Y.; Li, X.; Pan, J.; Lai, Y.; Lin, Y.; Jin, Y.; Roy, G.; Zhao, A.; et al. Adiponectin Deficiency Leads to Female Subfertility and Ovarian Dysfunctions in Mice. *Endocrinology* **2016**, *157*, 4875–4887. [CrossRef] [PubMed]

55. Guillod-Maximin, E.; Roy, A.F.; Vacher, C.M.; Aubourg, A.; Bailleux, V.; Lorsignol, A.; Penicaud, L.; Parquet, M.; Taouis, M. Adiponectin receptors are expressed in hypothalamus and colocalized with proopiomelanocortin and neuropeptide Y in rodent arcuate neurons. *J. Endocrinol.* **2009**, *200*, 93–105. [CrossRef] [PubMed]

56. Kaminski, T.; Smolinska, N.; Maleszka, A.; Kiezun, M.; Dobrzyn, K.; Czerwinska, J.; Szeszko, K.; Nitkiewicz, A. Expression of adiponectin and its receptors in the porcine hypothalamus during the oestrous cycle. *Reprod. Domest. Anim.* **2014**, *49*, 378–386. [CrossRef]

57. Kusminski, C.M.; McTernan, P.G.; Schraw, T.; Kos, K.; O'Hare, J.P.; Ahima, R.; Kumar, S.; Scherer, P.E. Adiponectin complexes in human cerebrospinal fluid: Distinct complex distribution from serum. *Diabetologia* **2007**, *50*, 634–642. [CrossRef]

58. Neumeier, M.; Weigert, J.; Buettner, R.; Wanninger, J.; Schaffler, A.; Muller, A.M.; Killian, S.; Sauerbruch, S.; Schlachetzki, F.; Steinbrecher, A.; et al. Detection of adiponectin in cerebrospinal fluid in humans. *Am. J. Physiol. Endocrinol. Metab.* **2007**, *293*, E965–E969. [CrossRef]

59. Qi, Y.; Takahashi, N.; Hileman, S.M.; Patel, H.R.; Berg, A.H.; Pajvani, U.B.; Scherer, P.E.; Ahima, R.S. Adiponectin acts in the brain to decrease body weight. *Nat. Med.* **2004**, *10*, 524–529. [CrossRef]

60. Cheng, X.B.; Wen, J.P.; Yang, J.; Yang, Y.; Ning, G.; Li, X.Y. GnRH secretion is inhibited by adiponectin through activation of AMP-activated protein kinase and extracellular signal-regulated kinase. *Endocrine* **2011**, *39*, 6–12. [CrossRef]

61. Wen, J.P.; Liu, C.; Bi, W.K.; Hu, Y.T.; Chen, Q.; Huang, H.; Liang, J.X.; Li, L.T.; Lin, L.X.; Chen, G. Adiponectin inhibits KISS1 gene transcription through AMPK and specificity protein-1 in the hypothalamic GT1-7 neurons. *J. Endocrinol.* **2012**, *214*, 177–189. [CrossRef] [PubMed]

62. Wen, J.P.; Lv, W.S.; Yang, J.; Nie, A.F.; Cheng, X.B.; Yang, Y.; Ge, Y.; Li, X.Y.; Ning, G. Globular adiponectin inhibits GnRH secretion from GT1-7 hypothalamic GnRH neurons by induction of hyperpolarization of membrane potential. *Biochem. Biophys. Res. Commun.* **2008**, *371*, 756–761. [CrossRef]

63. Klenke, U.; Taylor-Burds, C.; Wray, S. Metabolic influences on reproduction: Adiponectin attenuates GnRH neuronal activity in female mice. *Endocrinology* **2014**, *155*, 1851–1863. [CrossRef] [PubMed]

64. Rodriguez-Pacheco, F.; Martinez-Fuentes, A.J.; Tovar, S.; Pinilla, L.; Tena-Sempere, M.; Dieguez, C.; Castano, J.P.; Malagon, M.M. Regulation of pituitary cell function by adiponectin. *Endocrinology* **2007**, *148*, 401–410. [CrossRef]

65. Ramachandran, R.; Ocon-Grove, O.M.; Metzger, S.L. Molecular cloning and tissue expression of chicken AdipoR1 and AdipoR2 complementary deoxyribonucleic acids. *Domest. Anim. Endocrinol.* **2007**, *33*, 19–31. [CrossRef] [PubMed]

66. Kiezun, M.; Smolinska, N.; Maleszka, A.; Dobrzyn, K.; Szeszko, K.; Kaminski, T. Adiponectin expression in the porcine pituitary during the estrous cycle and its effect on LH and FSH secretion. *Am. J. Physiol. Endocrinol. Metab.* **2014**, *307*, E1038–E1046. [CrossRef]

67. Lu, M.; Tang, Q.; Olefsky, J.M.; Mellon, P.L.; Webster, N.J. Adiponectin activates adenosine monophosphate-activated protein kinase and decreases luteinizing hormone secretion in LbetaT2 gonadotropes. *Mol. Endocrinol.* **2008**, *22*, 760–771. [CrossRef]

68. Sarmento-Cabral, A.; Peinado, J.R.; Halliday, L.C.; Malagon, M.M.; Castano, J.P.; Kineman, R.D.; Luque, R.M. Adipokines (Leptin, Adiponectin, Resistin) Differentially Regulate All Hormonal Cell Types in Primary Anterior Pituitary Cell Cultures from Two Primate Species. *Sci. Rep.* **2017**, *7*, 43537. [CrossRef]

69. Rak, A.; Mellouk, N.; Froment, P.; Dupont, J. Adiponectin and resistin: Potential metabolic signals affecting hypothalamo-pituitary gonadal axis in females and males of different species. *Reproduction* **2017**, *153*, R215–R226. [CrossRef]

70. Kawwass, J.F.; Summer, R.; Kallen, C.B. Direct effects of leptin and adiponectin on peripheral reproductive tissues: A critical review. *Mol. Hum. Reprod.* **2015**, *21*, 617–632. [CrossRef]

71. Chabrolle, C.; Tosca, L.; Rame, C.; Lecomte, P.; Royere, D.; Dupont, J. Adiponectin increases insulin-like growth factor I-induced progesterone and estradiol secretion in human granulosa cells. *Fertil. Steril.* **2009**, *92*, 1988–1996. [CrossRef] [PubMed]

72. Bersinger, N.A.; Wunder, D.M. Adiponectin isoform distribution in serum and in follicular fluid of women undergoing treatment by ICSI. *Acta Obstet. Gynecol. Scand.* **2010**, *89*, 782–788. [CrossRef]

73. Li, L.; Ferin, M.; Sauer, M.V.; Lobo, R.A. Ovarian adipocytokines are associated with early in vitro human embryo development independent of the action of ovarian insulin. *J. Assist. Reprod. Genet.* **2012**, *29*, 1397–1404. [CrossRef]

74. Bersinger, N.A.; Birkhauser, M.H.; Wunder, D.M. Adiponectin as a marker of success in intracytoplasmic sperm injection/embryo transfer cycles. *Gynecol. Endocrinol.* **2006**, *22*, 479–483. [CrossRef] [PubMed]

75. Cao, Z.; Meng, B.; Fan, R.; Liu, M.; Gao, M.; Xing, Z.; Luan, X. Comparative proteomic analysis of ovaries from Huoyan geese between pre-laying and laying periods using an iTRAQ-based approach. *Poult. Sci.* **2018**, *97*, 2170–2182. [CrossRef]

76. Mellouk, N.; Rame, C.; Marchand, M.; Staub, C.; Touze, J.L.; Venturi, E.; Mercerand, F.; Travel, A.; Chartrin, P.; Lecompte, F.; et al. Effect of different levels of feed restriction and fish oil fatty acid supplementation on fat deposition by using different techniques, plasma levels and mRNA expression of several adipokines in broiler breeder hens. *PLoS ONE* **2018**, *13*, e0191121. [CrossRef]

77. Tabandeh, M.R.; Hosseini, A.; Saeb, M.; Kafi, M.; Saeb, S. Changes in the gene expression of adiponectin and adiponectin receptors (AdipoR1 and AdipoR2) in ovarian follicular cells of dairy cow at different stages of development. *Theriogenology* **2010**, *73*, 659–669. [CrossRef] [PubMed]

78. Wyskida, K.; Franik, G.; Wikarek, T.; Owczarek, A.; Delroba, A.; Chudek, J.; Sikora, J.; Olszanecka-Glinianowicz, M. The levels of adipokines in relation to hormonal changes during the menstrual cycle in young, normal-weight women. *Endocr. Connect.* **2017**, *6*, 892–900. [CrossRef] [PubMed]

79. Galvan, R.E.; Basurto, L.; Saucedo, R.; Campos, S.; Hernandez, M.; Zarate, A. Adiponectin concentrations during menstrual cycle. *Ginecol. Obstet. Mexico* **2007**, *75*, 435–438.

80. Gutman, G.; Barak, V.; Maslovitz, S.; Amit, A.; Lessing, J.B.; Geva, E. Recombinant luteinizing hormone induces increased production of ovarian follicular adiponectin in vivo: Implications for enhanced insulin sensitivity. *Fertil. Steril.* **2009**, *91*, 1837–1841. [CrossRef]

81. Ledoux, S.; Campos, D.B.; Lopes, F.L.; Dobias-Goff, M.; Palin, M.F.; Murphy, B.D. Adiponectin induces periovulatory changes in ovarian follicular cells. *Endocrinology* **2006**, *147*, 5178–5186. [CrossRef]

82. Lagaly, D.V.; Aad, P.Y.; Grado-Ahuir, J.A.; Hulsey, L.B.; Spicer, L.J. Role of adiponectin in regulating ovarian theca and granulosa cell function. *Mol. Cell. Endocrinol.* **2008**, *284*, 38–45. [CrossRef]

83. Pierre, P.; Froment, P.; Negre, D.; Rame, C.; Barateau, V.; Chabrolle, C.; Lecomte, P.; Dupont, J. Role of adiponectin receptors, AdipoR1 and AdipoR2, in the steroidogenesis of the human granulosa tumor cell line, KGN. *Hum. Reprod.* **2009**, *24*, 2890–2901. [CrossRef] [PubMed]

84. Maillard, V.; Uzbekova, S.; Guignot, F.; Perreau, C.; Rame, C.; Coyral-Castel, S.; Dupont, J. Effect of adiponectin on bovine granulosa cell steroidogenesis, oocyte maturation and embryo development. *Reprod. Biol. Endocrinol.* **2010**, *8*, 23. [CrossRef] [PubMed]

85. Comim, F.V.; Gutierrez, K.; Bridi, A.; Bochi, G.; Chemeris, R.; Rigo, M.L.; Dau, A.M.; Cezar, A.S.; Moresco, R.N.; Goncalves, P.B. Effects of Adiponectin Including Reduction of Androstenedione Secretion and Ovarian Oxidative Stress Parameters In Vivo. *PLoS ONE* **2016**, *11*, e0154453. [CrossRef] [PubMed]

86. Sepilian, V.; Nagamani, M. Adiponectin levels in women with polycystic ovary syndrome and severe insulin resistance. *J. Soc. Gynecol. Investig.* **2005**, *12*, 129–134. [CrossRef] [PubMed]

87. Thomas, S.; Kratzsch, D.; Schaab, M.; Scholz, M.; Grunewald, S.; Thiery, J.; Paasch, U.; Kratzsch, J. Seminal plasma adipokine levels are correlated with functional characteristics of spermatozoa. *Fertil. Steril.* **2013**, *99*, 1256–1263e3. [CrossRef] [PubMed]

88. Civitarese, A.E.; Jenkinson, C.P.; Richardson, D.; Bajaj, M.; Cusi, K.; Kashyap, S.; Berria, R.; Belfort, R.; DeFronzo, R.A.; Mandarino, L.J.; et al. Adiponectin receptors gene expression and insulin sensitivity in non-diabetic Mexican Americans with or without a family history of Type 2 diabetes. *Diabetologia* **2004**, *47*, 816–820. [CrossRef]

89. Caminos, J.E.; Nogueiras, R.; Gaytan, F.; Pineda, R.; Gonzalez, C.R.; Barreiro, M.L.; Castano, J.P.; Malagon, M.M.; Pinilla, L.; Toppari, J.; et al. Novel expression and direct effects of adiponectin in the rat testis. *Endocrinology* **2008**, *149*, 3390–3402. [CrossRef] [PubMed]

90. Martin, L.J. Implications of adiponectin in linking metabolism to testicular function. *Endocrine* **2014**, *46*, 16–28. [CrossRef] [PubMed]

91. Bjursell, M.; Ahnmark, A.; Bohlooly, Y.M.; William-Olsson, L.; Rhedin, M.; Peng, X.R.; Ploj, K.; Gerdin, A.K.; Arnerup, G.; Elmgren, A.; et al. Opposing effects of adiponectin receptors 1 and 2 on energy metabolism. *Diabetes* **2007**, *56*, 583–593. [CrossRef] [PubMed]

92. Choubey, M.; Ranjan, A.; Bora, P.S.; Baltazar, F.; Martin, L.J.; Krishna, A. Role of adiponectin as a modulator of testicular function during aging in mice. *Biochim. Biophys. Acta Mol. Basis Dis.* **2019**, *1865*, 413–427. [CrossRef] [PubMed]

93. Ocon-Grove, O.M.; Krzysik-Walker, S.M.; Maddineni, S.R.; Hendricks, G.L., 3rd; Ramachandran, R. Adiponectin and its receptors are expressed in the chicken testis: Influence of sexual maturation on testicular ADIPOR1 and ADIPOR2 mRNA abundance. *Reproduction* **2008**, *136*, 627–638. [CrossRef] [PubMed]

94. Pfaehler, A.; Nanjappa, M.K.; Coleman, E.S.; Mansour, M.; Wanders, D.; Plaisance, E.P.; Judd, R.L.; Akingbemi, B.T. Regulation of adiponectin secretion by soy isoflavones has implication for endocrine function of the testis. *Toxicol. Lett.* **2012**, *209*, 78–85. [CrossRef]

95. Gui, Y.; Silha, J.V.; Murphy, L.J. Sexual dimorphism and regulation of resistin, adiponectin, and leptin expression in the mouse. *Obes. Res.* **2004**, *12*, 1481–1491. [CrossRef]

96. Yarrow, J.F.; Beggs, L.A.; Conover, C.F.; McCoy, S.C.; Beck, D.T.; Borst, S.E. Influence of androgens on circulating adiponectin in male and female rodents. *PLoS ONE* **2012**, *7*, e47315. [CrossRef] [PubMed]

97. Lanfranco, F.; Zitzmann, M.; Simoni, M.; Nieschlag, E. Serum adiponectin levels in hypogonadal males: Influence of testosterone replacement therapy. *Clin. Endocrinol. (Oxf.)* **2004**, *60*, 500–507. [CrossRef] [PubMed]

98. Kadooka, K.; Sato, M.; Matsumoto, T.; Kuhara, S.; Katakura, Y.; Fujimura, T. Pig testis extract augments adiponectin expression and secretion through the peroxisome proliferator-activated receptor signaling pathway in 3T3-L1 adipocytes. *Cytotechnology* **2018**, *70*, 983–992. [CrossRef]

99. Choubey, M.; Ranjan, A.; Bora, P.S.; Baltazar, F.; Krishna, A. Direct actions of adiponectin on changes in reproductive, metabolic, and anti-oxidative enzymes status in the testis of adult mice. *Gen. Comp. Endocrinol.* **2018**. [CrossRef]

100. Ahn, S.W.; Gang, G.T.; Tadi, S.; Nedumaran, B.; Kim, Y.D.; Park, J.H.; Kweon, G.R.; Koo, S.H.; Lee, K.; Ahn, R.S.; et al. Phosphoenolpyruvate carboxykinase and glucose-6-phosphatase are required for steroidogenesis in testicular Leydig cells. *J. Biol. Chem.* **2012**, *287*, 41875–41887. [CrossRef]

101. Carmina, E.; Chu, M.C.; Moran, C.; Tortoriello, D.; Vardhana, P.; Tena, G.; Preciado, R.; Lobo, R. Subcutaneous and omental fat expression of adiponectin and leptin in women with polycystic ovary syndrome. *Fertil. Steril.* **2008**, *89*, 642–648. [CrossRef] [PubMed]

102. Banerjee, D.; Mazumder, S.; Bhattacharya, S.; Sinha, A.K. The sex specific effects of extraneous testosterone on ADP induced platelet aggregation in platelet-rich plasma from male and female subjects. *Int. J. Lab. Hematol.* **2014**, *36*, e74–e77. [CrossRef] [PubMed]

103. Wu, L.; Xu, B.; Fan, W.; Zhu, X.; Wang, G.; Zhang, A. Adiponectin protects Leydig cells against proinflammatory cytokines by suppressing the nuclear factor-kappaB signaling pathway. *FEBS J.* **2013**, *280*, 3920–3927. [CrossRef] [PubMed]

104. Chappaz, E.; Albornoz, M.S.; Campos, D.; Che, L.; Palin, M.F.; Murphy, B.D.; Bordignon, V. Adiponectin enhances in vitro development of swine embryos. *Domest. Anim. Endocrinol.* **2008**, *35*, 198–207. [CrossRef]

105. Gomes, E.T.; Costa, J.A.S.; Silva, D.M.F.; Al Shebli, W.; Azevedo, M.L.; Monteiro, P.L.J., Jr.; Araujo Silva, R.A.J.; Santos Filho, A.S.; Guerra, M.M.P.; Bartolomeu, C.C.; et al. Effects of adiponectin during in vitro maturation of goat oocytes: MEK 1/2 pathway and gene expression pattern. *Reprod. Domest. Anim.* **2018**, *53*, 1323–1329. [CrossRef] [PubMed]

106. Richards, J.S.; Liu, Z.; Kawai, T.; Tabata, K.; Watanabe, H.; Suresh, D.; Kuo, F.T.; Pisarska, M.D.; Shimada, M. Adiponectin and its receptors modulate granulosa cell and cumulus cell functions, fertility, and early embryo development in the mouse and human. *Fertil. Steril.* **2012**, *98*, 471–479. [CrossRef]

107. Oliveira, B.S.P.; Costa, J.A.S.; Gomes, E.T.; Silva, D.M.F.; Torres, S.M.; Monteiro, P.L.J., Jr.; Santos Filho, A.S.; Guerra, M.M.P.; Carneiro, G.F.; Wischral, A.; et al. Expression of adiponectin and its receptors (AdipoR1 and AdipoR2) in goat ovary and its effect on oocyte nuclear maturation in vitro. *Theriogenology* **2017**, *104*, 127–133. [CrossRef]

108. Wang, Q.; Tang, S.B.; Song, X.B.; Deng, T.F.; Zhang, T.T.; Yin, S.; Luo, S.M.; Shen, W.; Zhang, C.L.; Ge, Z.J. High-glucose concentrations change DNA methylation levels in human IVM oocytes. *Hum. Reprod.* **2018**, *33*, 474–481. [CrossRef] [PubMed]

109. Kasimanickam, V.R.; Kasimanickam, R.K.; Kastelic, J.P.; Stevenson, J.S. Associations of adiponectin and fertility estimates in Holstein bulls. *Theriogenology* **2013**, *79*, 766–777.e3. [CrossRef]

110. Kadivar, A.; Heidari Khoei, H.; Hassanpour, H.; Golestanfar, A.; Ghanaei, H. Correlation of Adiponectin mRNA Abundance and Its Receptors with Quantitative Parameters of Sperm Motility in Rams. *Int. J. Fertil. Steril.* **2016**, *10*, 127–135. [PubMed]

111. Mellouk, N.; Rame, C.; Delaveau, J.; Rat, C.; Maurer, E.; Froment, P.; Dupont, J. Adipokines expression profile in liver, adipose tissue and muscle during chicken embryo development. *Gen. Comp. Endocrinol.* **2018**, *267*, 146–156. [CrossRef] [PubMed]

112. Nishio, S.; Gibert, Y.; Bernard, L.; Brunet, F.; Triqueneaux, G.; Laudet, V. Adiponectin and adiponectin receptor genes are coexpressed during zebrafish embryogenesis and regulated by food deprivation. *Dev. Dyn.* **2008**, *237*, 1682–1690. [CrossRef] [PubMed]

113. Kim, S.T.; Marquard, K.; Stephens, S.; Louden, E.; Allsworth, J.; Moley, K.H. Adiponectin and adiponectin receptors in the mouse preimplantation embryo and uterus. *Hum. Reprod.* **2011**, *26*, 82–95. [CrossRef] [PubMed]

114. Cikos, S.; Burkus, J.; Bukovska, A.; Fabian, D.; Rehak, P.; Koppel, J. Expression of adiponectin receptors and effects of adiponectin isoforms in mouse preimplantation embryos. *Hum. Reprod.* **2010**, *25*, 2247–2255. [CrossRef]

115. Zglejc-Waszak, K.; Waszkiewicz, E.M.; Franczak, A. Periconceptional undernutrition affects the levels of DNA methylation in the peri-implantation pig endometrium and in embryos. *Theriogenology* **2019**, *123*, 185–193. [CrossRef]

116. Sturmey, R.G.; Reis, A.; Leese, H.J.; McEvoy, T.G. Role of fatty acids in energy provision during oocyte maturation and early embryo development. *Reprod. Domest. Anim.* **2009**, *44* (Suppl. 3), 50–58. [CrossRef]

117. Stubbs, C.D.; Smith, A.D. The modification of mammalian membrane polyunsaturated fatty acid composition in relation to membrane fluidity and function. *Biochim. Biophys. Acta* **1984**, *779*, 89–137. [CrossRef]

118. Schindler, M.; Pendzialek, M.; Grybel, K.J.; Seeling, T.; Gurke, J.; Fischer, B.; Navarrete Santos, A. Adiponectin stimulates lipid metabolism via AMPK in rabbit blastocysts. *Hum. Reprod.* **2017**, *32*, 1382–1392. [CrossRef] [PubMed]

119. Benaitreau, D.; Dos Santos, E.; Leneveu, M.C.; Alfaidy, N.; Feige, J.J.; de Mazancourt, P.; Pecquery, R.; Dieudonne, M.N. Effects of adiponectin on human trophoblast invasion. *J. Endocrinol.* **2010**, *207*, 45–53. [CrossRef] [PubMed]

120. Benaitreau, D.; Dos Santos, E.; Leneveu, M.C.; De Mazancourt, P.; Pecquery, R.; Dieudonne, M.N. Adiponectin promotes syncytialisation of BeWo cell line and primary trophoblast cells. *Reprod. Biol. Endocrinol.* **2010**, *8*, 128. [CrossRef] [PubMed]

121. Mazaki-Tovi, S.; Kanety, H.; Pariente, C.; Hemi, R.; Wiser, A.; Schiff, E.; Sivan, E. Maternal serum adiponectin levels during human pregnancy. *J. Perinatol.* **2007**, *27*, 77–81. [CrossRef] [PubMed]

122. Mazaki-Tovi, S.; Romero, R.; Kusanovic, J.P.; Erez, O.; Vaisbuch, E.; Gotsch, F.; Mittal, P.; Than, G.N.; Nhan-Chang, C.; Chaiworapongsa, T.; et al. Adiponectin multimers in maternal plasma. *J. Matern. Fetal Neonatal Med.* **2008**, *21*, 796–815. [CrossRef] [PubMed]

123. Takemura, Y.; Osuga, Y.; Yamauchi, T.; Kobayashi, M.; Harada, M.; Hirata, T.; Morimoto, C.; Hirota, Y.; Yoshino, O.; Koga, K.; et al. Expression of adiponectin receptors and its possible implication in the human endometrium. *Endocrinology* **2006**, *147*, 3203–3210. [CrossRef] [PubMed]

124. Dos Santos, E.; Pecquery, R.; de Mazancourt, P.; Dieudonne, M.N. Adiponectin and reproduction. *Vitam. Horm.* **2012**, *90*, 187–209. [CrossRef]

125. Bohlouli, S.; Khazaei, M.; Teshfam, M.; Hassanpour, H. Adiponectin effect on the viability of human endometrial stromal cells and mRNA expression of adiponectin receptors. *Int. J. Fertil. Steril.* **2013**, *7*, 43–48.

126. McDonald, E.A.; Wolfe, M.W. The pro-inflammatory role of adiponectin at the maternal-fetal interface. *Am. J. Reprod. Immunol.* **2011**, *66*, 128–136. [CrossRef] [PubMed]

127. Lappas, M.; Permezel, M.; Rice, G.E. Leptin and adiponectin stimulate the release of proinflammatory cytokines and prostaglandins from human placenta and maternal adipose tissue via nuclear factor-kappaB, peroxisomal proliferator-activated receptor-gamma and extracellularly regulated kinase 1/2. *Endocrinology* **2005**, *146*, 3334–3342. [CrossRef]

128. Benaitreau, D.; Dieudonne, M.N.; Dos Santos, E.; Leneveu, M.C.; Mazancourt, P.; Pecquery, R. Antiproliferative effects of adiponectin on human trophoblastic cell lines JEG-3 and BeWo. *Biol. Reprod.* **2009**, *80*, 1107–1114. [CrossRef]

129. Chen, H.; Chen, H.; Wu, Y.; Liu, B.; Li, Z.; Wang, Z. Adiponectin exerts antiproliferative effect on human placenta via modulation of the JNK/c-Jun pathway. *Int. J. Clin. Exp. Pathol.* **2014**, *7*, 2894–2904. [PubMed]

130. McDonald, E.A.; Wolfe, M.W. Adiponectin attenuation of endocrine function within human term trophoblast cells. *Endocrinology* **2009**, *150*, 4358–4365. [CrossRef]

131. Li, W.; Geng, L.; Liu, X.; Gui, W.; Qi, H. Recombinant adiponectin alleviates abortion in mice by regulating Th17/Treg imbalance via p38MAPK-STAT5 pathway. *Biol. Reprod.* **2018**. [CrossRef] [PubMed]

132. Duval, F.; Dos Santos, E.; Maury, B.; Serazin, V.; Fathallah, K.; Vialard, F.; Dieudonne, M.N. Adiponectin regulates glycogen metabolism at the human fetal-maternal interface. *J. Mol. Endocrinol.* **2018**, *61*, 139–152. [CrossRef]

133. Rosario, F.J.; Schumacher, M.A.; Jiang, J.; Kanai, Y.; Powell, T.L.; Jansson, T. Chronic maternal infusion of full-length adiponectin in pregnant mice down-regulates placental amino acid transporter activity and expression and decreases fetal growth. *J. Physiol.* **2012**, *590*, 1495–1509. [CrossRef]

134. Aye, I.L.; Powell, T.L.; Jansson, T. Review: Adiponectin—The missing link between maternal adiposity, placental transport and fetal growth? *Placenta* **2013**, *34*, S40–S45. [CrossRef]

135. Jones, H.N.; Jansson, T.; Powell, T.L. Full-length adiponectin attenuates insulin signaling and inhibits insulin-stimulated amino Acid transport in human primary trophoblast cells. *Diabetes* **2010**, *59*, 1161–1170. [CrossRef]

136. Caminos, J.E.; Nogueiras, R.; Gallego, R.; Bravo, S.; Tovar, S.; Garcia-Caballero, T.; Casanueva, F.F.; Dieguez, C. Expression and regulation of adiponectin and receptor in human and rat placenta. *J. Clin. Endocrinol. Metab.* **2005**, *90*, 4276–4286. [CrossRef] [PubMed]

137. Aye, I.L.; Gao, X.; Weintraub, S.T.; Jansson, T.; Powell, T.L. Adiponectin inhibits insulin function in primary trophoblasts by PPARalpha-mediated ceramide synthesis. *Mol. Endocrinol.* **2014**, *28*, 512–524. [CrossRef]

138. Aye, I.L.; Rosario, F.J.; Powell, T.L.; Jansson, T. Adiponectin supplementation in pregnant mice prevents the adverse effects of maternal obesity on placental function and fetal growth. *Proc. Natl. Acad. Sci. USA* **2015**, *112*, 12858–12863. [CrossRef] [PubMed]

139. Wang, J.; Shang, L.X.; Dong, X.; Wang, X.; Wu, N.; Wang, S.H.; Zhang, F.; Xu, L.M.; Xiao, Y. Relationship of adiponectin and resistin levels in umbilical serum, maternal serum and placenta with neonatal birth weight. *Aust. N. Z. J. Obstet. Gynaecol.* **2010**, *50*, 432–438. [CrossRef] [PubMed]

140. Nanda, S.; Yu, C.K.; Giurcaneanu, L.; Akolekar, R.; Nicolaides, K.H. Maternal serum adiponectin at 11-13 weeks of gestation in preeclampsia. *Fetal Diagn. Ther.* **2011**, *29*, 208–215. [CrossRef]

141. Worda, C.; Leipold, H.; Gruber, C.; Kautzky-Willer, A.; Knofler, M.; Bancher-Todesca, D. Decreased plasma adiponectin concentrations in women with gestational diabetes mellitus. *Am. J. Obstet. Gynecol.* **2004**, *191*, 2120–2124. [CrossRef]

142. Maayan-Metzger, A.; Schushan-Eisen, I.; Strauss, T.; Globus, O.; Leibovitch, L. Gestational weight gain and body mass indexes have an impact on the outcomes of diabetic mothers and infants. *Acta Paediatr.* **2015**, *104*, 1150–1155. [CrossRef]

143. Qiao, L.; Wattez, J.S.; Lee, S.; Guo, Z.; Schaack, J.; Hay, W.W., Jr.; Zita, M.M.; Parast, M.; Shao, J. Knockout maternal adiponectin increases fetal growth in mice: Potential role for trophoblast IGFBP-1. *Diabetologia* **2016**, *59*, 2417–2425. [CrossRef]

144. Teede, H.; Deeks, A.; Moran, L. Polycystic ovary syndrome: A complex condition with psychological, reproductive and metabolic manifestations that impacts on health across the lifespan. *BMC Med.* **2010**, *8*, 41. [CrossRef] [PubMed]

145. Teede, H.J.; Misso, M.L.; Boyle, J.A.; Garad, R.M.; McAllister, V.; Downes, L.; Gibson, M.; Hart, R.J.; Rombauts, L.; Moran, L.; et al. Translation and implementation of the Australian-led PCOS guideline: Clinical summary and translation resources from the International Evidence-based Guideline for the Assessment and Management of Polycystic Ovary Syndrome. *Med. J. Aust.* **2018**, *209*, S3–S8. [CrossRef]

146. Toulis, K.A.; Goulis, D.G.; Farmakiotis, D.; Georgopoulos, N.A.; Katsikis, I.; Tarlatzis, B.C.; Papadimas, I.; Panidis, D. Adiponectin levels in women with polycystic ovary syndrome: A systematic review and a meta-analysis. *Hum. Reprod. Update* **2009**, *15*, 297–307. [CrossRef] [PubMed]

147. Benrick, A.; Chanclon, B.; Micallef, P.; Wu, Y.; Hadi, L.; Shelton, J.M.; Stener-Victorin, E.; Wernstedt Asterholm, I. Adiponectin protects against development of metabolic disturbances in a PCOS mouse model. *Proc. Natl. Acad. Sci. USA* **2017**, *114*, E7187–E7196. [CrossRef] [PubMed]

148. Azziz, R.; Carmina, E.; Dewailly, D.; Diamanti-Kandarakis, E.; Escobar-Morreale, H.F.; Futterweit, W.; Janssen, O.E.; Legro, R.S.; Norman, R.J.; Taylor, A.E.; et al. Positions statement: Criteria for defining polycystic ovary syndrome as a predominantly hyperandrogenic syndrome: An Androgen Excess Society guideline. *J. Clin. Endocrinol. Metab.* **2006**, *91*, 4237–4245. [CrossRef] [PubMed]

149. Groth, S.W. Adiponectin and polycystic ovary syndrome. *Biol. Res. Nurs.* **2010**, *12*, 62–72. [CrossRef] [PubMed]

150. Liu, Z.; Wang, Z.; Hao, C.; Tian, Y.; Fu, J. Effects of ADIPOQ polymorphisms on PCOS risk: A meta-analysis. *Reprod. Biol. Endocrinol.* **2018**, *16*, 120. [CrossRef] [PubMed]

151. Li, S.; Huang, X.; Zhong, H.; Peng, Q.; Chen, S.; Xie, Y.; Qin, X.; Qin, A. Low circulating adiponectin levels in women with polycystic ovary syndrome: An updated meta-analysis. *Tumour Biol.* **2014**, *35*, 3961–3973. [CrossRef]

152. O'Connor, A.; Phelan, N.; Tun, T.K.; Boran, G.; Gibney, J.; Roche, H.M. High-molecular-weight adiponectin is selectively reduced in women with polycystic ovary syndrome independent of body mass index and severity of insulin resistance. *J. Clin. Endocrinol. Metab.* **2010**, *95*, 1378–1385. [CrossRef] [PubMed]

153. Panidis, D.; Kourtis, A.; Farmakiotis, D.; Mouslech, T.; Rousso, D.; Koliakos, G. Serum adiponectin levels in women with polycystic ovary syndrome. *Hum. Reprod.* **2003**, *18*, 1790–1796. [CrossRef] [PubMed]

154. Orio, F., Jr.; Palomba, S.; Cascella, T.; Milan, G.; Mioni, R.; Pagano, C.; Zullo, F.; Colao, A.; Lombardi, G.; Vettor, R. Adiponectin levels in women with polycystic ovary syndrome. *J. Clin. Endocrinol. Metab.* **2003**, *88*, 2619–2623. [CrossRef]

155. Lecke, S.B.; Mattei, F.; Morsch, D.M.; Spritzer, P.M. Abdominal subcutaneous fat gene expression and circulating levels of leptin and adiponectin in polycystic ovary syndrome. *Fertil. Steril.* **2011**, *95*, 2044–2049. [CrossRef]

156. Svendsen, P.F.; Christiansen, M.; Hedley, P.L.; Nilas, L.; Pedersen, S.B.; Madsbad, S. Adipose expression of adipocytokines in women with polycystic ovary syndrome. *Fertil. Steril.* **2012**, *98*, 235–241. [CrossRef] [PubMed]

157. Tao, T.; Xu, B.; Liu, W. Ovarian HMW adiponectin is associated with folliculogenesis in women with polycystic ovary syndrome. *Reprod. Biol. Endocrinol.* **2013**, *11*, 99. [CrossRef] [PubMed]

158. Artimani, T.; Saidijam, M.; Aflatoonian, R.; Ashrafi, M.; Amiri, I.; Yavangi, M.; SoleimaniAsl, S.; Shabab, N.; Karimi, J.; Mehdizadeh, M. Downregulation of adiponectin system in granulosa cells and low levels of HMW adiponectin in PCOS. *J. Assist. Reprod. Genet.* **2016**, *33*, 101–110. [CrossRef] [PubMed]

159. Inal, H.A.; Yilmaz, N.; Gorkem, U.; Oruc, A.S.; Timur, H. The impact of follicular fluid adiponectin and ghrelin levels based on BMI on IVF outcomes in PCOS. *J. Endocrinol. Investig.* **2016**, *39*, 431–437. [CrossRef] [PubMed]

160. Dehghan, R.; Saidijam, M.; Mehdizadeh, M.; Shabab, N.; Yavangi, M.; Artimani, T. Evidence for decreased expression of APPL1 associated with reduced insulin and adiponectin receptors expression in PCOS patients. *J. Endocrinol. Investig.* **2016**, *39*, 1075–1082. [CrossRef]

161. Xu, A.; Chan, K.W.; Hoo, R.L.; Wang, Y.; Tan, K.C.; Zhang, J.; Chen, B.; Lam, M.C.; Tse, C.; Cooper, G.J.; et al. Testosterone selectively reduces the high molecular weight form of adiponectin by inhibiting its secretion from adipocytes. *J. Biol. Chem.* **2005**, *280*, 18073–18080. [CrossRef]

162. Tan, B.K.; Chen, J.; Digby, J.E.; Keay, S.D.; Kennedy, C.R.; Randeva, H.S. Upregulation of adiponectin receptor 1 and 2 mRNA and protein in adipose tissue and adipocytes in insulin-resistant women with polycystic ovary syndrome. *Diabetologia* **2006**, *49*, 2723–2728. [CrossRef] [PubMed]

163. Campos, D.B.; Palin, M.F.; Bordignon, V.; Murphy, B.D. The 'beneficial' adipokines in reproduction and fertility. *Int. J. Obes. (Lond.)* **2008**, *32*, 223–231. [CrossRef]

164. Ranjzad, F.; Mahmoudi, T.; Irani Shemirani, A.; Mahban, A.; Nikzamir, A.; Vahedi, M.; Ashrafi, M.; Gourabi, H. A common variant in the adiponectin gene and polycystic ovary syndrome risk. *Mol. Biol. Rep.* **2012**, *39*, 2313–2319. [CrossRef] [PubMed]

165. Alfaqih, M.A.; Khader, Y.S.; Al-Dwairi, A.N.; Alzoubi, A.; Al-Shboul, O.; Hatim, A. Lower Levels of Serum Adiponectin and the T Allele of rs1501299 of the ADIPOQ Gene Are Protective against Polycystic Ovarian Syndrome in Jordan. *Korean J. Fam. Med.* **2018**, *39*, 108–113. [CrossRef] [PubMed]

166. Mohammadi, E.; Rafraf, M.; Farzadi, L.; Asghari-Jafarabadi, M.; Sabour, S. Effects of omega-3 fatty acids supplementation on serum adiponectin levels and some metabolic risk factors in women with polycystic ovary syndrome. *Asia Pac. J. Clin. Nutr.* **2012**, *21*, 511–518. [PubMed]

167. Yang, K.; Zeng, L.; Bao, T.; Ge, J. Effectiveness of Omega-3 fatty acid for polycystic ovary syndrome: A systematic review and meta-analysis. *Reprod. Biol. Endocrinol.* **2018**, *16*, 27. [CrossRef] [PubMed]

168. Singh, A.; Bora, P.; Krishna, A. Direct action of adiponectin ameliorates increased androgen synthesis and reduces insulin receptor expression in the polycystic ovary. *Biochem. Biophys. Res. Commun.* **2017**, *488*, 509–515. [CrossRef]

169. Singh, A.; Bora, P.; Krishna, A. Systemic adiponectin treatment reverses polycystic ovary syndrome-like features in an animal model. *Reprod. Fertil. Dev.* **2017**. [CrossRef]

170. Torre, L.A.; Bray, F.; Siegel, R.L.; Ferlay, J.; Lortet-Tieulent, J.; Jemal, A. Global cancer statistics, 2012. *CA Cancer J. Clin.* **2015**, *65*, 87–108. [CrossRef] [PubMed]

171. Otsuka, I.; Kameda, S.; Hoshi, K. Early detection of ovarian and fallopian tube cancer by examination of cytological samples from the endometrial cavity. *Br. J. Cancer* **2013**, *109*, 603–609. [CrossRef] [PubMed]

172. Romero, I.; Bast, R.C., Jr. Minireview: Human ovarian cancer: Biology, current management, and paths to personalizing therapy. *Endocrinology* **2012**, *153*, 1593–1602. [CrossRef] [PubMed]

173. Dong, X.; Men, X.; Zhang, W.; Lei, P. Advances in tumor markers of ovarian cancer for early diagnosis. *Indian J. Cancer* **2014**, *51* (Suppl. 3), e72–e76. [CrossRef] [PubMed]

174. Miyoshi, Y.; Funahashi, T.; Kihara, S.; Taguchi, T.; Tamaki, Y.; Matsuzawa, Y.; Noguchi, S. Association of serum adiponectin levels with breast cancer risk. *Clin. Cancer Res.* **2003**, *9*, 5699–5704. [PubMed]

175. Goktas, S.; Yilmaz, M.I.; Caglar, K.; Sonmez, A.; Kilic, S.; Bedir, S. Prostate cancer and adiponectin. *Urology* **2005**, *65*, 1168–1172. [CrossRef] [PubMed]

176. Yokota, T.; Oritani, K.; Takahashi, I.; Ishikawa, J.; Matsuyama, A.; Ouchi, N.; Kihara, S.; Funahashi, T.; Tenner, A.J.; Tomiyama, Y.; et al. Adiponectin, a new member of the family of soluble defense collagens, negatively regulates the growth of myelomonocytic progenitors and the functions of macrophages. *Blood* **2000**, *96*, 1723–1732.

177. Brakenhielm, E.; Veitonmaki, N.; Cao, R.; Kihara, S.; Matsuzawa, Y.; Zhivotovsky, B.; Funahashi, T.; Cao, Y. Adiponectin-induced antiangiogenesis and antitumor activity involve caspase-mediated endothelial cell apoptosis. *Proc. Natl. Acad. Sci. USA* **2004**, *101*, 2476–2481. [CrossRef]

178. Hoffmann, M.; Gogola, J.; Ptak, A. Adiponectin Reverses the Proliferative Effects of Estradiol and IGF-1 in Human Epithelial Ovarian Cancer Cells by Downregulating the Expression of Their Receptors. *Horm. Cancer* **2018**, *9*, 166–174. [CrossRef]

179. Li, X.; Yu, Z.; Fang, L.; Liu, F.; Jiang, K. Expression of Adiponectin Receptor-1 and Prognosis of Epithelial Ovarian Cancer Patients. *Med. Sci. Monit.* **2017**, *23*, 1514–1521. [CrossRef]

180. Nagaraju, G.P.; Rajitha, B.; Aliya, S.; Kotipatruni, R.P.; Madanraj, A.S.; Hammond, A.; Park, D.; Chigurupati, S.; Alam, A.; Pattnaik, S. The role of adiponectin in obesity-associated female-specific carcinogenesis. *Cytokine Growth Factor Rev.* **2016**, *31*, 37–48. [CrossRef]

181. Takemura, Y.; Osuga, Y.; Harada, M.; Hirata, T.; Koga, K.; Yoshino, O.; Hirota, Y.; Morimoto, C.; Yano, T.; Taketani, Y. Concentration of adiponectin in peritoneal fluid is decreased in women with endometriosis. *Am. J. Reprod. Immunol.* **2005**, *54*, 217–221. [CrossRef] [PubMed]

182. Soliman, P.T.; Wu, D.; Tortolero-Luna, G.; Schmeler, K.M.; Slomovitz, B.M.; Bray, M.S.; Gershenson, D.M.; Lu, K.H. Association between adiponectin, insulin resistance, and endometrial cancer. *Cancer* **2006**, *106*, 2376–2381. [CrossRef] [PubMed]

183. Yi, K.W.; Shin, J.H.; Park, H.T.; Kim, T.; Kim, S.H.; Hur, J.Y. Resistin concentration is increased in the peritoneal fluid of women with endometriosis. *Am. J. Reprod. Immunol.* **2010**, *64*, 318–323. [CrossRef] [PubMed]

184. Pandey, N.; Kriplani, A.; Yadav, R.K.; Lyngdoh, B.T.; Mahapatra, S.C. Peritoneal fluid leptin levels are increased but adiponectin levels are not changed in infertile patients with pelvic endometriosis. *Gynecol. Endocrinol.* **2010**, *26*, 843–849. [CrossRef] [PubMed]

185. Choi, Y.S.; Oh, H.K.; Choi, J.H. Expression of adiponectin, leptin, and their receptors in ovarian endometrioma. *Fertil. Steril.* **2013**, *100*, 135–141.e2. [CrossRef] [PubMed]

186. Ashizawa, N.; Yahata, T.; Quan, J.; Adachi, S.; Yoshihara, K.; Tanaka, K. Serum leptin-adiponectin ratio and endometrial cancer risk in postmenopausal female subjects. *Gynecol. Oncol.* **2010**, *119*, 65–69. [CrossRef] [PubMed]

187. Petridou, E.; Mantzoros, C.; Dessypris, N.; Koukoulomatis, P.; Addy, C.; Voulgaris, Z.; Chrousos, G.; Trichopoulos, D. Plasma adiponectin concentrations in relation to endometrial cancer: A case-control study in Greece. *J. Clin. Endocrinol. Metab.* **2003**, *88*, 993–997. [CrossRef] [PubMed]

188. Dal Maso, L.; Augustin, L.S.; Karalis, A.; Talamini, R.; Franceschi, S.; Trichopoulos, D.; Mantzoros, C.S.; La Vecchia, C. Circulating adiponectin and endometrial cancer risk. *J. Clin. Endocrinol. Metab.* **2004**, *89*, 1160–1163. [CrossRef] [PubMed]

189. Cust, A.E.; Kaaks, R.; Friedenreich, C.; Bonnet, F.; Laville, M.; Lukanova, A.; Rinaldi, S.; Dossus, L.; Slimani, N.; Lundin, E.; et al. Plasma adiponectin levels and endometrial cancer risk in pre- and postmenopausal women. *J. Clin. Endocrinol. Metab.* **2007**, *92*, 255–263. [CrossRef] [PubMed]

190. Moon, H.S.; Chamberland, J.P.; Aronis, K.; Tseleni-Balafouta, S.; Mantzoros, C.S. Direct role of adiponectin and adiponectin receptors in endometrial cancer: In vitro and ex vivo studies in humans. *Mol. Cancer Ther.* **2011**, *10*, 2234–2243. [CrossRef] [PubMed]

191. Taliaferro-Smith, L.; Nagalingam, A.; Zhong, D.; Zhou, W.; Saxena, N.K.; Sharma, D. LKB1 is required for adiponectin-mediated modulation of AMPK-S6K axis and inhibition of migration and invasion of breast cancer cells. *Oncogene* **2009**, *28*, 2621–2633. [CrossRef]

192. American Diabetes, A. 2. Classification and Diagnosis of Diabetes: Standards of Medical Care in Diabetes-2019. *Diabetes Care* **2019**, *42*, S13–S28. [CrossRef] [PubMed]

193. Plows, J.F.; Stanley, J.L.; Baker, P.N.; Reynolds, C.M.; Vickers, M.H. The Pathophysiology of Gestational Diabetes Mellitus. *Int. J. Mol. Sci.* **2018**, *19*, 3342. [CrossRef] [PubMed]

194. Parsons, J.A.; Brelje, T.C.; Sorenson, R.L. Adaptation of islets of Langerhans to pregnancy: Increased islet cell proliferation and insulin secretion correlates with the onset of placental lactogen secretion. *Endocrinology* **1992**, *130*, 1459–1466. [CrossRef]

195. Retnakaran, R. Adiponectin and beta-Cell Adaptation in Pregnancy. *Diabetes* **2017**, *66*, 1121–1122. [CrossRef]

196. Buckley, B.S.; Harreiter, J.; Damm, P.; Corcoy, R.; Chico, A.; Simmons, D.; Vellinga, A.; Dunne, F.; Group, D.C.I. Gestational diabetes mellitus in Europe: Prevalence, current screening practice and barriers to screening. A review. *Diabet. Med.* **2012**, *29*, 844–854. [CrossRef]

197. Catalano, P.M.; Hoegh, M.; Minium, J.; Huston-Presley, L.; Bernard, S.; Kalhan, S.; Hauguel-De Mouzon, S. Adiponectin in human pregnancy: Implications for regulation of glucose and lipid metabolism. *Diabetologia* **2006**, *49*, 1677–1685. [CrossRef]

198. Lara-Castro, C.; Luo, N.; Wallace, P.; Klein, R.L.; Garvey, W.T. Adiponectin multimeric complexes and the metabolic syndrome trait cluster. *Diabetes* **2006**, *55*, 249–259. [CrossRef] [PubMed]

199. Qiao, L.; Wattez, J.S.; Lee, S.; Nguyen, A.; Schaack, J.; Hay, W.W., Jr.; Shao, J. Adiponectin Deficiency Impairs Maternal Metabolic Adaptation to Pregnancy in Mice. *Diabetes* **2017**, *66*, 1126–1135. [CrossRef]

200. Pala, H.G.; Ozalp, Y.; Yener, A.S.; Gerceklioglu, G.; Uysal, S.; Onvural, A. Adiponectin levels in gestational diabetes mellitus and in pregnant women without glucose intolerance. *Adv. Clin. Exp. Med.* **2015**, *24*, 85–92. [CrossRef]

201. Kajantie, E.; Hytinantti, T.; Hovi, P.; Andersson, S. Cord plasma adiponectin: A 20-fold rise between 24 weeks gestation and term. *J. Clin. Endocrinol. Metab.* **2004**, *89*, 4031–4036. [CrossRef]

202. Chan, T.F.; Chung, Y.F.; Chen, H.S.; Su, J.H.; Yuan, S.S. Elevated amniotic fluid leptin levels in early second trimester are associated with earlier delivery and lower birthweight in twin pregnancy. *Acta Obstet. Gynecol. Scand.* **2004**, *83*, 707–710. [CrossRef] [PubMed]

203. Chen, J.; Tan, B.; Karteris, E.; Zervou, S.; Digby, J.; Hillhouse, E.W.; Vatish, M.; Randeva, H.S. Secretion of adiponectin by human placenta: Differential modulation of adiponectin and its receptors by cytokines. *Diabetologia* **2006**, *49*, 1292–1302. [CrossRef] [PubMed]

204. Ategbo, J.M.; Grissa, O.; Yessoufou, A.; Hichami, A.; Dramane, K.L.; Moutairou, K.; Miled, A.; Grissa, A.; Jerbi, M.; Tabka, Z.; et al. Modulation of adipokines and cytokines in gestational diabetes and macrosomia. *J. Clin. Endocrinol. Metab.* **2006**, *91*, 4137–4143. [CrossRef]

205. Horosz, E.; Bomba-Opon, D.A.; Szymanska, M.; Wielgos, M. Third trimester plasma adiponectin and leptin in gestational diabetes and normal pregnancies. *Diabetes Res. Clin. Pract.* **2011**, *93*, 350–356. [CrossRef] [PubMed]

206. Retnakaran, R.; Qi, Y.; Connelly, P.W.; Sermer, M.; Hanley, A.J.; Zinman, B. Low adiponectin concentration during pregnancy predicts postpartum insulin resistance, beta cell dysfunction and fasting glycaemia. *Diabetologia* **2010**, *53*, 268–276. [CrossRef]

207. Radaelli, T.; Varastehpour, A.; Catalano, P.; Hauguel-de Mouzon, S. Gestational diabetes induces placental genes for chronic stress and inflammatory pathways. *Diabetes* **2003**, *52*, 2951–2958. [CrossRef] [PubMed]

208. Ruan, H.; Lodish, H.F. Insulin resistance in adipose tissue: Direct and indirect effects of tumor necrosis factor-alpha. *Cytokine Growth Factor Rev.* **2003**, *14*, 447–455. [CrossRef]

209. Kern, P.A.; Di Gregorio, G.B.; Lu, T.; Rassouli, N.; Ranganathan, G. Adiponectin expression from human adipose tissue: Relation to obesity, insulin resistance, and tumor necrosis factor-alpha expression. *Diabetes* **2003**, *52*, 1779–1785. [CrossRef]

210. Bao, W.; Baecker, A.; Song, Y.; Kiely, M.; Liu, S.; Zhang, C. Adipokine levels during the first or early second trimester of pregnancy and subsequent risk of gestational diabetes mellitus: A systematic review. *Metabolism* **2015**, *64*, 756–764. [CrossRef] [PubMed]

211. Iliodromiti, S.; Sassarini, J.; Kelsey, T.W.; Lindsay, R.S.; Sattar, N.; Nelson, S.M. Accuracy of circulating adiponectin for predicting gestational diabetes: A systematic review and meta-analysis. *Diabetologia* **2016**, *59*, 692–699. [CrossRef] [PubMed]

212. Williams, M.A.; Qiu, C.; Muy-Rivera, M.; Vadachkoria, S.; Song, T.; Luthy, D.A. Plasma adiponectin concentrations in early pregnancy and subsequent risk of gestational diabetes mellitus. *J. Clin. Endocrinol. Metab.* **2004**, *89*, 2306–2311. [CrossRef] [PubMed]

213. Lain, K.Y.; Daftary, A.R.; Ness, R.B.; Roberts, J.M. First trimester adipocytokine concentrations and risk of developing gestational diabetes later in pregnancy. *Clin. Endocrinol. (Oxf.)* **2008**, *69*, 407–411. [CrossRef]

214. Lacroix, M.; Battista, M.C.; Doyon, M.; Menard, J.; Ardilouze, J.L.; Perron, P.; Hivert, M.F. Lower adiponectin levels at first trimester of pregnancy are associated with increased insulin resistance and higher risk of developing gestational diabetes mellitus. *Diabetes Care* **2013**, *36*, 1577–1583. [CrossRef] [PubMed]

215. Pawlik, A.; Teler, J.; Maciejewska, A.; Sawczuk, M.; Safranow, K.; Dziedziejko, V. Adiponectin and leptin gene polymorphisms in women with gestational diabetes mellitus. *J. Assist. Reprod. Genet.* **2017**, *34*, 511–516. [CrossRef]

216. Beltcheva, O.; Boyadzhieva, M.; Angelova, O.; Mitev, V.; Kaneva, R.; Atanasova, I. The rs266729 single-nucleotide polymorphism in the adiponectin gene shows association with gestational diabetes. *Arch. Gynecol. Obstet.* **2014**, *289*, 743–748. [CrossRef] [PubMed]

217. Han, Y.; Zheng, Y.L.; Fan, Y.P.; Liu, M.H.; Lu, X.Y.; Tao, Q. Association of adiponectin gene polymorphism 45TG with gestational diabetes mellitus diagnosed on the new IADPSG criteria, plasma adiponectin levels and adverse pregnancy outcomes. *Clin. Exp. Med.* **2015**, *15*, 47–53. [CrossRef] [PubMed]

218. Takhshid, M.A.; Haem, Z.; Aboualizadeh, F. The association of circulating adiponectin and + 45 T/G polymorphism of adiponectin gene with gestational diabetes mellitus in Iranian population. *J. Diabetes Metab. Disord.* **2015**, *14*, 30. [CrossRef]

219. Low, C.F.; Mohd Tohit, E.R.; Chong, P.P.; Idris, F. Adiponectin SNP45TG is associated with gestational diabetes mellitus. *Arch. Gynecol. Obstet.* **2011**, *283*, 1255–1260. [CrossRef]

220. Ye, R.; Wang, M.; Wang, Q.A.; Scherer, P.E. Adiponectin-mediated antilipotoxic effects in regenerating pancreatic islets. *Endocrinology* **2015**, *156*, 2019–2028. [CrossRef]

221. Retnakaran, R.; Connelly, P.W.; Maguire, G.; Sermer, M.; Zinman, B.; Hanley, A.J. Decreased high-molecular-weight adiponectin in gestational diabetes: Implications for the pathophysiology of Type 2 diabetes. *Diabet. Med.* **2007**, *24*, 245–252. [CrossRef]

222. Retnakaran, R.; Hanley, A.J.; Raif, N.; Hirning, C.R.; Connelly, P.W.; Sermer, M.; Kahn, S.E.; Zinman, B. Adiponectin and beta cell dysfunction in gestational diabetes: Pathophysiological implications. *Diabetologia* **2005**, *48*, 993–1001. [CrossRef]

223. Abalos, E.; Cuesta, C.; Grosso, A.L.; Chou, D.; Say, L. Global and regional estimates of preeclampsia and eclampsia: A systematic review. *Eur. J. Obstet. Gynecol. Reprod. Biol.* **2013**, *170*, 1–7. [CrossRef] [PubMed]

224. Mayrink, J.; Costa, M.L.; Cecatti, J.G. Preeclampsia in 2018: Revisiting Concepts, Physiopathology, and Prediction. *Sci. World J.* **2018**, *2018*, 6268276. [CrossRef]

225. Song, Y.; Gao, J.; Qu, Y.; Wang, S.; Wang, X.; Liu, J. Serum levels of leptin, adiponectin and resistin in relation to clinical characteristics in normal pregnancy and preeclampsia. *Clin. Chim. Acta* **2016**, *458*, 133–137. [CrossRef]

226. Demir, B.C.; Atalay, M.A.; Ozerkan, K.; Doster, Y.; Ocakoglu, G.; Kucukkomurcu, S. Maternal adiponectin and visfatin concentrations in normal and complicated pregnancies. *Clin. Exp. Obstet. Gynecol.* **2013**, *40*, 261–267.

227. Miehle, K.; Stepan, H.; Fasshauer, M. Leptin, adiponectin and other adipokines in gestational diabetes mellitus and pre-eclampsia. *Clin. Endocrinol. (Oxf.)* **2012**, *76*, 2–11. [CrossRef] [PubMed]

228. Mannisto, T.; Mendola, P.; Vaarasmaki, M.; Jarvelin, M.R.; Hartikainen, A.L.; Pouta, A.; Suvanto, E. Elevated blood pressure in pregnancy and subsequent chronic disease risk. *Circulation* **2013**, *127*, 681–690. [CrossRef] [PubMed]

229. Ramsay, J.E.; Jamieson, N.; Greer, I.A.; Sattar, N. Paradoxical elevation in adiponectin concentrations in women with preeclampsia. *Hypertension* **2003**, *42*, 891–894. [CrossRef]

230. Naruse, K.; Yamasaki, M.; Umekage, H.; Sado, T.; Sakamoto, Y.; Morikawa, H. Peripheral blood concentrations of adiponectin, an adipocyte-specific plasma protein, in normal pregnancy and preeclampsia. *J. Reprod. Immunol.* **2005**, *65*, 65–75. [CrossRef]

231. Haugen, F.; Ranheim, T.; Harsem, N.K.; Lips, E.; Staff, A.C.; Drevon, C.A. Increased plasma levels of adipokines in preeclampsia: Relationship to placenta and adipose tissue gene expression. *Am. J. Physiol. Endocrinol. Metab.* **2006**, *290*, E326–E333. [CrossRef] [PubMed]

232. Eleuterio, N.M.; Palei, A.C.; Rangel Machado, J.S.; Tanus-Santos, J.E.; Cavalli, R.C.; Sandrim, V.C. Relationship between adiponectin and nitrite in healthy and preeclampsia pregnancies. *Clin. Chim. Acta* **2013**, *423*, 112–115. [CrossRef]

233. Hendler, I.; Blackwell, S.C.; Mehta, S.H.; Whitty, J.E.; Russell, E.; Sorokin, Y.; Cotton, D.B. The levels of leptin, adiponectin, and resistin in normal weight, overweight, and obese pregnant women with and without preeclampsia. *Am. J. Obstet. Gynecol.* **2005**, *193*, 979–983. [CrossRef] [PubMed]

234. Takemura, Y.; Osuga, Y.; Koga, K.; Tajima, T.; Hirota, Y.; Hirata, T.; Morimoto, C.; Harada, M.; Yano, T.; Taketani, Y. Selective increase in high molecular weight adiponectin concentration in serum of women with preeclampsia. *J. Reprod. Immunol.* **2007**, *73*, 60–65. [CrossRef]

235. D'Anna, R.; Baviera, G.; Corrado, F.; Giordano, D.; De Vivo, A.; Nicocia, G.; Di Benedetto, A. Adiponectin and insulin resistance in early- and late-onset pre-eclampsia. *BJOG* **2006**, *113*, 1264–1269. [CrossRef]

236. Cortelazzi, D.; Corbetta, S.; Ronzoni, S.; Pelle, F.; Marconi, A.; Cozzi, V.; Cetin, I.; Cortelazzi, R.; Beck-Peccoz, P.; Spada, A. Maternal and foetal resistin and adiponectin concentrations in normal and complicated pregnancies. *Clin. Endocrinol. (Oxf.)* **2007**, *66*, 447–453. [CrossRef] [PubMed]

237. Dalamaga, M.; Srinivas, S.K.; Elovitz, M.A.; Chamberland, J.; Mantzoros, C.S. Serum adiponectin and leptin in relation to risk for preeclampsia: Results from a large case-control study. *Metabolism* **2011**, *60*, 1539–1544. [CrossRef]

238. Mazaki-Tovi, S.; Romero, R.; Vaisbuch, E.; Kusanovic, J.P.; Erez, O.; Gotsch, F.; Chaiworapongsa, T.; Than, N.G.; Kim, S.K.; Nhan-Chang, C.L.; et al. Maternal serum adiponectin multimers in preeclampsia. *J. Perinat. Med.* **2009**, *37*, 349–363. [CrossRef] [PubMed]

239. Machado, J.S.; Palei, A.C.; Amaral, L.M.; Bueno, A.C.; Antonini, S.R.; Duarte, G.; Tanus-Santos, J.E.; Sandrim, V.C.; Cavalli, R.C. Polymorphisms of the adiponectin gene in gestational hypertension and pre-eclampsia. *J. Hum. Hypertens.* **2014**, *28*, 128–132. [CrossRef]

240. Saarela, T.; Hiltunen, M.; Helisalmi, S.; Heinonen, S.; Laakso, M. Adiponectin gene haplotype is associated with preeclampsia. *Genet. Test.* **2006**, *10*, 35–39. [CrossRef] [PubMed]

241. Zhu, W.; Cheng, K.K.; Vanhoutte, P.M.; Lam, K.S.; Xu, A. Vascular effects of adiponectin: Molecular mechanisms and potential therapeutic intervention. *Clin. Sci. (Lond.)* **2008**, *114*, 361–374. [CrossRef] [PubMed]

242. Miller, S.L.; Huppi, P.S.; Mallard, C. The consequences of fetal growth restriction on brain structure and neurodevelopmental outcome. *J. Physiol.* **2016**, *594*, 807–823. [CrossRef]

243. Malhotra, A.; Allison, B.J.; Castillo-Melendez, M.; Jenkin, G.; Polglase, G.R.; Miller, S.L. Neonatal Morbidities of Fetal Growth Restriction: Pathophysiology and Impact. *Front. Endocrinol. (Lausanne)* **2019**, *10*, 55. [CrossRef]

244. Ghidini, A. Idiopathic fetal growth restriction: A pathophysiologic approach. *Obstet. Gynecol. Surv.* **1996**, *51*, 376–382. [CrossRef]

245. Sharp, A.N.; Heazell, A.E.; Crocker, I.P.; Mor, G. Placental apoptosis in health and disease. *Am. J. Reprod. Immunol.* **2010**, *64*, 159–169. [CrossRef]

246. Straszewski-Chavez, S.L.; Abrahams, V.M.; Mor, G. The role of apoptosis in the regulation of trophoblast survival and differentiation during pregnancy. *Endocr. Rev.* **2005**, *26*, 877–897. [CrossRef] [PubMed]

247. Gaccioli, F.; Lager, S. Placental Nutrient Transport and Intrauterine Growth Restriction. *Front. Physiol.* **2016**, *7*, 40. [CrossRef]

248. Gardosi, J.; Kady, S.M.; McGeown, P.; Francis, A.; Tonks, A. Classification of stillbirth by relevant condition at death (ReCoDe): Population based cohort study. *BMJ* **2005**, *331*, 1113–1117. [CrossRef] [PubMed]

249. Sharma, D.; Shastri, S.; Sharma, P. Intrauterine Growth Restriction: Antenatal and Postnatal Aspects. *Clin. Med. Insights Pediatr.* **2016**, *10*, 67–83. [CrossRef]

250. Goto, E. Blood adiponectin concentration at birth in small for gestational age neonates: A meta-analysis. *Diabetes Metab. Syndr.* **2019**, *13*, 183–188. [CrossRef]

251. Evagelidou, E.N.; Giapros, V.I.; Challa, A.S.; Kiortsis, D.N.; Tsatsoulis, A.A.; Andronikou, S.K. Serum adiponectin levels, insulin resistance, and lipid profile in children born small for gestational age are affected by the severity of growth retardation at birth. *Eur. J. Endocrinol.* **2007**, *156*, 271–277. [CrossRef] [PubMed]

252. Buke, B.; Topcu, H.O.; Engin-Ustun, Y.; Danisman, N. Comparison of serum maternal adiponectin concentrations in women with isolated intrauterine growth retardation and intrauterine growth retardation concomitant with pre-eclampsia. *J. Turk. Ger. Gynecol. Assoc.* **2014**, *15*, 173–176. [CrossRef]

253. Kyriakakou, M.; Malamitsi-Puchner, A.; Militsi, H.; Boutsikou, T.; Margeli, A.; Hassiakos, D.; Kanaka-Gantenbein, C.; Papassotiriou, I.; Mastorakos, G. Leptin and adiponectin concentrations in intrauterine growth restricted and appropriate for gestational age foetuses, neonates, and their mothers. *Eur. J. Endocrinol.* **2008**, *158*, 343–348. [CrossRef]

254. Visentin, S.; Lapolla, A.; Londero, A.P.; Cosma, C.; Dalfra, M.; Camerin, M.; Faggian, D.; Plebani, M.; Cosmi, E. Adiponectin levels are reduced while markers of systemic inflammation and aortic remodelling are increased in intrauterine growth restricted mother-child couple. *Biomed. Res. Int.* **2014**, *2014*, 401595. [CrossRef] [PubMed]

255. Lekva, T.; Roland, M.C.P.; Michelsen, A.E.; Friis, C.M.; Aukrust, P.; Bollerslev, J.; Henriksen, T.; Ueland, T. Large Reduction in Adiponectin During Pregnancy Is Associated with Large-for-Gestational-Age Newborns. *J. Clin. Endocrinol. Metab.* **2017**, *102*, 2552–2559. [CrossRef] [PubMed]

256. Duval, F.; Santos, E.D.; Poidatz, D.; Serazin, V.; Gronier, H.; Vialard, F.; Dieudonne, M.N. Adiponectin Inhibits Nutrient Transporters and Promotes Apoptosis in Human Villous Cytotrophoblasts: Involvement in the Control of Fetal Growth. *Biol. Reprod.* **2016**, *94*, 111. [CrossRef] [PubMed]

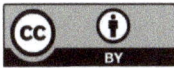

International Journal of
Molecular Sciences

MDPI

Article

Transcriptomic Analysis of Porcine Endometrium during Implantation after In Vitro Stimulation by Adiponectin

Nina Smolinska *, Karol Szeszko, Kamil Dobrzyn, Marta Kiezun, Edyta Rytelewska, Katarzyna Kisielewska, Marlena Gudelska, Kinga Bors, Joanna Wyrebek, Grzegorz Kopij, Barbara Kaminska and Tadeusz Kaminski

Department of Animal Anatomy and Physiology, Faculty of Biology and Biotechnology, University of Warmia and Mazury in Olsztyn, Oczapowskiego 1A, 10-719 Olsztyn-Kortowo, Poland; karol.szeszko@uwm.edu.pl (K.S.); kamil.dobrzyn@uwm.edu.pl (K.D.); marta.kiezun@uwm.edu.pl (M.K.); edyta.rytelewska@uwm.edu.pl (E.R.); katarzyna.kisielewska@uwm.edu.pl (K.K.); marlena.gudelska@uwm.edu.pl (M.G.); kinga.bors@uwm.edu.pl (K.B.); joanna.wyrebek@uwm.edu.pl (J.W.); grzegorz.kopij@student.uwm.edu.pl (G.K.); barbara.kaminska@uwm.edu.pl (B.K.); tkam@uwm.edu.pl (T.K.)
* Correspondence: nina.smolinska@uwm.edu.pl

Received: 26 February 2019; Accepted: 13 March 2019; Published: 16 March 2019

Abstract: Comprehensive understanding of the regulatory mechanism of the implantation process in pigs is crucial for reproductive success. The endometrium plays an important role in regulating the establishment and maintenance of gestation. The goal of the current study was to determine the effect of adiponectin on the global expression pattern of genes and relationships among differentially expressed genes (DE-genes) in the porcine endometrium during implantation using microarrays. Diverse transcriptome analyses including gene ontology (GO), biological pathway, networks, and DE-gene analyses were performed. Adiponectin altered the expression of 1286 genes with fold-change (FC) values greater than 1.2 ($p < 0.05$). The expression of 560 genes were upregulated and 726 downregulated in the endometrium treated with adiponectin. Thirteen genes were selected for real-time PCR validation of differential expression based on a known role in metabolism, steroid and prostaglandin synthesis, interleukin and growth factor action, and embryo implantation. Functional analysis of the relationship between DE-genes indicated that adiponectin interacts with genes that are involved in the processes of cell proliferation, programmed cell death, steroid and prostaglandin synthesis/metabolism, cytokine production, and cell adhesion that are critical for reproductive success. The presented results suggest that adiponectin signalling may play a key role in the implantation of pig.

Keywords: endometrium; implantation; transcriptome; microarray; adiponectin; pig

---

1. Introduction

Understanding the mechanisms controlling energy homeostasis and reproduction creates the foundation and opens a way towards future effective modification of these processes in farm animals. Most authors agree that 20% to 30% of porcine embryos are lost between days 12 to 30 of pregnancy (reviewed by Reference [1]). This critical period for embryos is not yet fully understood. Establishment and maintenance of pregnancy require reciprocal interactions between the conceptus and endometrium. The embryos migrating within the uterus about days 10 to 11 of pregnancy synthesize and secrete oestradiol (E2) and prostaglandin E2 (PGE2), the key hormonal components of the process of maternal recognition of pregnancy (days 12 to 13). On the other hand, the endometrium undergoes hormonally regulated (mainly by progesterone (P4) and E2) alteration of receptivity in order to attach and implant the embryo, which occurs around days 15 to 16 of gestation. The period of uterine receptivity, called the "window of implantation", is also related to the presence of growth factors, multiple adhesion molecules, such as integrins, or proteolytic enzymes, such as metalloproteinases, which are essential for embryo implantation. During this period, the endometrium produces prostaglandins, chemokines, and cytokines, which are responsible for the proper course of the implantation process [2–4]. During the peri-implantation period, properly synchronized expression of genes for many factors, e.g., steroid hormones, prostaglandins, cytokines, angiogenic factors, apoptosis-related substances, integrins, and metalloproteinases in the uteri, conceptuses, and trophoblasts are important for effective maternal recognition of pregnancy and implantation, and consequently it is essential for embryo survival and development. Adiponectin, which is a member of adipokine family, could belong to the group of hormones that affect the processes/mechanisms related to the peri-implantation period directly or indirectly by controlling the synthesis of the above factors.

Adiponectin is a 30 kDa cytokine, predominantly synthesized and secreted by the adipose tissue and circulating at high levels in the bloodstream [5,6]. In the plasma, adiponectin can be found in the form of a trimer (low molecular weight, LMW), a combination of two trimers (middle molecular weight, MMW) or a structure of six trimers (high molecular weight, HMW) [7]. Adiponectin levels in the blood and in the adipose tissue are negatively associated with obesity [6,8]. Adiponectin exerts its effect by binding to two transmembrane receptors, adiponectin receptor type 1 (AdipoR1) and adiponectin receptor type 2 (AdipoR2). Adiponectin receptor type 1 demonstrates a higher affinity for the trimeric form of adiponectin, and it is found at the highest concentrations in skeletal muscles, whereas AdipoR2, found mainly in the liver, shows greater affinity for MMW and HMW forms. Adiponectin regulates energy homeostasis by fatty-acid oxidation, stimulation of glucose uptake, and inhibition of gluconeogenesis. The above leads to intensified thermogenesis, weight loss, and increased insulin sensitivity in tissues [9]. This adipokine possesses anti-atherogenic, anti-inflammatory, anti-proliferative, anti-angiogenic, and pro-apoptotic properties (for review see Reference [10]).

Accumulating evidence suggests the involvement of adiponectin in reproduction control (for review see References [11,12]). Adiponectin and its receptors (the adiponectin system) have been found in the female reproductive tract of different species such as human, rat, mouse, and pig [13–18]. Our previous findings show that the concentrations of adiponectin system transcripts and proteins in the porcine endometrium and myometrium fluctuated during different phases of the oestrous cycle and pregnancy, which indicates that females' hormonal status influences the expression of adiponectin system components and the sensitivity of the examined structures to the adipokine [19,20]. Our study revealed that adiponectin regulates the expression of steroidogenic enzymes genes and the secretion of steroid hormones by *in vitro* incubated porcine endometrial and myometrial explants during early pregnancy and on days 10 to 11 of the oestrous cycle [21]. Based on our observations, we hypothesized that adiponectin may be an important factor in the regulation of processes taking place in the uterus. Thus, the aim of the present study was to investigate the comprehensive effect of adiponectin on the transcriptome of the porcine endometrial cells during the implantation period, on days 15 to 16 of pregnancy. The proposed study will help to identify genes and the processes modified by adiponectin, and thereby provide further evidence that adiponectin plays a role in reproduction.

2. Results

2.1. Microarray Data Analysis

2.1.1. Identification of Differentially Expressed (DE) Genes

Transcriptome analyses were carried out to compare the gene expression between the control endometrial tissue explants and endometrial tissue explants treated with 10 µg/mL of adiponectin. A complete list of DE-genes recognized during this study is presented in table format in the Table S1. The table includes a probe set name, gene ID, fold change, *p*-value, the direction of change (up or down), as well as function and accession number. The whole number of DE-genes generated by GeneSpring was 1494, among which 1286 genes had a FC values greater than 1.2 ($p < 0.05$). The expression of 560 genes was upregulated and 726 downregulated in the endometrium treated with adiponectin.

2.1.2. Gene Ontology Analysis

Gene ontology enrichment analysis was used to perform a functional categorisation of the DE-genes. As a result of the analysis prepared in DAVID (Database for Annotation, Visualization and Integrated Discovery), three GO categories were specified: biological process (BP), metabolic function (MF), and cell component (CC). The results for the entire DE-gene list (up- and downregulated; modified Fisher's exact test $p < 0.1$) are summarized in the Table S2. The most significantly enriched genes ontologies were obtained under the BP category. Furthermore, two additional BP lists were generated from upregulated and downregulated DE-genes (Supplementary Materials Table S3). These results allowed us to choose 102 of the most important processes for endometrium functioning, including 35 and 67 processes connected to up- and downregulated DE-genes, respectively (Supplementary Materials Table S4). In the analysis conducted on the basis of the upregulated DE-gene list, we observed a group of 47 gene products associated with GO terms related to *gene expression* (GO:0010467). Most of these gene products (26) were involved in *transcription, DNA-templated* (GO:0006351), which suggests that adiponectin induces transcription in the endometrial cells. The next group of 39 gene products was involved in the *RNA metabolic processes* (GO:0016070), including 30 engaged in *RNA biosynthetic processes* (GO:0032774) and *nucleic acid-templated transcription* (GO:0097659). Adiponectin also had an effect on the *regulation of gene expression* (GO:0010468), *regulation of transcription, DNA-templated* (GO:0006355), and the *positive regulation of pri-miRNA transcription from RNA polymerase II promoter* (GO:1902895) by increasing the expression of 33, 24, and 2 DE-genes, respectively. The next group of 33 gene products was involved in the *regulation of nitrogen compound metabolic processes* (GO:0051171): 27 of these gene products were connected with the *regulation of nucleobase-containing compound metabolic processes* (GO:0019219), 25 with the *regulation of RNA metabolic processes* (GO:0051252), 24 with the *regulation of RNA biosynthetic processes* (GO:2001141), and also 24 with the *regulation of nucleic acid-templated transcription* (GO:1903506).

Another biological process modulated by the studied hormone were the *regulation of macromolecule biosynthetic processes* (GO:0010556) and *regulation of cellular macromolecule biosynthetic processes* (GO:2000112). We identified 31 and 29 upregulated DE-genes related to these GO terms, respectively. The adipokine increased the expression of 15 genes, whose products were involved in the *cellular catabolic processes* (GO:0044248). Another 14 gene products were associated with the *vesicle-mediated transport* (GO:0016192). The next group of 12 gene products was involved in the *DNA metabolic processes* (GO:0006259) including seven and five engaged in *DNA repair* (GO:0006281) and *DNA recombination* (GO:0006310), respectively. Another biological process modulated by the adiponectin was the *protein modification by small protein conjugation or removal* (GO:0070647). Moreover, nine DE-genes were involved in the regulation of the *response to abiotic stimulus* (GO:0009628) and three of these in the *cellular response to light stimulus* (GO:0071482). The next group of eight gene products was involved in the *ribonucleoprotein complex biogenesis* (GO:0022613) and three in *ribosome biogenesis* (GO:0042254). Another biological process modulated by the studied hormone was the *nucleoside metabolic processes* (GO:0009116; 6 DE-genes). The same group of six gene products was also involved in *purine nucleoside metabolic process* (GO:0042278) and *purine ribonucleotide metabolic process* (GO:0046128). Another group of six gene products was involved in *glycosyl compound metabolic processes* (GO:1901657). The last five significant results were related to *nucleoside triphosphate metabolic processes* (GO:0009141; 5 DE-genes), *positive regulation of cell projection organization* (GO:0031346; 5 DE-genes), *cell–matrix adhesion* (GO:0007160; 4 DE-genes), *translational initiation* (GO:0006413; 4 DE-genes), and *regulation of mRNA 3'-end processing* (GO:0031440; 2 DE-genes). In the group of genes connected to *positive regulation of cell projection organization*, four gene products were also involved in *positive regulation of neuron projection development* (GO:0010976).

In the case of GO analysis of downregulated DE-genes, the most significant group consisted of 85 genes whose products were involved in the *regulation of gene expression* (GO:0010468); 41 of these gene products were connected with the *positive regulation of gene expression* (GO:0010628), 36 with the *negative regulation of gene expression* (GO:0010629) and six with *gene silencing* (GO:0016458). Another 56 gene products were associated with *the negative regulation of metabolic processes* (GO:0009892), including 53 involved in the *negative regulation of cellular metabolic processes* (GO:0031324), and 23 in the *negative regulation of cellular protein metabolic processes* (GO:0032269). The next group of 41 gene products was involved in 19 GO terms related to the *regulation of immune system processes* (GO:0002682), including *positive regulation of immune system processes* (GO:0002684; 27 DE-genes), *regulation of immune response* (GO:0050776; 15 DE-genes), *positive regulation of immune response* (GO:0050778; 13 DE-genes), *activation of immune response* (GO:0002253; 10 DE-genes), *regulation of hemopoiesis* (GO:1903706; 13 DE-genes), *positive regulation of hemopoiesis* (GO:1903708; 7 DE-genes), *negative regulation of hemopoiesis* (GO:1903707; 7 DE-genes), *regulation of myeloid cell differentiation* (GO:0045637; 10 DE-genes), *positive regulation of myeloid cell differentiation* (GO:0045639; 5 DE-genes), *negative regulation of myeloid cell differentiation* (GO:0045638; 5 DE-genes), *regulation of erythrocyte differentiation* (GO:0045646; 6 DE-genes), *negative regulation of erythrocyte differentiation* (GO:0045647; 3 DE-genes), *regulation of innate immune response* (GO:0045088; 8 DE-genes), *positive regulation of innate immune response* (GO:0045089; 7 DE-genes), *regulation of leukocyte migration* (GO:0002685; 8 DE-genes), *leukocyte tethering or rolling* (GO:0050901; 3 DE-genes), *regulation of neutrophil migration* (GO:1902622; 3 DE-genes), and *regulation of neutrophil chemotaxis* (GO:0090022; 3 DE-genes). Another biological process modulated by the studied adipokine were the *regulation of cell proliferation* (GO:0042127; 38 DE-genes) and *negative regulation of cell proliferation* (GO:0008285; 17 DE-genes). The next group of 36 gene products was involved in *cell proliferation* (GO:0008283). The studied hormone also had an effect on *programmed cell death* (GO:0012501) by decreasing the expression of 35 DE-genes. Additionally, we identified 29 downregulated DE-genes related to *biological adhesion* (GO:0022610), 29 of these DE-genes affect *cell adhesion* (GO:0007155), 24 with *single organism cell adhesion* (GO:0098602), 23 with *single organismal cell–cell adhesion* (GO:0016337), 23 with *cell–cell adhesion* (GO:0098609), 17 with *leukocyte cell–cell adhesion* (GO:0007159), four with *leukocyte adhesion to vascular endothelial cell* (GO:0061756), and seven affect *cell–matrix adhesion* (GO:0007160). Moreover, 28 DE-genes were involved in *immune system development* (GO:0002520) and *hematopoietic or lymphoid organ development* (GO:0048534), 26 of these DE-genes in the *hemopoiesis* (GO:0030097) including the *myeloid cell differentiation* (GO:0030099; 17 DE-genes), *erythrocyte differentiation* (GO:0030218; 8 DE-genes), and *myeloid cell development* (GO:0061515; 4 DE-genes).

Adiponectin also downregulated 18 DE-genes associated with the *multicellular organism reproduction* (GO:0032504) and *multicellular organismal reproductive processes* (GO:0048609). The group of 17 of these genes was related to *sexual reproduction* (GO:0019953), 14 to *gamete generation* (GO:0007276), three to the *ovulation* (GO:0030728) and four to *ovulation cycle processes* (GO:0022602). The next group of 17 gene products was involved in *developmental processes involved in reproduction* (GO:0003006) including eight engaged in *development of primary sexual characteristics* (GO:0045137) and *development of primary female sexual characteristics* (GO:0046545), five DE-genes in the *female sex differentiation* (GO:0046660) processes. Other biological processes modulated by the studied adipokine were *cytokine production* (GO:0001816; 16 DE-genes), *cytokine metabolic processes* (GO:0042107; 5 DE-genes), and *cytokine biosynthetic processes* (GO:0042089; 5 DE-genes). Next, the biological process worth emphasizing was the *regulation of cell adhesion* (GO:0030155), which was represented by 16 DE-genes. Moreover, 13 of these DE-genes affected the *regulation of cell–cell adhesion* (GO:0022407), 10 affected the *regulation of leukocyte cell–cell adhesion* (GO:1903037), and 11 affected the *positive regulation of cell adhesion* (GO:0045785). Adiponectin had also an effect on the *reproductive system development* (GO:0061458) by decreasing the expression of 12 DE-genes. Most of these were involved in *reproductive structure development* (GO:0048608), *gonad development* (GO:0008406), and *female gonad development* (GO:0008585). The next group of 12 gene products was involved in the *negative regulation of cell cycle* (GO:0045786). The last two processes affected by adiponectin were the *regulation of haemostasis* (GO:1900046; 5 DE-genes) and *positive regulation of cytokine biosynthetic processes* (GO:0042108; 4 DE-genes).

2.1.3. Biological Pathway Analysis

Forty-four biological pathways were generated using the KEGG (Kyoto Encyclopedia of Genes) database (Table 1). The pathways with the largest number of involved genes were *pathways in cancer* (21 DE-genes). The other pathways indicated by the DAVID tool that were affected by adiponectin treatment were as follows: *cytokine–cytokine receptor interaction* (18 DE-genes), *Jak–STAT signalling pathway* (16 DE-genes), *regulation of actin cytoskeleton* (15 DE-genes), *HTLV-I infection* (15 DE-genes), *transcriptional misregulation in cancer* (14 DE-genes), *herpes simplex infection* (14 DE-genes), *viral carcinogenesis* (14 DE-genes), *insulin signalling pathway* (13 DE-genes), *chemokine signalling pathway* (13 DE-genes), *Epstein–Barr virus infection* (12 DE-genes), *measles* (11 DE-genes), *ubiquitin mediated proteolysis* (11 DE-genes), *prolactin signalling pathway* (10 DE-genes), *Salmonella infection* (10 DE-genes), *NF-kappa B signalling pathway* (10 DE-genes), *TNF signalling pathway* (10 DE-genes), *hepatitis C* (10 DE-genes), and *osteoclast differentiation* (10 DE-genes). Less significant pathways included the i.a. *ErbB signalling pathway (9 DE-genes), toll-like receptor signalling pathway (9 DE-genes), insulin resistance (9 DE-genes), ribosome biogenesis in eukaryotes (8 DE-genes), bacterial invasion of epithelial cells (7 DE-genes), peroxisome (7 DE-genes), small-cell lung cancer (7 DE-genes), phosphatidylinositol signalling system (7 DE-genes), systemic lupus erythematosus (7 DE-genes), NOD-like receptor signalling pathway (5 DE-genes), ovarian steroidogenesis (5 DE-genes), pentose phosphate pathway (4 DE-genes), intestinal immune network for IgA production (4 DE-genes), fatty-acid biosynthesis (3 DE-genes), glycosaminoglycan biosynthesis–chondroitin sulfate/dermatan sulfate (3 DE-genes), nicotinate, and nicotinamide metabolism (3 DE-genes).*

2.1.4. Network between Differentially Expressed Genes

Analysis of the interaction network was performed between 13 selected genes involved in metabolism, steroid and prostaglandin synthesis, interleukin and growth factor action, and embryo implantation. GeneMania was used to predict the relations between the chosen genes (query genes) in three different types of interaction as follows: co-expression (Figure 1A), co-localization and pathways (Figure 1B), as well as physical interactions and shared protein domains (Figure 1C). The analysis considered an additional 19 automatically generated genes, which were necessary to indicate the observed networks (interacting genes). Moreover, using different colours, we indicated the contribution of genes in specific biological functions related to female reproduction: female pregnancy (red), embryo implantation (blue), steroid biosynthetic process (yellow), prostaglandin biosynthetic process (purple), and angiogenesis (green; refer to the key in the Figure 1). Co-expression of the genes was found in 57 interactions and co-localization was observed in 41 interactions. In 21 cases, the genes participated in common pathways. Physical interactions were present in 37 cases, and in 19 cases interactions were based on the shared protein domains. The complete list of gene interactions is presented in Table S5.

Table 1. Analysis of pathways significantly enriched in the list of differentially expressed genes.

Analysis Name	Gene Number	p-Value	KEGG Pathway Analysis — Altered Genes
Pathways in cancer	21	1.00×10^{-1}	CEBPA, STAT5A, CBL, CXCL8, NFKBIA, GNG12, APPL1, CBLB, CDKN1A, EP300, GNAQ, CXCR4, NCOA4, TGFA, PIK3R5, LAMC2, RARB, NOS2, CRK, CHUK, TRAF3
Cytokine–cytokine receptor interaction	18	3.60×10^{-3}	CSF3, IL9, CXCL8, CCL28, TNFRSF4, CCL4, IFNAR1, TNFRSF1B, TNFSF13B, PRLR, TNFSF13B, IL10RB, CXCR4, IL4R, IL13RA1, IFNGR2, BMPR1A
Jak–STAT signalling pathway	16	1.60×10^{-4}	CSF3, STAT5A, SOCS1, IL9, SOCS4, IL24, IFNAR1, EP300, PRLR, IL10RB, IL4R, PIK3R5, JAK3, IL13RA1, IFNGR2
Regulation of actin cytoskeleton	15	1.40×10^{-2}	ITGAL, SSH1, DIAPH1, SSH2, ARPC5, GNG12, PPP1CC, NCKAP1, ARPC1B, ITGB7, PIK3R5, MSN, PIP4K2A, CRK, MYLK
HTLV-I infection	15	8.30×10^{-2}	ITGAL, TLN1, KAT2B, STAT5A, NFKBIA, MYBL2, ATM, SLA-8, CDKN1A, EP300, ETS1, PIK3R5, JAK3, NFATC3, CHUK
Transcriptional misregulation in cancer	14	3.80×10^{-3}	CEBPA, CEBPB, KMT2A, CEBPE, LDB1, CCNT1, ELANE, CXCL8, ATM, HHEX, CDKN1A, ITGB7, GOLPH3L
Herpes simplex infection	14	1.60×10^{-2}	CSNK2A2, CFP, EP300, HNRNPK, TAF5, EIF2S1, NFKBIA, HCFC2, PPP1CC, IFNGR2, CHUK, IFNAR1, SLA-8, TRAF3
Viral carcinogenesis	14	1.90×10^{-2}	LOC100156127, KAT2B, UBE3A, STAT5A, NFKBIA, PMAIP1, SLA-8, CDKN1A, HNRNPK, EP300, PIK3R5, JAK3, LOC100621389, TRAF3
Insulin signalling pathway	13	2.40×10^{-3}	SOCS1, CBL, ACACA, FBP1, RPS6KB1, SOCS4, PPP1CC, CBLB, PYGM, PYGL, PIK3R5, CRK, INSR
Chemokine signalling pathway	13	2.30×10^{-2}	AMCF-II, CXCR4, CXCL2, CXCL8, NFKBIA, PIK3R5, FOXO3, GNG12, JAK3, CCL4, CCL28, CRK, CHUK
Epstein–Barr virus infection	12	7.90×10^{-2}	CSNK2A2, ITGAL, CDKN1A, EP300, IL10RB, NFKBIA, PIK3R5, JAK3, TNFAIP3, CHUK, SLA-8, TRAF3
Measles	11	1.80×10^{-2}	CSNK2A2, EIF2S1, STAT5A, NFKBIA, PIK3R5, JAK3, MSN, TNFAIP3, IFNGR2, CHUK, IFNAR1
Ubiquitin-mediated proteolysis	11	2.00×10^{-2}	CUL5, CBLB, UBE3A, UBR5, WWP1, SOCS1, CBL, RHOBTB1, KEAP1, LOC780419, TRIP12
Prolactin signalling pathway	10	2.90×10^{-4}	CGA, PRLR, STAT5A, SOCS1, IRF1, SOCS4, PIK3R5, FOXO3, LHB, CSN2
Salmonella infection	10	1.50×10^{-3}	ARPC1B, CXCL2, PKN2, CXCL8, ARPC5, NOS2, DYNC1H1, CASP1, CCL4, IFNGR2

Table 1. *Cont.*

Analysis Name	Gene Number	p-Value	KEGG Pathway Analysis — Altered Genes
NF-kappa B signalling pathway	10	3.10×10^{-3}	CSNK2A2, TNFSF13B, LY96, CXCL8, NFKBIA, TNFAIP3, CCL4, ATM, CHUK, TRAF3
TNF signalling pathway	10	1.20×10^{-2}	LOC100736836, TNFRSF1B, CEBPB, CXCL2, NFKBIA, PIK3R5, TNFAIP3, CHUK, TRAF3
Hepatitis C	10	3.30×10^{-2}	CDKN1A, EIF2S1, IRF1, CXCL8, NFKBIA, PIK3R5, CHUK, IFNAR1, PPP2R2A, TRAF3
Osteoclast differentiation	10	4.30×10^{-2}	CYLD, TNFRSF11B, CTSK, SOCS1, NFKBIA, PIK3R5, IFNGR2, SIRPA, CHUK, IFNAR1
ErbB signalling pathway	9	7.20×10^{-3}	CBLB, CDKN1A, STAT5A, CBL, TGFA, PIK3R5, RPS6KB1, ABL2, CRK
Toll-like receptor signalling pathway	9	2.10×10^{-2}	CTSK, LY96, CXCL8, NFKBIA, PIK3R5, CCL4, CHUK, IFNAR1, TRAF3
Chagas disease (American trypanosomiasis)	9	2.90×10^{-2}	GNAQ, CD247, CXCL8, NFKBIA, PIK3R5, NOS2, IFNGR2, CHUK, PPP2R2A
Insulin resistance	9	3.80×10^{-2}	RPS6KA3, PYGM, PYGL, NFKBIA, PIK3R5, RPS6KB1, PPP1CC, SLC27A2, INSR
Toxoplasmosis	9	4.10×10^{-2}	LY96, IL10RB, SOCS1, NFKBIA, LAMC2, PIK3R5, NOS2, IFNGR2, CHUK
AMPK signalling pathway	9	4.70×10^{-2}	EEF2K, ACACA, FBP1, RAB14, PIK3R5, RPS6KB1, FOXO3, INSR, PPP2R2A
Chronic myeloid leukemia	8	6.50×10^{-3}	CBLB, CDKN1A, STAT5A, CBL, NFKBIA, PIK3R5, CRK, CHUK
Ribosome biogenesis in eukaryotes	8	1.80×10^{-2}	CSNK2A2, RN18S, MPHOSPH10, NOP58, WDR3, NOP56, BMS1, GNL3
HIF-1 signalling pathway	8	5.20×10^{-2}	PDK1, CDKN1A, EP300, PIK3R5, RPS6KB1, NOS2, IFNGR2, INSR
Bacterial invasion of epithelial cells	7	3.40×10^{-2}	ARPC1B, CBLB, CBL, PIK3R5, ARPC5, CRK, ARHGAP10
Peroxisome	7	4.80×10^{-2}	ACSL1, NUDT12, NOS2, SLC27A2, ACSL3, CROT, SOD2
Small cell lung cancer	7	5.90×10^{-2}	NFKBIA, LAMC2, PIK3R5, NOS2, RARB, CHUK, TRAF3
Phosphatidylinositol signalling system	7	9.40×10^{-2}	MTMR14, PI4KA, PIK3R5, DGKH, INPP4A, PIP4K2A, INPP5B
Systemic lupus erythematosus	7	9.80×10^{-2}	LOC100156127, LOC100157763, LOC100158121, ELANE, LOC100154071, LOC100153329, LOC100621389
Pertussis	6	7.50×10^{-2}	AMCF-II, LY96, IRF1, CXCL8, NOS2, CASP1
NOD-like receptor signalling pathway	5	5.10×10^{-2}	CXCL8, NFKBIA, TNFAIP3, CASP1, CHUK
Ovarian steroidogenesis	5	5.40×10^{-2}	CGA, PLA2G4A, HSD3B1, LHB, INSR
Malaria	5	5.80×10^{-2}	CSF3, ITGAL, SELP, CXCL8
Acute myeloid leukemia	5	6.70×10^{-2}	CEBPA, STAT5A, PIK3R5, RPS6KB1, CHUK
Pentose phosphate pathway	4	1.10×10^{-2}	FBP1, TKT, RPIA, PRPS2

Table 1. *Cont.*

	KEGG Pathway Analysis		
Analysis Name	Gene Number	*p*-Value	Altered Genes
Intestinal immune network for IgA production	4	9.50×10^{-2}	*TNFSF13B, CXCR4, ITGB7, CCL28*
Fatty acid biosynthesis	3	1.40×10^{-2}	*ACSL1, ACACA, ACSL3*
Glycosaminoglycan biosynthesis-chondroitin sulphate/dermatan sulphate	3	5.10×10^{-2}	*CSGALNACT2, CHST3, CHSY1*
Nicotinate and nicotinamide metabolism	3	9.40×10^{-2}	*ENPP1, NUDT12, NMRK1*
Dorso-ventral axis formation	3	9.40×10^{-2}	*CPEB2, ETS1, CPEB4*

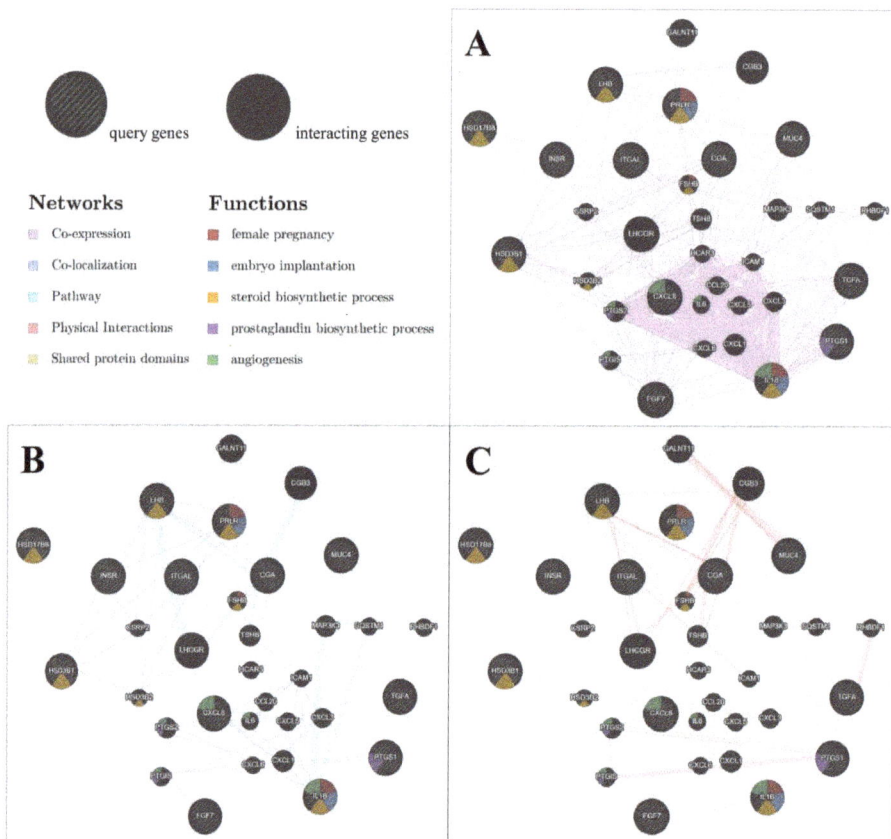

Figure 1. Gene interaction networks created in GeneMania for selected genes. The relations between the chosen genes based on their known participation in female reproduction and metabolism (query genes, striped circles) and additionally automatically generated genes mediating in the biological processes (interacting genes, non-striped circles). Colours on the circles indicate the contribution of the genes in the specific biological functions. The size of the circle indicates the importance of the gene in the specific interactions. The colour of the lines connecting the genes denotes the type of interaction: co-expression (**A**), co-localization and pathways (**B**), as well as physical interactions and shared protein domains (**C**), while the width of lines indicates the weight of interaction between genes (refer to the key).

2.2. Validation of the Microarray Results by Real-Time PCR (qPCR).

Real-time PCR method was used to verify the differential expression of 13 genes that were detected by the 4 × 44 Porcine (V2) Two-Colour Gene Expression Microarray kit (Agilent, Santa Clara, CA, USA). Only genes with an FC greater than 1.2 and *p*-values under 0.05 were selected. The protein products of selected genes were involved in processes important for endometrium functions during early pregnancy, such as metabolism of lipids, carbohydrates, and proteins (insulin receptor—*INSR*), gonadotropin metabolism and action (alpha polypeptide of glycoprotein hormones—*CGA*, luteinizing hormone beta polypeptide—*LHB*, prolactin receptor—*PRLR*), steroid hormone and prostaglandin synthesis and metabolism (hydroxy-delta-5-steroid dehydrogenase—*HSD3B1*, hydroxysteroid (17-beta) dehydrogenase 8—*HSD17B8*, prostaglandin-endoperoxide synthase 1—*PTGS1*), interleukin and growth factor action (C-X-C motif chemokine ligand 8—*CXCL8*, fibroblast growth factor 7—*FGF7*, interleukin 1 beta—*IL1B*, transforming growth factor alpha—*TGFA*), and embryo implantation (integrin, alpha L—*ITGAL*, mucin 4—*MUC4*). All changes in the gene expression determined by the microarray analysis were confirmed by qPCR (Figure 2).

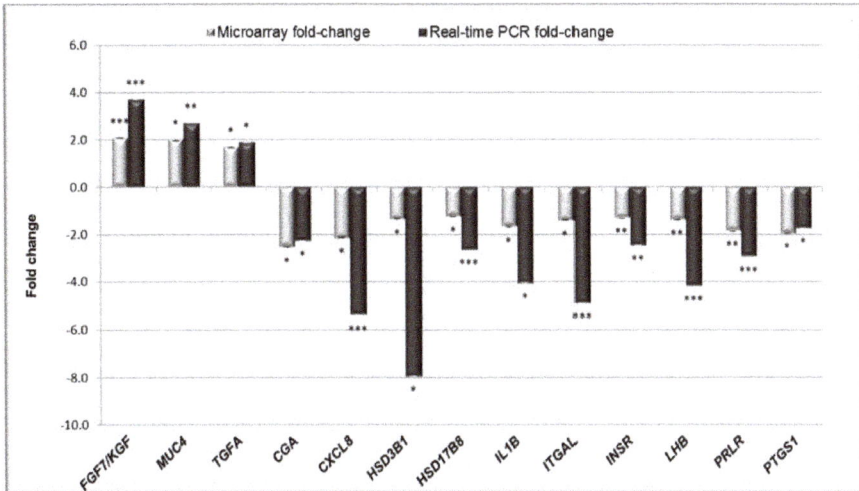

Figure 2. Real-time PCR validation of the microarray experiment. Light-grey bars represent fold changes for microarray data; dark-grey bars represent fold changes for qPCR data. Data are presented as means ± SEM from four different observations; * $p < 0.05$; ** $p < 0.01$; *** $p < 0.001$.

3. Discussion

In mammals, conceptus implantation in the endometrium is of critical importance for reproductive success; in pigs this process takes place on days 15 to 16 of gestation. Consequently, physiological mechanisms and cellular signal pathways related to implantation have long been a research interest. The highest conceptus mortality in pigs occurs between days 12 to 30 of pregnancy (reviewed by Reference [1]). Establishing the interface between the developing embryos, appropriate remodelling of maternal endometrium, and uterine receptivity involves a number of complex signalling networks. Periodic expression of numerous genes essential for embryo survival and development occurs during implantation. In the present study, in-depth genomic analysis demonstrates for the first time, the effect of adiponectin on global gene expression in the porcine endometrium during implantation period. The obtained list of DE-genes was used to analyse specific genes ontologies, biological pathways, and possible interaction networks. In our present study, 1494 DE-genes were identified among which 1286 genes had FC values greater than 1.2. The expression of 560 genes was upregulated and 726 downregulated in the endometrium treated with adiponectin relative to the control group. It is important to note that, of the 13 genes selected for interaction analysis, six genes were directly involved in the steroid hormone biosynthesis or embryo implantation, two genes were engaged in the angiogenesis, and one gene was involved in the prostaglandin biosynthetic process.

The adiponectin system (adiponectin and its receptors) has been found in the uterus of many species, including pig, human, mouse, and rabbit [14,19,20,22]. Adiponectin concentrations in the porcine serum and uterine luminal fluid were the highest on days 15 to 16 and 27 to 28 of gestation, i.e., the beginning and the end of implantation period [23]. Only a few previous studies indicated adiponectin's effect on endometrial gene expression; however, these concerned pre-determined genes and did not analyse the whole transcriptome. According to the study by Brochu-Gaudreau et al. [24], adiponectin regulates the endometrial expression of genes associated with placental formation, cyclooxygenase-2 (*COX-2*), vascular endothelial growth factor (*VEGF*), and peroxisome proliferator-activated receptor gamma (*PPARγ*). Our earlier study revealed that adiponectin modulates the expression of key enzymes in the synthesis of the steroids: steroidogenic acute regulatory protein (*StAR*), P450 side-chain cleavage enzyme (*CYP11A1*), and 3β-hydroxysteroid dehydrogenase (*HSD3B1*), as well as P4 and androstenedione (A4) secretion by the porcine uterus during early pregnancy [21]. Although the above studies have significantly helped us understand the role of adiponectin in the uterus, a genome-wide approach using a microarray analysis allows us to more efficiently investigate the effect of adiponectin on global gene expression in the endometrium during critical period for embryo survival and development. Understanding the processes/mechanisms that occur in the endometrium during the peri-implantation period will provide more avenues to influence conceptus growth and litter size. Moreover, the domestic pig is not only an economically important species but also a good experimental model for understanding human health and diseases. It is much more similar to humans than the more frequently-used laboratory rodents because of profound changes in rodents and other small mammals caused by redistribution of purifying selection [25,26]. Thus, results from the present study will also significantly contribute to a better understanding of human physiology.

In the constructed network of interactions, the gene encoding interleukin 1 beta (*IL1B*) was the node with the largest number of co-expression, co-localization, pathways, and functions. We demonstrated that *IL1B* gene expression was significantly downregulated in the porcine endometrium treated with adiponectin during implantation. This pro-inflammatory cytokine has been reported to play important roles in the implantation process, mediating conceptus–endometrial interactions in a number of mammalian species (for review see Reference [27]). During the period of implantation, the porcine embryos (and endometrium) produced IL1B [28,29]. Conceptus IL1B mRNA and protein expression is rapidly increased during porcine trophoblast elongation but rapidly declines immediately following the completion of the elongation process [29]. Therefore, IL1B was proposed as a candidate for initiating the cellular signalling pathway for the remodelling of conceptus and might be involved in the successful establishment of pregnancy in pigs. The result of the gene ontology analysis showed that adiponectin affects the expression of genes involved in the regulation of *cell proliferation* (GO:0042127), *negative regulation of cell proliferation* (GO:0008285), *cell proliferation* (GO:0008283), and *programmed cell death* (GO:0012501). Adiponectin decreased human endometrial stromal cell proliferation in dose- and time-dependent manners and caused cell death. Therefore, it is suggested that the adipokine is an anti-endometriosis factor [30]. This finding has been confirmed by subsequent studies by the same group of authors indicating the inhibitory effect of adiponectin on the proliferation of endometriotic stromal cells [31]. Evidence has revealed that adiponectin concentrations were decreased in the plasma and peritoneal fluid of women with endometriosis [32,33]. Plasma adiponectin concentrations were also decreased in genital cancers, such as oestrogen-related cancer as well as endometrial cancer [34,35]. Furthermore, high levels of circulating adiponectin are associated with reduced endometrial cancer risk [36]. The above studies correspond with findings reported by Cong et al. [37] implying the direct anti-proliferative impact of adiponectin on human endometrial cancer cell lines by inducing cell cycle arrest and apoptosis. On the other hand, the latest studies revealed that adiponectin significantly stimulated proliferation and suppressed apoptosis of porcine uterine luminal epithelial cells (LEc) which would enhance uterine receptivity for embryo implantation. The mentioned adiponectin-stimulated proliferation of LEc was related to activation of the phosphatidylinositol 3-kinase (PI3K) and mitogen-activated protein kinase signal transduction pathways [38]. This finding supports the hypothesis that adiponectin signalling is necessary for the establishment and maintenance of conceptus–uterine cross-talk during early pregnancy. However, further research is required to support the suggestion of adiponectin involvement in the implantation process and its utilization as prognostic markers and/or therapeutic targets in endometrial cancer.

The analysis of DE-genes indicated that adiponectin stimulated *MUC4* gene expression. Mucin 4 is a member of the family of membrane mucins and it is expressed at the apical surface of most epithelia including the endometrium [39,40]. Mucins are able to form gels and they are proposed to protect the surface of most epithelia [41]. Studies carried out in various species imply that MUC4 is involved in embryo implantation. In the normal cycling rodent, uterine luminal epithelium (LE) expression of MUC4 is high during oestrous stages corresponding with high oestrogen concentrations and low during stages characterised by high P4 levels [42]. In rats with the invasive type of implantation, loss of MUC4 in the uterine LE occurs at the beginning of the period of receptivity for implantation. Mucin 4 has anti-adhesive properties; therefore, it is assumed to make a barrier in the uterus to block blastocyst implantation during the pre-receptive period. The absence of MUC4 during implantation implies that this glycoprotein must be lost from the apical surface of the rat uterine LE to create the receptive state for uterine implantation [43]. However, in gilts with the non-invasive, epitheliochorial implantation, endometrial MUC4 expression increased during the period of trophoblastic attachment to the uterine luminal surface. It is suggested that maintenance of MUC4 on the uterine surface epithelium could play a role in modulating the proteolytic activity of porcine conceptuses to prevent erosion of the glandular and surface epithelia [44]. It would be interesting to check whether the expression of MUC4 in the porcine uterine LE, similar to the regulation proposed in the rodents, is regulated by steroid hormones. It would also be interesting to explain the mechanism of adiponectin action in this regulation. Our previous studies indicated the effect of adiponectin on steroids production and steroid hormones on adiponectin expression in the porcine uterus during early pregnancy [21,45,46]. In the current studies, treatment with adiponectin inhibited the expression of *HSD3B1* which is responsible for P4 and A4 production, and *HSD17B8* which selectively catalyses the conversion of E2 to biologically less-active oestrone [47]. Therefore, it cannot be excluded that adiponectin affects luminal uterine expression of MUC4 through steroid hormones or the other way around.

Adiponectin also affects the following groups of genes that encode *biological adhesion* (GO:0022610), *cell adhesion* (GO:0007155), *cell–cell adhesion* (GO:0098609), and *cell–matrix adhesion* (GO:0007160). In all of these processes, the *ITGAL* gene is involved. The results from the analysis of DE-genes revealed that adiponectin inhibited the expression of *ITGAL* coding integrin subunit alpha. In pigs, implantation follows an extended pre-attachment period of 8 to 15 days [48]. Adhesion and signal transduction events that occur during prolonged periods of apposition and attachment include the modulation of number adhesion molecules. Conceptus attachment to the uterine LE does not take place until hormonally regulated events change the non-adhesive (pre-receptive) uterine wall to mutually adhesive receptive epithelial surface [49]. Integrins are a family of glycoconjugates that are heterodimeric intrinsic membrane proteins composed of non-covalently linked α and β subunits that interact with various extracellular matrix (ECM) components and cell adhesion molecules [50]. Integrins play a dominant role in the attachment and implantation of the blastocyst to the uterine LE. They have been recognised as critical molecules involved in the implantation adhesion cascade that possess the ability to bind ECM and other ligands to mediate adhesion, migration, invasion, and cause cytoskeletal reorganization and transduce cellular signals [51]. In the pig, the constitutive and cycle-dependent expression of integrin subunits including $\alpha1$, $\alpha3$, $\alpha4$, $\alpha5$, αv, $\beta1$, $\beta3$, and $\beta5$ has been found on the surface of uterine LE and conceptuses. Of these, the $\alpha4$, $\alpha5$, αv, $\beta1$, $\beta3$, and $\beta5$ subunits were indicated at sites of initial attachment between uterine LE and trophectoderm on days 12 to 15 of gestation. During the peri-implantation period, P4 stimulated the expression of integrins that may partially define "the window of implantation" in this species [49]. It seems that the endometrium is the only tissue known to exhibit hormone-dependent integrin expression. In humans, three integrins are considered as markers of uterine receptivity for implantation and occur when the uterus is influenced by P4. The expression of $\alpha v \beta3$ correlates with conceptus attachment and loss of the $\alpha4$ integrin subunits is coincident with closure of the window of receptivity. Furthermore, the presence of both $\alpha v \beta3$ and $\alpha4\beta1$ on the apical surface of uterine LE suggests a role of these integrins in initial trophectoderm–LE interaction during implantation [52]. It is possible that adiponectin also participates in the implantation adhesion cascade. As a continuation of the present work, we intend to investigate the expression patterns of integrins in the porcine endometrium during the peri-implantation period under the influence of adiponectin.

4. Materials and Methods

4.1. Experimental Animals and Tissue Collection

Four mature gilts (Large White × Polish Landrace; 7 to 8 months of age, body weight of 120 to 130 kg) descended from a private breeding farm were used in the study. The gilts used in the study were on days 15 to 16 of pregnancy. Females were monitored daily for oestrus behaviour in the presence of an intact boar. The day of onset of the second oestrus was designated as day 0 of the oestrous cycle. Insemination was performed on days 1 to 2 of the oestrous cycle. Uteri collected after slaughter from pregnant gilts were immediately placed in ice-cold PBS supplemented with 100 IU/mL penicillin and 100 μg/mL streptomycin and transported to the laboratory on ice within 1 h for in vitro explant tissue culture. Pregnancy was confirmed by the presence of conceptuses. All slices of the endometrium on days 15 to 16 of gestation were collected at the implantation sites. The experiments were carried out in accordance with the ethical standards of the Animal Ethics Committee at the University of Warmia and Mazury in Olsztyn (Ethical approval: 113/2011/DTN; 14.12.2011).

4.2. Endometrial Explant Culture

Uteri collected from gilts on days 15 to 16 of pregnancy were washed three times in sterile PBS. Endometrial explant cultures were performed according to Smolinska et al. [21]. The endometrial tissues from the uterine horns were dissected and cut into small, irregular slices (3-mm thick, 100 mg ± 10%) and then washed three times in medium M199 (Sigma–Aldrich Co., Saint Louis, MO, USA). Individual endometrial explants were placed into culture glass vials with 2-mL medium M199 containing 0.1% BSA (MP Biomedicals, Santa Ana, CA, USA), 5% dextran/charcoal-stripped new-born calf serum (Sigma–Aldrich Co.), penicillin (100 IU/mL), and streptomycin (100 μg/mL). The tissue cultures were preincubated in a shaking water bath for 2 h at 37 °C in an atmosphere of 95% O_2 and 5% CO_2. After preincubation, to examine the impact of adiponectin on the global gene expression in the endometrium, the slices were treated for 24 h with recombinant human adiponectin (10 μg/mL, BioVendor, Brno, Czech Republic). The doses of adiponectin were established based on Ledoux et al. [53] and Maleszka et al. [17,18]. Control slices were incubated without any treatment. All cultures were performed in duplicates in four independent experiments ($n = 4$). The viability of tissue explants was monitored by measuring lactate dehydrogenase (LDH) activity in medium at 2 h of preincubation as well as at the end of the treatment period. The release of LDH was performed using a Liquick Cor-LDH kit (Cormay, Lomianki, Poland) following the manufacturer's instructions. The activity of LDH during the culture of tissue explants was compared to its activity in medium obtained after destruction of endometrial cells by homogenization (positive control for causing cell death and the maximal release of LDH). Mean activity of LDH in cultured slices after treatment period was 55.1 ± 4.5 U/L (1.8% of maximal release of LDH after total endometrial cell destruction).

4.3. Total RNA Isolation and Quality Control

Total RNA was isolated from 8 endometrium samples (4 endometrium slices treated with adiponectin and 4 control endometrium) using the RNeasy Mini Kit (Qiagen, Germantown, MD, USA). The DNA was removed by on-column DNase I digestion as recommended by Qiagen (Germantown, MD, USA). The quality of the RNA was checked using an Agilent 2100 Bioanalyzer (Agilent Technologies, Santa Clara, CA, USA) and an RNA 6000 Nano Assay Kit (Agilent Technologies, Santa Clara, CA, USA). The RNA quantity was determined spectrophotometrically (Infinite 200 PRO plate reader with NanoQuant plates, Tecan Group, Mannedorf, Switzerland). In order to ensure the most reliable results from the microarray and quantitative real-time PCR (qPCR) validation experiments, only samples with an RNA integrity number (RIN) above 8 were used. The RNA samples were stored at −80 °C.

4.4. Microarray Hybridization

The porcine genome microarrays were purchased from Agilent Technologies (Porcine (V2) Gene Expression Microarray 4 × 44; Agilent Technologies, Santa Clara, CA, USA). The microarray experiment was performed as previously described by Szeszko et al. [54] and Dobrzyn et al. [55]. The RNA from the four endometrium slices treated with adiponectin and four control endometria was used to generate Cyanine-3 (Cy3) and Cyanine-5 (Cy5) labelled cRNA with a Low Input Quick Amp, Two-Colour kit (Agilent Technologies, Santa Clara, CA, USA) according to the manufacturer's instructions. Quantification of cRNA and cyanine dye incorporation were measured with Infinite 200 PRO plate reader with NanoQuant plates (Tecan Group, Mannedorf, Switzerland). For each microarray, 825 ng of the Cy3 and 825 ng of the Cy5 labelled cRNA were mixed together. The dual-labelled cRNA samples (obtained from treated and control samples) were fragmented and placed on each array ($n = 4$, one slide) in a balanced block design with dye swaps (Figure S1). To discount the dye bias effect observed in the dual-colour experiments, the study design included the alternate use of both dyes (dye swap), namely, in two microarrays the control probes were dyed by Cy-3 and the adiponectin-treated samples with Cy-5, whereas in another two microarrays, the control probes were dyed with Cy-5 and the adiponectin-treated with Cy-3. Hybridization was carried out according to the manufacturer's instructions at 60 °C for 17 h in an Agilent hybridization oven. After hybridization, slides were washed and scanned on an Agilent's High-Resolution C Microarray Scanner at a 5 μm resolution. In the next step, the images' raw data was acquired by Feature Extraction Software (Agilent Technologies, Santa Clara, CA, USA) for filtering of outlier spots, background subtraction from features, dye normalizations (linear and LOWESS), and expression data extraction and detailed analysis. All the microarray raw data files were uploaded on the National Centre for Biotechnology Information Gene Expression Omnibus (GEO) server (https://www.ncbi.nlm.nih.gov/geo/; accession number: GSE122400).

4.5. Bioinformatic Analysis

In order to identify DE-genes between control and treated by adiponectin endometrial explants, FC rule was used. The FC of DE-genes was obtained by analysis of previously generated expression data using the GeneSpring GX 12 software (Agilent Technologies, Santa Clara, CA, USA). The results obtained through the normalization of fluorescence intense were log-transformed, and then analysed using Student's *t*-test. The threshold set for up- and downregulated genes was if they had an FC greater than 1.2 and a *p*-value ≤ 0.05. The 1.2 FC cut-off was selected based on previous studies, which used the microarray technology [54–57]. To compare the normalized fluorescence intense for adiponectin treated versus control samples Student's *t*-test was applied. The FC was estimated based on the mean values of the treated/control gene expression levels of four biological replicates. Additionally, the Basic Local Alignment Search Tool (BLAST) was used to align the unknown gene probe sequences with the whole porcine transcriptome deposited in the database, which resulted in manual enrichment of the DE-genes list. For DE-genes represented on the Agilent's Porcine V2 microarray by multiple probes, the FC mean value for all the probes was calculated.

4.5.1. Gene Ontology Analysis

The functional analysis of these DE-genes was performed by utilizing the DAVID tool (http://david.abcc.ncifcrf.gov) to explore functional class scoring in the resulting gene list by means of GO term enrichment analysis [58]. Performed gene ontology analysis was limited to *Sus scrofa*, furthermore the genome of this species was used as a background. The level of significance was determined by the modified Fisher's exact test, incorporating gene-enrichment analysis, which modifies the original *p*-value by the threshold of maximum probability (EASE Score Threshold, $p \leq 0.1$).

4.5.2. Biological Pathways Analysis

The biological pathways analysis was also conducted based on the DE-genes resulting list by the DAVID tool. The software was able to categorize DE-transcripts into different biological functions and pathways, using information from each individual gene and computing a total over-representation value for each pathway represented in the KEGG. Like in the case of GO analysis, this analysis was limited to *Sus scrofa*, and also a genome of this species was used as a background. Values at $p \leq 0.05$ were considered statistically significant.

4.5.3. Interaction Network of Differentially Expressed Genes

An interaction network between DE-genes was performed with the GeneMania Prediction Server [59]. From the DE-genes list, there were 13 genes selected with fold change > 1.2: *CGA, FGF7, HSD3B1, HSD17B8, IL1B, CXCL8, INSR, LHB, PRLR, PTGS1, TGFA, ITGAL,* and *MUC4*. Products of the selected genes are known to be involved in the regulation of female reproduction and metabolism. GeneMania was used to predict the functions of selected genes and define possible interaction networks between them based on known interplay such as co-expression, co-localization, genetic interactions, signalling pathways, physical interactions, and shared protein domains.

4.6. Real-Time PCR Validations

Complementary DNA (cDNA) synthesis and qPCR were conducted by using the same total RNA ($n = 4$, for both, the treated and the control samples) as for the microarray experiment, as described previously by Szeszko et al. [54] and Dobrzyn et al. [55]. One microgram of total RNA was reverse transcribed into cDNA using the Omniscript RT Kit (Qiagen, Germantown, MD, USA) in a total volume of 20 μL with 0.5 μg oligo(dt)15 Primer (Roche, Basel, Switzerland). The reverse transcription reaction was carried out at 37 °C for 1 h and finally were heat-inactivated by incubation at 93 °C for 5 min. Real-time PCR analyses were performed in two technical repeats for each sample using a 7300 Real-Time PCR system and Power SYBR® Green PCR Master Mix (Life Technologies, Carlsbad, CA, USA). Real-Time PCR reaction mix included: 20 ng cDNA, 1 of 13 primer pairs (forward and reverse) at various concentrations, 12.5 μL SYBR® Green PCR Master Mix (Applied Biosystems, Waltham, MA, USA), and RNase free water to a final volume of 25 μL. The specificity of amplification was tested at the end of the qPCR by melting-curve analysis. Product purity was confirmed by agarose gel electrophoresis. The negative controls were performed in which cDNA was substituted by water, or reverse transcription was not performed before qPCR. The negative controls gave non-detectable signals in all samples, confirming the high specificity of the assay. To validate microarray results by qPCR, we chose the same thirteen genes as in the interaction network analysis. Selected forward and reverse primers sequences, qPCR conditions, and concentrations of primers are presented in Table 2. Calculation of the relative expression levels of the genes was conducted based on the comparative cycle threshold method (ΔΔCT) and normalised using the geometrical means of reference gene expression levels: β-actin (*ACTB*) and glyceraldehyde 3-phosphate dehydrogenase (*GAPDH*). During the preliminary studies it was found that the expression of both constitutively expressed genes did not differ significantly between the treated and control sample; therefore, these genes were suitable housekeeping genes for this experiment. Presented data are means ± SEM from four different biological replicates. Differences between treated samples and controls were analysed by one-way ANOVA followed by the least significant differences (LSD) post-hoc test using Statistica Software (StatSoft Inc., Tulsa, OK, USA). Values of $p < 0.05$ were considered as statistically significant. The Ct values for all non-template controls were under the detection threshold.

Table 2. Primers used for the validation of microarray results.

Gene Symbol	Primers Sequences	Reaction Conditions		Primer (nM)	Target Sequence Accession Number	References
CGA	F: 5′-CTCCAGAGCGTACCCAACTC-3′ R: 5′-ACTGTGGCCTTGGTAAATGC-3′	Activation: 50 °C, 30 min; 95 °C 15 min, 1. Denaturation: 94 °C, 15 s 2. Annealing: 55 °C, 30 s 3. Extension: 72 °C, 30 s 77 °C, 15 s	40 cycles	500 nM	XM_005659277.1	[60]
CXCL8	F: 5′-GGCAGTTTTCCTGCTTTCT-3′ R: 5′-CAGTGGGGTCCACTCTCAAT-3′	Activation: 95 °C, 15 min 1. Denaturation: 94 °C, 15 s 2. Annealing: 58 °C, 30 s 3. Extension: 72 °C, 30 s	40 cycles	400 nM	X61151.1	[61]
FGF7/KGF	F: 5′-GCTTCCACATTATCTGTCTGGTG-3′ R: 5′-GTCCCTTTGACTTTGCCTCG-3′	Activation: 95 °C, 10 min 1. Denaturation: 95 °C, 15 s 2. Annealing: 60 °C, 1 min 3. Extension: 72 °C, 1 min	40 cycles	500 nM	AF217463.1	This study
HSD3B1	F: 5′-AGGTTCGCCCGCTCATC-3′ R: 5′-CTGGGCACCGAGAAATACTTG-3′	Activation: 95 °C, 10 min 1. Denaturation: 95 °C, 15 s 2. Annealing: 61 °C, 1 min 3. Extension: 72 °C, 1 min	40 cycles	300 nM	NM_001004049.1	[62]
HSD17B8	F: 5′-TTCTGCTCCGCATGTCTGAAG-3′ R: 5′-CCATGTTTCCCACCTTCCCTA-3′	Activation: 95 °C, 10 min 1. Denaturation: 95 °C, 15 s 2. Annealing: 60 °C, 1 min 3. Extension: 72 °C, 1 min	40 cycles	500 nM	NM_001130730.1	This study
IL1B	F: 5′-TGCCAACGTGCAGTCTATGG-3′ R: 5′-TGGGCCAGCCAGCACTAG-3′	Activation: 95 °C, 10 min 1. Denaturation: 95 °C, 15 s 2. Annealing: 60 °C, 1 min 3. Extension: 72 °C, 1 min	40 cycles	100 nM	NM_214055	[29]
INSR	F: 5′-AAAACGCCAGGACATCGTCAAGG-3′ R: 5′-CCGCAGGGAACGCAGGTAACTCT-3′	Activation: 95 °C-10 min 1. Denaturation: 95 °C, 15 s 2. Annealing: 60 °C, 1 min 3. Extension: 72 °C, 1 min	40 cycles	200 nM	XM_005654749.1	[63]

Table 2. *Cont.*

Gene Symbol	Primers Sequences	Reaction Conditions		Primer (nM)	Target Sequence Accession Number	References
ITGAL	F: 5′-CTTGTCGAGCTGAAGGCTGA-3′ R: 5′-TTCCTGGTCCTTGGTGAGGA-3′	Activation: 95 °C, 10 min 1. Denaturation: 95 °C, 15 s 2. Annealing: 60 °C, 1 min 3. Extension: 72 °C, 1 min	40 cycles	500 nM	NM_001044608.1	This study
LHB	F: 5′-TTCACCACCAGCATCTGTTGC-3′ R: 5′-AAGAGGAGGCCTGGGAGTAG-3′	Activation: 95 °C, 10 min 1. Denaturation: 95 °C, 15 s 2. Annealing: 60 °C, 1 min 3. Extension: 72 °C, 1 min	40 cycles	500 nM	XM_005664700.1	This study
MUC4	F: 5′-GATGCCCTGGCCACAGAA-3′ R: 5′-TGATTCAAGGTAGCATTCATTTGC-3′	Activation: 95 °C, 10 min 1. Denaturation: 95 °C, 15 s 2. Annealing: 60 °C, 1 min	40 cycles	500 nM	NM_001206344.2	[64]
PRLR	F: 5′-CCAGATACCTAATGACTTCTCAATG-3′ R: 5′-TCCAACAGATGGGTGTCAAA-3′	Activation: 50 °C, 30 min; 95 °C, 15 min 1. Denaturation: 94 °C, 15 s 2. Annealing: 55 °C, 30 s 3. Extension: 72 °C, 30 s 77 °C, 15 s	40 cycles	500 nM	NM_214084	[63]
PTGS1	F: 5′-CAACACTTCACCCACCAGTTCTTC-3′ R: 5′-TCCATAAATGTGGCCGAGGTCTAC-3′	Activation: 95 °C, 10 min 1. Denaturation: 95 °C, 15 s 2. Annealing: 60 °C, 1 min 3. Extension: 72 °C, 1 min	40 cycles	500 nM	AF207823.1	[65]
TGFA	F: 5′-CGCGCCTGGGTATCTTGTTG-3′ R: 5′-GTGGGAATCTGGGCAGTCAT-3′	Activation: 50 °C, 2 min; 95 °C, 10 min 1. Denaturation: 95 °C, 3 s 2. Annealing: 60 °C, 30 s 3. Extension: 72 °C, 1 min	40 cycles	200 nM	NM_214251.1	[66]
ACTB	F: 5′-ACATCAAGGAGAAGCTCTGCTACG-3′ R: 5′-GAGGGGCGATGATCTTGATCTTCA-3′	Activation: 95 °C, 10 min 1. Denaturation: 95 °C, 15 s 2. Annealing: 61 °C, 1 min 3. Extension: 72 °C, 1 min	40 cycles	500 nM	U07786	[67]
GAPDH	F: 5′-CCTTCATTGACCTCCACTACATGG-3′ R: 5′-CCACAACATACGTAGCACCAGCATC-3′	Activation: 95 °C, 10 min 1. Denaturation: 95 °C, 15 s 2. Annealing: 59 °C, 1 min	40 cycles	500 nM	U48832	[68]

5. Conclusions

Conceptuses loss during early gestation can be a critical determinant of litter size. Identification of genes/proteins of many factors involved in different molecular pathways may contribute to successful pregnancy establishment and embryo development. This is the first global microarray-based study analysing differentially regulated genes by adiponectin in the endometrium of pregnant gilts during the implantation period. The present work indicates that adiponectin affects a number of genes and processes that are engaged in i.a. cell proliferation, programmed cell death, immune system response, metabolism of lipids, carbohydrates, and proteins, steroid hormone and prostaglandin synthesis and metabolism, interleukin and growth factor action, and cell adhesion. The above processes are critical for reproductive success; therefore, adiponectin may be an important regulator of implantation in pigs. Nevertheless, understanding the relationship between transcriptome and proteome, and further functional studies are required to explain the role and mechanism of adiponectin action in the porcine endometrium during peri-implantation period.

Supplementary Materials: Supplementary materials can be found at http://www.mdpi.com/1422-0067/20/6/1335/s1.

Author Contributions: Conceptualization: N.S., T.K.; methodology, N.S., K.S., and K.D.; validation, K.K., M.K., and E.R.; formal analysis, N.S., K.S., and M.G.; investigation, N.S., K.S., and K.D.; resources, K.B., J.W., and G.K.; data curation, K.S., M.K., and B.K.; writing—original draft preparation, N.S.; writing—review and editing, N.S., K.S., T.K., B.K., and K.D.; supervision, N.S., T.K.; project administration, N.S.; funding acquisition, N.S.

Funding: This research was supported by the National Science Centre (Project no.: 2011/03/B/NZ9/04187).

Conflicts of Interest: The authors declare no conflict of interest.

References

1. Geisert, R.D.; Schmitt, R.A.M. Early embryonic survival in the pig: Can it be improved? *J. Anim. Sci.* **2002**, *80*, E54–E65. [CrossRef]
2. Bazer, F.W.; Johnson, G.A. Pig blastocyst-uterine interactions. *Differentiation* **2014**, *87*, 52–65. [CrossRef] [PubMed]
3. Viganò, P.; Mangioni, S.; Pompei, F.; Chiodo, I. Maternal-conceptus cross talk-a review. *Placenta* **2003**, *24*, S56–S61. [CrossRef]
4. Ziecik, A.J.; Waclawik, A.; Kaczmarek, M.M.; Blitek, A.; Jalali, B.M.; Andronowska, A. Mechanisms for the establishment of pregnancy in the pig. *Reprod. Domest. Anim.* **2011**, *46* (Suppl. 3), 31–41. [CrossRef] [PubMed]
5. Scherer, P.E.; Williams, S.; Fogliano, M.; Baldini, G.; Lodish, H.F. A novel serum protein similar to C1q, produced exclusively in adipocytes. *J. Biol. Chem.* **1995**, *270*, 11259–11263. [CrossRef]
6. Maeda, K.; Okubo, K.; Shimomura, I.; Funahashi, T.; Matsuzawa, Y.; Matsubara, K. cDNA cloning and expression of a novel adipose specific collagen-like factor, apM1 (AdiPose Most abundant Gene transcript 1). *Biochem. Biophys. Res. Commun.* **1996**, *221*, 286–289. [CrossRef]
7. Nakano, Y.; Tobe, T.; Choi-Miura, N.H.; Mazda, T.; Tomita, M. Isolation and characterization of GBP28, a novel gelatin-binding protein purified from human plasma. *J. Biochem.* **1996**, *120*, 803–812. [CrossRef] [PubMed]
8. Hu, E.; Liang, P.; Spiegelman, B.M. AdipoQ is a novel adipose-specific gene dysregulated in obesity. *J. Biol. Chem.* **1996**, *271*, 10697–10703. [CrossRef]
9. Yamauchi, T.; Kamon, J.; Waki, H.; Terauchi, Y.; Kubota, N.; Hara, K.; Mori, Y.; Ide, T.; Murakami, K.; Tsuboyama-Kasaoka, N.; et al. The fat-derived hormone adiponectin reverses insulin resistance associated with both lipoatrophy and obesity. *Nat. Med.* **2001**, *7*, 941–946. [CrossRef]
10. Kadowaki, T.; Yamauchi, T. Adiponectin and adiponectin receptors. *Endocr. Rev.* **2005**, *26*, 439–451. [CrossRef]
11. Palin, M.F.; Bordignon, V.V.; Murphy, B.D. Adiponectin and the control of female reproductive functions. *Vitam. Horm.* **2012**, *90*, 239–287. [CrossRef] [PubMed]

12. Dobrzyn, K.; Smolinska, N.; Kiezun, M.; Szeszko, K.; Rytelewska, E.; Kisielewska, K.; Gudelska, M.; Kaminski, T. Adiponectin: A New Regulator of Female Reproductive System. *Int. J. Endocrinol.* **2018**, *2018*, 7965071. [CrossRef] [PubMed]

13. Lord, E.; Ledoux, S.; Murphy, B.D.; Beaudry, D.; Palin, M.F. Expression of adiponectin and its receptors in swine. *J. Anim. Sci.* **2005**, *83*, 565–578. [CrossRef] [PubMed]

14. Takemura, Y.; Osuga, Y.; Yamauchi, T.; Kobayashi, M.; Harada, M.; Hirata, T.; Morimoto, C.; Hirota, Y.; Yoshino, O.; Koga, K.; et al. Expression of Adipoq receptors and its possible implication in the human endometrium. *Endocrinology* **2006**, *147*, 3203–3210. [CrossRef] [PubMed]

15. Kim, S.T.; Marquard, K.; Stephens, S.; Louden, E.; Allsworth, J.; Moley, K.H. Adipoq and Adipoq receptors in the mouse preimplantation embryo and uterus. *Hum. Reprod.* **2011**, *26*, 82–95. [CrossRef] [PubMed]

16. Chabrolle, C.; Tosca, L.; Dupont, J. Regulation of Adipoq and its receptors in rat ovary by human chorionic gonadotrophin treatment and potential involvement of Adipoq in granulosa cell steroidogenesis. *Reproduction* **2007**, *133*, 719–731. [CrossRef]

17. Maleszka, A.; Smolinska, N.; Nitkiewicz, A.; Kiezun, M.; Dobrzyn, K.; Czerwinska, J.; Szeszko, K.; Kaminski, T. Expression of Adipoq receptors 1 and 2 in the ovary and concentration of plasma Adipoq during the oestrous cycle of the pig. *Acta Vet. Hung.* **2014**, *62*, 386–396. [CrossRef]

18. Maleszka, A.; Smolinska, N.; Nitkiewicz, A.; Kiezun, M.; Chojnowska, K.; Dobrzyn, K.; Szwaczek, H.; Kaminski, T. Adipoq Expression in the Porcine Ovary during the Oestrous Cycle and Its Effect on Ovarian Steroidogenesis. *Int. J. Endocrinol.* **2014**, *2014*, 9570–9576. [CrossRef]

19. Smolinska, N.; Maleszka, A.; Dobrzyn, K.; Kiezun, M.; Szeszko, K.; Kaminski, T. Expression of Adipoq and Adipoq receptors 1 and 2 in the porcine uterus, conceptus, and trophoblast during early pregnancy. *Theriogenology* **2014**, *82*, 951–965. [CrossRef]

20. Smolinska, N.; Dobrzyn, K.; Maleszka, A.; Kiezun, M.; Szeszko, K.; Kaminski, T. Expression of Adipoq and Adipoq receptors 1 (AdipoR1) and 2 (AdipoR2) in the porcine uterus during the oestrous cycle. *Anim. Reprod. Sci.* **2014**, *146*, 42–54. [CrossRef]

21. Smolinska, N.; Dobrzyn, K.; Kiezun, M.; Szeszko, K.; Maleszka, A.; Kaminski, T. Effect of adiponectin on the steroidogenic acute regulatory protein, P450 side chain cleavage enzyme and 3β-hydroxysteroid dehydrogenase genes expression, progesterone and androstenedione production by the porcine uterus during early pregnancy. *J. Physiol. Pharmacol.* **2016**, *67*, 443–456.

22. Gamundi-Segura, S.; Serna, J.; Oehninger, S.; Horcajadas, J.A.; Arbones-Mainar, J.M. Effects of adipocyte-secreted factors on decidualized endometrial cells: Modulation of endometrial receptivity in vitro. *J. Physiol. Biochem.* **2015**, *71*, 537–546. [CrossRef]

23. Smolinska, N.; Kiezun, M.; Dobrzyn, K.; Szeszko, K.; Maleszka, A.; Kaminski, T. Adiponectin, orexin A and orexin B concentrations in the serum and uterine luminal fluid during early pregnancy of pigs. *Anim. Reprod. Sci.* **2017**, *178*, 1–8. [CrossRef]

24. Brochu-Gaudreau, K.; Beaudry, D.; Blouin, R.; Bordignon, V.; Murphy, B.D.; Palin, M.F. Adiponectin Regulates Gene Expression in the Porcine Uterus. *Biol. Reprod.* **2008**, *78*, 210–211. [CrossRef]

25. Demetrius, L. Of mice and men. When it comes to studying ageing and the means to slow it down, mice are not just small humans. *EMBO Rep.* **2005**, *6*, S39–S44. [CrossRef]

26. Vinogradov, A.E.; Anatskaya, O.V. Gene Golden Age paradox and its partial solution. *Genomics* **2018**. [CrossRef]

27. Geisert, R.; Fazleabas, A.; Lucy, M.; Mathew, D. Interaction of the conceptus and endometrium to establish pregnancy in mammals: Role of interleukin 1β. *Cell Tissue Res.* **2012**, *349*, 825–838. [CrossRef]

28. Tuo, W.; Harney, J.P.; Bazer, F.W. Developmentally regulated expression of interleukin-1β by periimplantation conceptuses in swine. *J. Reprod. Immunol.* **1996**, *31*, 185–198. [CrossRef]

29. Ross, J.W.; Malayer, J.R.; Ritchey, J.W.; Geisert, R.D. Characterization of the interleukin-1beta system during porcine trophoblastic elongation and early placental attachment. *Biol. Reprod.* **2003**, *69*, 1251–1259. [CrossRef]

30. Bohlouli, S.; Khazaei, M.; Teshfam, M.; Hassanpour, H. Adiponectin effect on the viability of human endometrial stromal cells and mRNA expression of adiponectin receptors. *Int. J. Fertil. Steril.* **2013**, *7*, 43–48.

31. Bohlouli, S.; Rabzia, A.; Sadeghi, E.; Chobsaz, F.; Khazaei, M. In vitro Anti-Proliferative Effect of Adiponectin on Human Endometriotic Stromal Cells through AdipoR1 and AdipoR2 Gene Receptor Expression. *Iran. Biomed. J.* **2016**, *20*, 12–17. [CrossRef] [PubMed]

32. Bråkenhielm, E.; Veitonmäki, N.; Cao, R.; Kihara, S.; Matsuzawa, Y.; Zhivotovsky, B.; Funahashi, T.; Cao, Y. Adiponectin-induced antiangiogenesis and antitumor activity involve caspase-mediated endothelial cell apoptosis. *Proc. Natl. Acad. Sci. USA* **2004**, *101*, 2476–2481. [CrossRef] [PubMed]

33. Yi, K.W.; Shin, J.H.; Park, H.T.; Kim, T.; Kim, S.H.; Hur, J.Y. Resistin concentration is increased in the peritoneal fluid of women with endometriosis. *Am. J. Reprod. Immunol.* **2010**, *64*, 318–323. [CrossRef] [PubMed]

34. Soliman, P.T.; Wu, D.; Tortolero-Luna, G.; Schmeler, K.M.; Slomovitz, B.M.; Bray, M.S.; Gershenson, D.M.; Lu, K.H. Association between adiponectin, insulin resistance, and endometrial cancer. *Cancer* **2006**, *106*, 2376–2381. [CrossRef]

35. Dal Maso, L.; Augustin, L.S.; Karalis, A.; Talamini, R.; Franceschi, S.; Trichopoulos, D.; Mantzoros, C.S.; La Vecchia, C. Circulating adiponectin and endometrial cancer risk. *J. Clin. Endocrinol. Metab.* **2004**, *89*, 1160–1163. [CrossRef]

36. Cust, A.E.; Kaaks, R.; Friedenreich, C.; Bonnet, F.; Laville, M.; Lukanova, A.; Rinaldi, S.; Dossus, L.; Slimani, N.; Lundin, E.; et al. Plasma adiponectin levels and endometrial cancer risk in pre- and postmenopausal women. *J. Clin. Endocrinol. Metab.* **2007**, *92*, 255–263. [CrossRef]

37. Cong, L.; Gasser, J.; Zhao, J.; Yang, B.; Li, F.; Zhao, A.Z. Human adiponectin inhibits cell growth and induces apoptosis in human endometrial carcinoma cells, HEC-1-A and RL95 2. *Endocr. Relat. Cancer* **2007**, *14*, 713–720. [CrossRef] [PubMed]

38. Lim, W.; Choi, M.J.; Bae, H.; Bazer, F.W.; Song, G. A critical role for adiponectin-mediated development of endometrial luminal epithelial cells during the peri-implantation period of pregnancy. *J. Cell. Physiol.* **2017**, *232*, 3146–3157. [CrossRef]

39. Audie, J.P.; Tetaert, D.; Pigny, P.; Buisine, M.P.; Janin, A.; Aubert, J.P.; Porchet, N.; Boersma, A. Mucin gene expression in the human endocervix. *Hum. Reprod.* **1995**, *10*, 98–102. [CrossRef]

40. Gipson, I.K.; Ho, S.B.; Spurr-Michaud, S.J.; Tisdale, A.S.; Zhan, Q.; Torlakovic, E.; Pudney, J.; Anderson, D.J.; Toribara, N.W.; Hill, J.A., 3rd. Mucin genes expressed by human female reproductive tract epithelia. *Biol. Reprod.* **1997**, *56*, 999–1011. [CrossRef]

41. Carraway, K.L.; Price-Schiavi, S.A.; Komatsu, M.; Idris, N.; Perez, A.; Li, P.; Jepson, S.; Zhu, X.; Carvajal, M.E.; Carraway, C.A. Multiple facets of sialomucin complex/MUC4, a membrane mucin and erbb2 ligand, in tumors and tissues (Y2K update). *Front. Biosci.* **2000**, *5*, D95–D107.

42. Idris, N.; Carraway, K.L. Sialomucin complex (Muc4) expression in the rat female reproductive tract. *Biol. Reprod.* **1999**, *61*, 1431–1438. [CrossRef]

43. McNeer, R.R.; Carraway, C.A.; Fregien, N.L.; Carraway, K.L. Characterization of the expression and steroid hormone control of sialomucin complex in the rat uterus: Implications for uterine receptivity. *J. Cell. Physiol.* **1998**, *176*, 110–119. [CrossRef]

44. Ferrell, A.D.; Malayer, J.R.; Carraway, K.L.; Geisert, R.D. Sialomucin complex (Muc4) expression in porcine endometrium during the oestrous cycle and early pregnancy. *Reprod. Domest. Anim.* **2003**, *38*, 63–65. [CrossRef]

45. Dobrzyn, K.; Smolinska, N.; Szeszko, K.; Kiezun, M.; Maleszka, A.; Rytelewska, E.; Kaminski, T. Effect of progesterone on adiponectin system in the porcine uterus during early pregnancy. *J. Anim. Sci.* **2017**, *95*, 338–352. [CrossRef]

46. Dobrzyn, K.; Smolinska, N.; Kiezun, M.; Szeszko, K.; Maleszka, A.; Kaminski, T. The effect of estrone and estradiol on the expression of the adiponectin system in the porcine uterus during early pregnancy. *Theriogenology* **2017**, *88*, 183–196. [CrossRef]

47. Villar, J.; Celay, J.; Alonso, M.M.; Rotinen, M.; de Miguel, C.; Migliaccio, M.; Encío, I. Transcriptional regulation of the human type 8 17beta-hydroxysteroid dehydrogenase gene by C/EBPbeta. *J. Steroid. Biochem. Mol. Biol.* **2007**, *105*, 131–139. [CrossRef]

48. Bazer, F.W.; Roberts, R.M. Biochemical aspects of conceptus—Endometrial interactions. *J. Exp. Zool.* **1983**, *228*, 373–383. [CrossRef]

49. Bowen, J.A.; Burghardt, R.C. Cellular mechanisms of implantation in domestic farm animals. *Semin. Cell Dev. Biol.* **2000**, *11*, 93–104. [CrossRef]

50. Hynes, R.O. Integrins: Versatility, modulation, and signaling in cell adhesion. *Cell* **1992**, *69*, 11–25. [CrossRef]

51. Burghardt, R.C.; Johnson, G.A.; Jaeger, L.A.; Ka, H.; Garlow, J.E.; Spencer, T.E.; Bazer, F.W. Integrins and extracellular matrix proteins at the maternal-fetal interface in domestic animals. *Cells Tissues Organs* **2002**, *172*, 202–217. [CrossRef]

52. Lessey, B.A. Endometrial integrins and the establishment of uterine receptivity. *Hum. Reprod.* **1998**, *13* (Suppl. 3), 247–258. [CrossRef] [PubMed]

53. Ledoux, S.; Campos, D.B.; Lopes, F.L.; Dobias-Goff, M.; Palin, M.F.; Murphy, B.D. Adiponectin induces periovulatory changes in ovarian follicular cells. *Endocrinology* **2006**, *147*, 5178–5186. [CrossRef] [PubMed]

54. Szeszko, K.; Smolinska, N.; Kiezun, M.; Dobrzyn, K.; Maleszka, A.; Kaminski, T. The influence of adiponectin on the transcriptomic profile of porcine luteal cells. *Funct. Integr. Genom.* **2016**, *16*, 101–114. [CrossRef]

55. Dobrzyn, K.; Szeszko, K.; Kiezun, M.; Kisielewska, K.; Rytelewska, E.; Gudelska, M.; Wyrebek, J.; Bors, K.; Kaminski, T.; Smolinska, N. In vitro effect of orexin A on the transcriptomic profile of the endometrium during early pregnancy in pigs. *Anim. Reprod. Sci.* **2019**, *200*, 31–42. [CrossRef] [PubMed]

56. Li, Z.; Pan, J.; Ma, J.; Zhang, Z.; Bai, Y. Microarray gene expression of periosteum in spontaneous bone regeneration of mandibular segmental defects. *Sci. Rep.* **2017**, *7*, 13535. [CrossRef] [PubMed]

57. Zglejc, K.; Martyniak, M.; Waszkiewicz, E.; Kotwica, G.; Franczak, A. Peri-conceptional under-nutrition alters transcriptomic profile in the endometrium during the peri-implantation period-The study in domestic pigs. *Reprod. Domest. Animal.* **2018**, *53*, 74–84. [CrossRef] [PubMed]

58. Huang, D.W.; Sherman, B.T.; Lempicki, R.A. Systematic and integrative analysis of large gene lists using DAVID bioinformatics resources. *Nat. Protoc.* **2009**, *4*, 44–57. [CrossRef]

59. Warde-Farley, D.; Donaldson, S.L.; Comes, O.; Zuberi, K.; Badrawi, R.; Chao, P.; Franz, M.; Grouios, C.; Kazi, F.; Lopes, C.T.; et al. The GeneMANIA prediction server: Biological network integration for gene prioritization and predicting gene function. *Nucleic Acids Res.* **2010**, *38*, W214–W220. [CrossRef]

60. Quilter, C.R.; Gilbert, C.L.; Oliver, G.L.; Jafer, O.; Furlong, R.A.; Blott, S.C.; Wilson, A.E.; Sargent, C.A.; Mileham, A.; Affara, N.A. Gene expression profiling in porcine maternal infanticide: A model for puerperal psychosis. *Am. J. Med. Genet. B Neuropsychiatr. Genet.* **2008**, *47*, 1126–1137. [CrossRef] [PubMed]

61. Ramsay, T.G.; Caperna, T.J. Ontogeny of adipokine expression in neonatal pig adipose tissue. *Comp. Biochem. Physiol. B Biochem. Mol. Biol.* **2009**, *152*, 72–78. [CrossRef]

62. Wojciechowicz, B.; Kotwica, G.; Kolakowska, J.; Franczak, A. The Activity and Localization of 3β-hydroxysteroid Dehydrogenase/Δ5-Δ4 Isomerase and Release of Androstenedione and Progesterone by Uterine Tissues During Early Pregnancy and the Estrous Cycle in Pigs. *J. Reprod. Dev.* **2013**, *59*, 49–58. [CrossRef]

63. Liu, G.M.; Wei, Y.; Wang, Z.S.; Wu, D.; Zhou, A.G.; Liu, G.L. Effects of herbal extract supplementation on growth performance and insulin-like growth factor (IGF)-I system in finishing pigs. *J. Anim. Feed Sci.* **2008**, *17*, 538–547. [CrossRef]

64. Smith, A.G.; O'Doherty, J.V.; Reilly, P.; Ryan, M.T.; Bahar, B.; Sweeney, T. The effects of laminarin derived from Laminaria digitata on measurements of gut health: Selected bacterial populations, intestinal fermentation, mucin gene expression and cytokine gene expression in the pig. *Br. J. Nutr.* **2011**, *105*, 669–677. [CrossRef] [PubMed]

65. Seo, H.; Choi, Y.; Shim, J.; Choi, Y.; Ka, H. Regulatory mechanism for expression of IL1B receptors in the uterine endometrium and effects of IL1B on prostaglandin synthetic enzymes during the implantation period in pigs. *Biol. Reprod.* **2012**, *87*, 31. [CrossRef] [PubMed]

66. Farmer, C.; Palin, M.F. Feeding flaxseed to sows during late-gestation and lactation affects mammary development but not mammary expression of selected genes in their offspring. *Can. J. Anim. Sci.* **2013**, *93*, 17. [CrossRef]

67. Spagnuolo-Weaver, M.; Fuerst, R.; Campbell, S.T.; Meehan, B.M.; Mcneilly, F.; Adair, B.; Allan, G. A fluorimeter-Based RT-PCR method for the detection and quantitation of porcine cytokines. *J. Immunol. Methods* **1999**, *230*, 19–27. [CrossRef]

68. Nitkiewicz, A.; Smolinska, N.; Przala, J.; Kaminski, T. Expression of orexin receptors 1 (OX1R) and 2 (OX2R) in the porcine ovary during the oestrous cycle. *Regul. Pept.* **2010**, *165*, 186–190. [CrossRef] [PubMed]

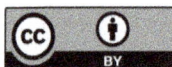

International Journal of
Molecular Sciences

MDPI

Review

Beneficial Effects of Adiponectin on Glucose and Lipid Metabolism and Atherosclerotic Progression: Mechanisms and Perspectives

Hidekatsu Yanai [1,*] and Hiroshi Yoshida [2,*]

1   Department of Internal Medicine, National Center for Global Health and Medicine Kohnodai Hospital, 1-7-1 Kohnodai, Chiba 272-8516, Japan
2   Department of Laboratory Medicine, The Jikei University Kashiwa Hospital, 163-1 Kashiwashita, Kashiwa, Chiba 277-8567, Japan
*   Correspondence: dyanai@hospk.ncgm.go.jp (H.Y.); hyoshida@jikei.ac.jp (H.Y.); Tel.: +81-473-72-3501 (H.Y.); +81-4-7164-1111 (ext. 2270) (H.Y.); Fax: +81-473-72-1858 (H.Y.); +81-4-7166-9374 (H.Y.)

Received: 6 February 2019; Accepted: 5 March 2019; Published: 8 March 2019

Abstract: Circulating adiponectin concentrations are reduced in obese individuals, and this reduction has been proposed to have a crucial role in the pathogenesis of atherosclerosis and cardiovascular diseases associated with obesity and the metabolic syndrome. We focus on the effects of adiponectin on glucose and lipid metabolism and on the molecular anti-atherosclerotic properties of adiponectin and also discuss the factors that increase the circulating levels of adiponectin. Adiponectin reduces inflammatory cytokines and oxidative stress, which leads to an improvement of insulin resistance. Adiponectin-induced improvement of insulin resistance and adiponectin itself reduce hepatic glucose production and increase the utilization of glucose and fatty acids by skeletal muscles, lowering blood glucose levels. Adiponectin has also β cell protective effects and may prevent the development of diabetes. Adiponectin concentration has been found to be correlated with lipoprotein metabolism; especially, it is associated with the metabolism of high-density lipoprotein (HDL) and triglyceride (TG). Adiponectin appears to increase HDL and decrease TG. Adiponectin increases ATP-binding cassette transporter A1 and lipoprotein lipase (LPL) and decreases hepatic lipase, which may elevate HDL. Increased LPL mass/activity and very low density lipoprotein (VLDL) receptor and reduced apo-CIII may increase VLDL catabolism and result in the reduction of serum TG. Further, adiponectin has various molecular anti-atherosclerotic properties, such as reduction of scavenger receptors in macrophages and increase of cholesterol efflux. These findings suggest that high levels of circulating adiponectin can protect against atherosclerosis. Weight loss, exercise, nutritional factors, anti-diabetic drugs, lipid-lowering drugs, and anti-hypertensive drugs have been associated with an increase of serum adiponectin level.

Keywords: adiponectin; atherosclerosis; cholesterol efflux; diabetes; inflammation

---

1. Introduction

Previously, the adipose tissue was considered a generally passive repository for stored triglycerides (TG). With the discovery of adiponectin, it has become clear that the adipose tissue carries out a large number of intricate metabolic, paracrine, and endocrine functions. The adiponectin gene was found to be the most abundantly expressed gene in the adipose tissue. It encodes a 244-amino-acid protein with a predicted size of 30 kDa [1]. Adiponectin contains a putative N-terminal signal sequence and a collagen-like domain and structurally belongs to the complement 1q (C1q) family, being characterized by a carboxyl-terminal globular domain and an amino-terminal collagenous domain highly homologous to collagen X, VIII, and C1q. Adiponectin is exclusively expressed and secreted into the circulation by the adipose tissue and appears to act as a hormone which could reduce inflammatory responses in vitro [2,3].

Circulating adiponectin can exist as a trimer, hexamer, or higher-order multimer with 12–18 subunits [4,5]. Adiponectin receptors include two similar transmembrane receptors which are known as AdipoR1 and AdipoR2, and another type of receptor without a transmembrane domain which may act as a co-receptor for the high-molecular weight (HMW) form of adiponectin on endothelial and smooth muscle cells [6,7]. Recent data indicate that the HMW form has the predominant action in metabolic tissues [8]. Adiponectin accounts for about 0.01% of all plasma proteins (5–10 µg/mL), and its plasma concentration was reported to be higher in women than in men [9,10].

Circulating adiponectin concentrations are reduced in obese individuals [10], and this reduction was proposed to have a crucial role in the pathogenesis of atherosclerosis and cardiovascular diseases associated with obesity and the metabolic syndrome [11,12]. Furthermore, this idea is supported by reports that adiponectin has effects considered to be protective against cardiovascular diseases [13,14].

Here, we focus on the effects of adiponectin on glucose and lipid metabolism and on its anti-atherosclerotic properties. Furthermore, we discuss the factors which increase circulating adiponectin levels.

2. Effects of Adiponectin on Glucose Metabolism

2.1. Possible Mechnisms for the Improvement of Glucose Metabolism by Adiponectin

2.1.1. Reduction of Inflammation and Oxidative Stress and Improvement of Insulin Resistance by Adiponectin

The adipose tissue is an active endocrine organ that secretes a variety of hormones known as adipokines. Adipokines are secreted into the circulation and participate in the regulation of insulin sensitivity and glucose and lipid metabolism [15]. In obesity and metabolic syndrome, a highly inflammatory status is induced by the infiltration of inflammatory cells into the adipose tissue, especially activated macrophages. Under these conditions, the adipose tissue produces proinflammatory adipokines, such as tumor necrosis factor-alpha (TNF-α), interleukin (IL)-6, monocyte chemoattractant protein-1 (MCP-1), lipocalin-2, and resistin, which induce atherosclerosis [16]. In these circumstances, the production of adiponectin is markedly reduced.

Chronically elevated levels of inflammatory cytokines could directly enhance insulin resistance and lead to disrupted insulin sensitivity, in turn impairing glucose and lipid metabolism. Epidemiological studies have reported that levels of pro-inflammatory and inflammatory cytokines such as C-reactive protein (CRP), TNF-α, IL-1β, and IL-6 were elevated in patients with type 2 diabetes and were associated with the development of type 2 diabetes [3,17–25].

Adiponectin could reduce inflammatory reactions [2,3], which may be associated with an improvement of insulin resistance. The anti-inflammatory properties of adiponectin are likely to be the major component of its beneficial effects for alleviating insulin resistance and vascular diseases [26]. Adiponectin has been reported to decrease CRP mRNA and protein [27] and inhibit the stimulation of nuclear factor-κB (NF-κB) signaling and TNF-α secretion from macrophages [28]. Adiponectin suppresses TNF-α-induced monocyte adhesion to human aortic endothelial cells and the expression of certain adhesion molecules [29]. Further, adiponectin reduces the expression of cell adhesion molecules and the activation of IL-8 and NFκB by decreasing TNF-α in endothelial cells [27,30]. Adiponectin also modulates macrophage function and phenotype [31]. IL-10 stimulation and IL-1 receptor antagonists are associated with the anti-inflammatory actions of adiponectin in human monocytes, monocyte-derived macrophages, and dendritic cells [32].

Adiponectin suppresses the generation of oxidative and nitrative stress by inhibiting inducible nitric oxide synthase (iNOS) and suppressing the expression of a nicotinamide adenine dinucleotide phosphate (NADPH) oxidase subunit [33], which improves insulin resistance. Further, adiponectin improves insulin resistance in the liver and skeletal muscle via adenosine monophosphate-activated protein kinase (AMPK) and peroxisome proliferator-activated receptor-α (PPAR-α) activation [34].

2.1.2. Pancreatic β Cell Protective Effect of Adiponectin

Adiponectin prevents ceramide- or inflammatory cytokine-induced apoptosis in cultured β cells [35,36] and maintains β cell mass and glucose homeostasis in *ob/ob* mice and in a mice model of type 1 diabetes [35,37]. Adiponectin-null mice are more susceptible to caspase-8-induced β cell apoptosis [36]. Via adiponectin receptors AdipoR1 and AdipoR2, adiponectin stimulates the de-acylation of ceramide, yielding sphingosine after conversion to sphingosine 1-phosphate (S1P) by sphingosine kinase. The resulting conversion from ceramide to S1P promotes the survival of functional β-cell mass [38].

2.1.3. Increase of Glucose Utilization and Fatty Acid Oxidation in Skeletal Muscles by Adiponectin

Adiponectin has been reported to improve glucose utilization and fatty acid (FA) oxidation in myocytes [39]. In addition, in mice fed with high fat/sucrose diet, adiponectin showed to increase energy expenditure by increasing FA oxidation and to increase glucose uptake in skeletal muscle [40]. Adiponectin increased glucose transporter-4 (GLUT-4) translocation and glucose uptake by rat skeletal muscle cells [41]. These beneficial effects of adiponectin on glucose metabolism were mainly via the activation of AMPK in skeletal muscles [42]. In addition, it has been suggested that adiponectin decreases insulin resistance by decreasing the muscular lipid content in obese mice [43].

2.1.4. Adiponectin Reduces Hepatic Glucose Production

In the liver, adiponectin improves hepatic and systemic insulin resistance through the activation of AMPK and PPAR-α pathways [34]. Adiponectin has been reported to suppress both glycogenolysis and gluconeogenesis [42] by reducing the rate-limiting enzymes for hepatic glucose production, such as glucose-6-phosphatase (G6Pase) and phosphoenolpyruvate carboxy kinase (PEPCK) [39,44–47]. Besides the suppression of G6Pase and PEPCK, adiponectin can suppress glucose production by reducing the availability of gluconeogenic substrates [47]. Adiponectin stimulates FA oxidation, which reduces gluconeogenic availability.

2.1.5. Adiponectin Increases Insulin-Stimulated Glucose Uptake by Adipocytes

Adiponectin treatment enhances insulin-stimulated glucose uptake via activation of AMPK in primary rat adipocytes [48]. Adiponectin directly targets insulin receptor substrate-1 (IRS-1) rather than the insulin receptor (IR) [49]. IRS-1 plays a crucial role in insulin mediation of glucose uptake in adipocytes [50]. Decreased levels of IRS-1 are significantly associated with insulin resistance and type 2 diabetes [51,52].

2.1.6. Summary of Anti-Diabetic Effects of Adiponectin

Possible mechanisms for the improvement of glucose metabolism by adiponectin are shown in Figure 1.

2.2. Adiponectin and Development of Type 2 Diabetes

In a case–control series which was performed in the Pima Indian population [53], at baseline, the serum adiponectin level was significantly lower in the cases ($n = 70$) than in the controls ($n = 70$), and individuals who showed high serum adiponectin levels were less likely to develop type 2 diabetes than individuals with low serum adiponectin levels (incidence rate ratio 0.63 (95% confidence intervals (CI) 0.43–0.92); $p = 0.02$) [54]. In the population-based Monitoring of Trends and Determinants in Cardiovascular Disease (MONICA)/Cooperative Health Research in the Region of Augsburg (KORA) cohort study between 1984 and 1995 with follow-up until 2002 (mean follow-up 10.9 ± 4.7 years) [55], low levels of adiponectin were associated with an increased type 2 diabetes risk. The multivariable adjusted hazard ratio (HR) with 95% CI comparing tertile extremes was 2.65 (1.88-3.76) for adiponectin (bottom vs. top tertile), respectively [54]. A systematic review and meta-analysis of prospective studies was conducted to assess the association of serum adiponectin level with risk of type 2 diabetes. This meta-analysis included 19 studies, comprising a total of 39,136 participants and 7924 cases, and showed that type 2 diabetes risk was strongly associated with low levels of adiponectin [55]. Furthermore, other observational studies showed that low levels of adiponectin are significantly associated with the development of type 2 diabetes [23,25,56–58].

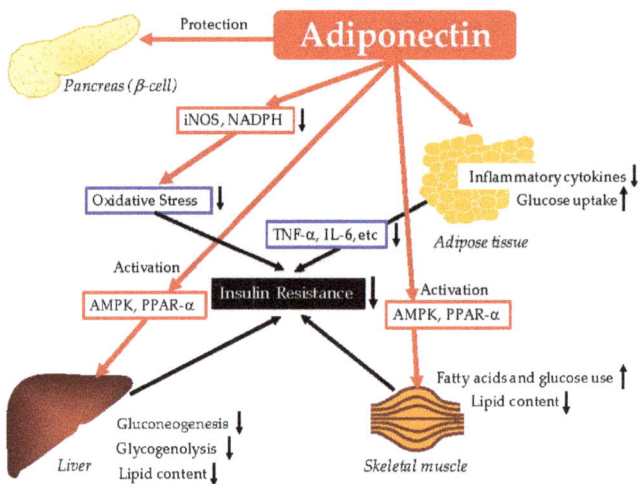

Figure 1. Possible mechanisms for the improvement of glucose metabolism by adiponectin. AMPK, adenosine monophosphate-activated protein kinase; IL-6, interleukin-6; iNOS, inducible nitric oxide synthase; NADPH, nicotinamide adenine dinucleotide phosphate; PPAR-α, peroxisome proliferator-activated receptor-α, TNF-α, tumor necrosis factor-α.

3. Effects of Adiponectin on Lipid Metabolism

3.1. Possible Mechanisms for the Improvement of Lipid Metabolism by Adiponectin

Adiponectin has been found to be correlated with various parameters of lipoprotein metabolism and, especially, it is associated with the metabolism of high-density lipoprotein (HDL) and TG. Adiponectin appears to induce an increase in serum HDL and, in addition, it lowers serum TG through the enhanced catabolism of TG-rich lipoproteins [59].

3.1.1. Possible Mechanism for the Increase of HDL by Adiponectin

Almost all of the previous studies reported that serum adiponectin is positively correlated with serum HDL-C level [60–66]. Especially, HDL-C has been shown to be positively correlated with HMW adiponectin, which is considered the most biologically active form of adiponectin [60,64,65], independently of adiposity and of insulin sensitivity [61,63–65,67–69]. We also found that adiponectin was independently and positively correlated with HDL-C in 174 subjects without diabetes [70].

Adiponectin has been shown to increase HDL-C via an increase in the hepatic production of apo-AI, which is the major apolipoprotein of HDL, and through an increase in the production of ATP-binding cassette transporter A1 (ABCA1), which induces HDL assembly through reverse cholesterol transport [71–76]. Adiponectin has been shown to enhance ABCA1 expression through the activation of nuclear receptors including liver X receptor α and PPAR-γ [75].

Adiponectin-induced increase in HDL-C involves the down-regulation of hepatic lipase (HL) activity, given the reported inverse association of serum adiponectin with HL activity, which appears to be independent of measures of adiposity and insulin resistance [77,78].

Another possible mechanism underlying the adiponectin-induced up-regulation of HDL-C is the activation of lipoprotein lipase (LPL) by adiponectin and/or the improvement of insulin resistance, which can also reduce TG.

3.1.2. Possible Mechanisms for TG reduction by Adiponectin

The majority of previous studies have demonstrated a negative association between circulating adiponectin and serum TG [60,61,63–69,78]. Very low density lipoprotein (VLDL), one of TG-rich lipoproteins, has been found to be correlated with serum HMW adiponectin [66,79–81]. We also found that VLDL-C levels were inversely correlated with adiponectin levels independently of age, body mass index (BMI), gender, and glycemic control in patients with type 2 diabetes [82] The reported association of circulating adiponectin with VLDL apoB100 fractional catabolic rate suggests that the regulation of serum VLDL-C by adiponectin may involve VLDL catabolism [79,83,84]. A plausible explanation for the adiponectin-induced increase in TG catabolism is the regulation of LPL activity by adiponectin. It is well known that LPL, which is translocated to the endothelial cell surface of the vessels of heart, muscles, and adipose tissue, hydrolyses TG in TG-rich lipoproteins including chylomicrons and VLDL [85]. Serum adiponectin has been reported to be positively correlated with post-heparin LPL concentration and activity in the fasting state, apparently independently of insulin resistance and inflammation [86,87]. As mice over-expressing adiponectin display increased LPL gene expression and LPL activity in skeletal muscle during fasting and in adipose tissue mainly during the well-fed state [74,88], adiponectin may have a direct role in inducing LPL expression and activation in both skeletal muscle and adipose tissue.

Another possible mechanism for TG reduction by adiponectin would be attributable to adiponectin-induced decrease in serum apo-CIII, a well-known inhibitor of LPL, as indicated by the reported negative association between circulating adiponectin and serum apo-CIII [89,90], and the down-regulation of apo-CIII-mRNA levels in adiponectin-treated human HepG2 hepatocytes [87]. In addition, the other mechanism of the adiponectin-induced up-regulation of VLDL catabolism involves the increased expression of VLDL receptor (VLDL-R) in skeletal muscle. Using adenovirus-mediated gene transduction, an increase of VLDL-R expression has been observed in adiponectin-treated myotubes, with an acute elevation of plasma adiponectin leading to the increased VLDL catabolism [87].

Insulin resistance increases activity and expression of hormone-sensitive lipase (HSL) in adipose tissue, which catalyzes the breakdown of TG, releasing free fatty acids (FFA) [91]. Increased FFA enter the liver and enhance the production of VLDL. Therefore, an improvement of insulin resistance by adiponectin may reduce HSL activity and result in a reduction of VLDL production.

Adiponectin has been also shown to be associated with apo-B48, which is an apolipoprotein of chylomicrons from the small intestine [89,90]. A plausible explanation for this relationship is the up-regulation of postprandial TG catabolism by adiponectin, as indicated by the reported association of circulating adiponectin with heparin-releasable LPL activity in subcutaneous adipose tissue, observed after a meal [77].

3.1.3. Effects of Adiponectin on LDL and Other Atherogenic Lipids

With regard to possible relationship between circulating adiponectin and low-density lipoprotein cholesterol (LDL-C), the majority of studies have shown no association [64,65,70,92–94]. Small dense LDL (sd-LDL) is considered an emerging risk factor for cardiovascular diseases (CVD). High sd-LDL levels have been reported to be associated with elevated TG levels and low HDL-C levels and constitute a common feature of type 2 diabetes and metabolic syndrome [95,96]. Oxidative modifications of LDL represent an early stage of atherosclerosis, and sd-LDL are more susceptible to oxidation than larger, more buoyant particles [96]. Adiponectin-mediated improvement of TG and HDL may reduce the atherogenic lipoprotein sd-LDL. Remnant lipoproteins, derived from VLDL and chylomicrons, have been considered to be atherogenic [97]. In patients with hypertriglyceridemia, TG-rich lipoproteins mainly increase during fasting and the postprandial state. Remnant lipoproteins directly and indirectly correlate to the enhancement of atherogenicity [98]. Therefore, the reduction of remnant lipoproteins due to the decrease of TG by adiponectin may contribute to the anti-atherogenic effects of adiponectin.

3.1.4. Summary of Mechanisms for the Improvement of Lipid Metabolism by Adiponectin.

Possible mechanisms for the improvement of lipid metabolism by adiponectin are shown in Figure 2.

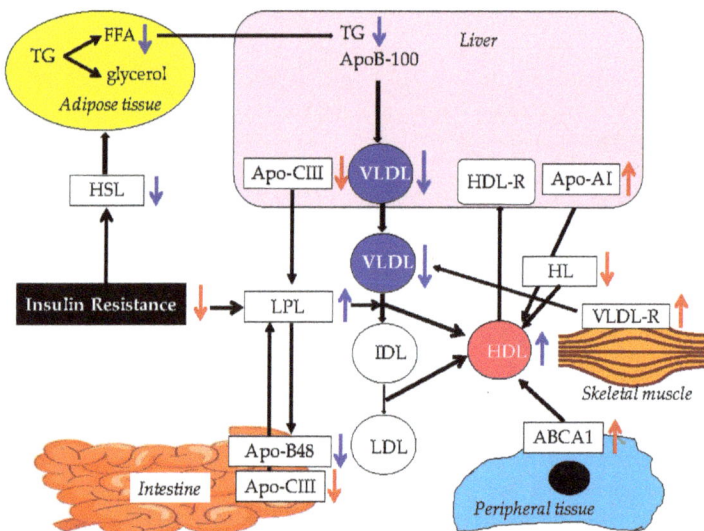

Figure 2. Possible mechanisms for the improvement of lipid metabolism by adiponectin. Red and blue arrows indicate direct and indirect lipid metabolism improving effects of adiponectin, respectively. ABCA1, ATP-binding cassette transporter A1; FFA, free fatty acids; HDL, high-density lipoprotein; HL, hepatic lipase; HSL, hormone-sensitive lipase; IDL, intermediate-density lipoprotein; LDL, low-density lipoprotein; TG, triglyceride; VLDL, very low density lipoprotein; VLDL-R, very low density lipoprotein-receptor.

Adiponectin increases HDL-C via an increase in the hepatic production of apo-AI, through an increase in the expression of ABCA1 in peripheral tissues. Down-regulation of HL activity by adiponectin may also increase HDL-C. Increased LPL expression and activity in skeletal muscle and adipose tissue contribute to the reduction of TG-rich lipoproteins and the elevation of HDL. Adiponectin-induced decrease of hepatic apo-CIII production and adiponectin-induced up-regulation of VLDL-R in skeletal muscle also lead to the decrease of TG. An improvement of insulin resistance by adiponectin may reduce HSL activity and result in the reduction of VLDL production due to a decreased release of FFA from the adipose tissue to the liver.

4. Anti-Atherosclerotic Effects of Adiponectin

4.1. Improvement of Endothelial Function and Interaction Between Monocyte and Endothelium by Adiponectin

There is a close relationship between hypoadiponectinemia and peripheral arterial dysfunction [99–101]. Adiponectin knockout mice showed significantly increased neointimal hyperplasia, disordered endothelium-dependent vasodilation, and increased blood pressure, compared with wild-type mice [99,102,103]. Flow-mediated dilation of the brachial artery has a significant relationship with plasma HMW adiponectin levels in young healthy men [104]. The biosynthesis of nitric oxide (NO) is performed by AMPK and is mediated by adiponectin-induced phosphorylation of endothelial nitric oxide synthase (eNOS). Adiponectin inhibits the interaction between leukocytes and endothelial cells by reducing E-selectin and vascular cell adhesion molecule-1 induced by TNF-α, resistin, and IL-8, and by increasing endothelial NO [105], which results in the attenuation of monocyte attachment to endothelial cells [31]. Serum adiponectin concentration also showed a significant negative correlation with serum MCP-1 concentration ($r = -0.244$, $p = 0.05$) in postmenopausal women [106]. Adiponectin also reduces irregular high glucose-induced apoptosis and oxidative stress in human umbilical vein endothelial cells [105,107].

Elevated serum TG levels are an independent predictor of endothelial dysfunction. Lowering circulating TG levels by adiponectin may improve the endothelial function [108]. The increase of TG and decrease of HDL reduce the activity and expression of eNOS and disrupt the integrity of the vascular endothelium due to oxidative stress [109]. Diabetes-induced endothelial dysfunction is a critical and initiating factor in the genesis of diabetic vascular complications [110]. Therefore, reduction of TG, elevation of HDL, and improvement of glucose metabolism may ameliorate the endothelial function.

4.2. Inhibition of Smooth Muscle Proliferation by Adiponectin

Rapid proliferation and migration of vascular smooth muscle cells (SMCs) toward the intima contribute to intimal thickening of arteries and atherosclerosis development. Adiponectin blocks the proliferation and migration of human aortic SMCs by inhibiting several atherogenic growth factors, including platelet-derived growth factor, basic fibroblast growth factor, and heparin-binding epidermal growth factor [111,112].

4.3. Increase of Macrophage Cholesterol Efflux and Suppression of Foam Cell Formation

Serum HDL-C levels are inversely correlated to the risk of atherosclerotic cardiovascular diseases. The reverse cholesterol transport is one of the major protective systems against atherosclerosis, in which HDL particles play a crucial role, carrying cholesterol derived from peripheral tissues to the liver. ABCA1 receptors has been identified as important membrane receptors to generate HDL by cholesterol efflux from foam cells. Adiponectin has been reported to up-regulate the expression of ABCA1 in human macrophages and enhance apo-AI-mediated cholesterol efflux from macrophages [75]. Recently, Marsche et al. investigated the association between cholesterol efflux capacity and metabolic parameters in 683 participants (281 youths, of whom 227 were overweight/obese; 402 adults, of whom 197 were overweight/obese). They found that hypoadiponectinemia is a robust predictor of reduced cholesterol efflux capacity in adults, irrespective of BMI and fat distribution [113]. Adiponectin markedly suppressed foam cell formation in oxidized LDL-treated macrophages from diabetic subjects, which was mainly attributed to an increase in cholesterol efflux [114]. In addition, a deletion of adipoR1 in macrophages from diabetic patients accelerated foam cell formation induced by oxidized LDL [114]. A strong positive correlation was noted between decreased serum adiponectin and impaired cholesterol efflux capacity, both before and after adjustment for HDL-C and apo-AI in diabetic patients (both $p < 0.001$) [114]. The adiponectin-treated macrophages contained fewer lipid droplets stained by oil red O [3]. The adipocyte-derived plasma protein adiponectin suppressed macrophage-to-foam cell transformation by reducing the expression of class A macrophage scavenger receptor at both mRNA and protein levels [3].

Kubota et al. carried out serum cholesterol efflux studies in individuals with glucose intolerance [115]. An inverse correlation was found between the cholesterol efflux capability and the extent of glucose intolerance in an oral glucose tolerance test. An improvement of glucose metabolism and insulin resistance may ameliorate cholesterol efflux. Interestingly, enhanced cholesterol efflux to HDL through the ABCA1 transporter was observed in hypertriglyceridemic patients with type 2 diabetes [116,117]. Further, enhanced efflux of cholesterol from ABCA1-expressing macrophages to serum was observed in patients with hypertriglyceridemia [118].

4.4. Putative Molecular Anti-Atherosclerotic Effects of Adiponectin

Possible anti-atherosclerotic effects of adiponectin are shown in Figure 3.

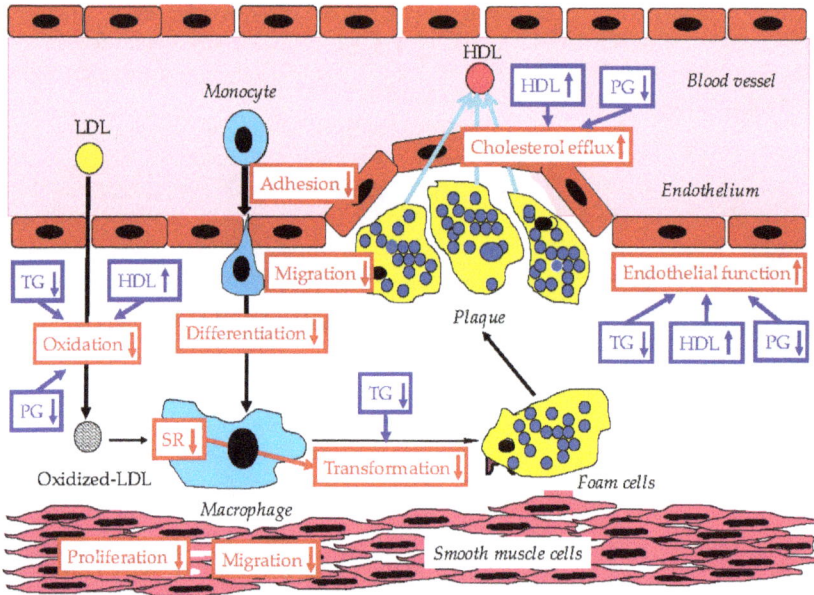

Figure 3. Possible anti-atherosclerotic effects of adiponectin and improvement of lipid/glucose metabolism by adiponectin. The red words in the red squares show the anti-arteriosclerotic effects of adiponectin. HDL, high-density lipoprotein; LDL, low-density lipoprotein; PG, plasma glucose; SR, scavenger receptor; TG, triglyceride.

5. How can We Increase Adiponectin?

5.1. Weight Loss

A systematic review which assessed the consequences of all types of obesity surgery showed that adiponectin was significantly increased after bariatric surgery [119]. Sibutramine is an anti-obesity medication whose effects on weight loss have been widely explored. A systematic review and meta-analysis of available evidence was conducted in order to calculate the effect size of sibutramine therapy on adipokines [120]. Random-effect meta-analysis evidenced a significant increase of adiponectin (weighted mean difference (WMD) 9.86%, 95%CI: 1.76, 17.96, $p = 0.017$) following sibutramine therapy. A systematic review and meta-analysis of clinical trials that assessed the effect of a low-calorie diet on adiponectin concentration showed that a weight-loss diet can substantially increase the overall adiponectin concentration (Hedges' $g = 0.34$, 95% CI:0.17–0.50, $p < 0.001$) [121].

5.2. Exercise

We examined the effects of supervised aerobic exercise on serum adiponectin and lipids in patients with moderate dyslipidemia. In this study, 25 patients (mean BMI, 24.6 kg/m^2; mean age, 39 years; mean total cholesterol, 226 mg/dL; mean TG, 149 mg/dL) without metabolic syndrome, diabetes, and hypertension underwent a 16-week supervised aerobic exercise program (60 min/day,

2 to 3 times/week) with moderate exercise intensity [122]. Adiponectin significantly increased by 51% at week 16, although changes in these parameters were not significant at week 8 [123]. Several meta-analyses have shown that the exercise increased serum adiponectin [124–127], supporting our study result.

5.3. Nutritional Factors

5.3.1. Vitamins

Vitamin D has been proposed to have anti-inflammatory properties. A meta-analysis was performed to examine the effect of vitamin D supplementation on adipocytokines in patients with type 2 diabetes [128]. In the meta-analysis of 20 randomized controlled trials (RCTs) (n = 1270 participants), vitamin D-supplemented groups had lower levels of CRP and TNF α and higher levels of leptin compared with control groups. However, no differences were observed for adiponectin. Also another meta-analysis did not indicate a significant effect of vitamin D supplementation on serum adiponectin levels [123].

A meta-analysis assessed the effects of vitamin K supplementation on a homeostasis model assessment of insulin resistance (HOMA-IR), fasting plasma glucose and insulin, CRP, adiponectin, leptin, or IL-6 levels [129]. A total of eight trials involving 1077 participants met the inclusion criteria. Vitamin K supplementation did not affect insulin sensitivity as measured by HOMA-IR, fasting plasma glucose and insulin, CRP, adiponectin, leptin, and IL-6 levels.

5.3.2. Polyphenols

Resveratrol is a non-flavonoid polyphenol that naturally occurs as phytoalexin. The shell and stem of *Vitis vinifera* L. (Vitaceae) are the richest sources of this compound. A variety of in vitro and in vivo studies suggested the effectiveness of resveratrol in diabetes [130]. A systematic review and a meta-analysis of available RCTs to elucidate the role of resveratrol supplementation on adipokines showed a significant change in serum adiponectin concentrations following resveratrol supplementation (WMD: 1.10 μg/mL, 95% CI: 0.88, 1.33, $p < 0.001$) [131].

5.3.3. Carotenoids

Astaxanthin is a naturally occurring red pigmented carotenoid classified as a xanthophyll, found in microalgae and seafood such as salmon, trout, and shrimp. Astaxanthin as a bioactive compound has a potential role in the prevention of atherosclerosis and a beneficial effect on adiponectin levels [132]. We performed an RCT of astaxanthin analyzing metabolic parameters. Placebo-controlled astaxanthin administration at doses of 0, 6, 12, 18 mg/day for 12 weeks was randomly allocated to 61 non-obese subjects with fasting serum TG of 120-200 mg/dL and without diabetes and hypertension, aged 25–60 years. Serum adiponectin was increased by astaxanthin (12 and 18 mg/day), and changes in adiponectin correlated positively with HDL-C changes, independent of age and BMI [133].

Carotenoids have been implicated in the regulation of adipocyte metabolism. Canas et al. compared the effects of mixed-carotenoid supplementation (MCS, which contains β-carotene, α-carotene, lutein, zeaxanthin, lycopene, astaxanthin, and γ-tocopherol) to those of a placebo on adipokines in children with obesity [134]. An RCT to evaluate the effects of MCS over 6 months was performed. Twenty children (6 male and 14 female) with simple obesity (BMI > 90%) and a mean age ($\pm$ SD) of 10.5 $\pm$ 0.4 years, were enrolled. MCS increased total adiponectin and HMW adiponectin compared with the placebo.

Another study assessed the effects of 280 mL of tomato juice (containing 32.5 mg of lycopene) consumed daily in addition to a normal diet and an exercise program for 2 months [135]. The tomato juice supplementation significantly reduced body weight, body fat, waist circumference, and BMI, and significantly increased serum adiponectin levels. The intervention included 10 weeks of consumption of a tomato-based diet ($\geq$25 mg lycopene daily) with an intermediate 2-week washout and was performed in 70 postmenopausal women with mean age of 57.2 years and mean BMI of 30.0 kg/m² [136]. After the tomato intervention, adiponectin concentration increased (ratio 1.09, 95%CI 1.00–1.18), with a stronger effect observed among nonobese women (ratio 1.13, 95% CI 1.02–1.25).

A positive association between concentrations of β-carotene and adiponectin independent of sex, age, smoking status, BMI, and waist circumference was observed in non-diabetic obese subjects. [137]. In this cross-sectional study which assessed whether serum carotenoids are associated with HMW adiponectin in 437 Japanese subjects (116 men and 321 women), serum β-carotene concentrations were significantly associated with serum HMW adiponectin concentrations in both sexes (standardized β coefficient = 0.197, p = 0.036 for men; standardized β coefficient = 0.146, p = 0.012 for women) [138].

Serum β-cryptoxanthin levels are lower in overweight subjects than in normal subjects. An intervention study consisted of a three-week long before-and-after controlled trial, where β-cryptoxanthin (4.7 mg/day) was given to 17 moderately obese postmenopausal women [139]. Serum HMW adiponectin levels significantly increased after this intervention. An RCT tested the effects of antioxidant (AOX) supplementation (vitamin E, 800 IU/day; vitamin C, 500 mg/day; β-carotene, 10 mg/day) on insulin sensitivity and adipokines in overweight and normal-weight individuals (n = 48, aged 18–30 years) [140]. The participants received either AOX or a placebo for 8 weeks. Adiponectin increased in both AOX groups. In another RCT by the same research group, overweight (BMI, 33.2 ± 1.9 kg/m²) and comparative normal-weight (BMI, 21.9 ± 0.5 kg/m²) adults, aged 18 to 30 years old (n = 48), were enrolled [141]. Either daily AOX treatment or placebo were administered for 8 weeks to the study subjects who completed a standardized 30-minute cycle exercise bout at baseline and week 8. Adiponectin was increased in both overweight and normal-weight AOX groups (22.1% vs. 3.1%; p < 0.05) but reduced in placebo groups.

5.3.4. Omega-3 FA

Fish oil, a source of omega-3 FAs, improves insulin sensitivity in animal experiments, but findings remain inconsistent in humans. A meta-analysis of RCTs determined the effect of omega-3 FA consumption on circulating adiponectin in humans [142]. Fourteen RCT arms evaluated fish oil (fish oil, n = 682; placebo, n = 641). Fish oil increased adiponectin by 0.37 µg/mL (95% CI 0.07; 0.67, p = 0.02). To determine the effects of omega-3 FA supplementation on adipocytokine levels in adult prediabetic and diabetic individuals, a meta-analysis of RCTs was performed [143]. Fourteen individual studies (n = 685) were included in the meta-analysis. Omega-3 FA supplementation increased adiponectin by 0.48 µg/mL (95% CI, 0.27 to 0.68; p < 0.00001). In the meta-analysis of RCTs which assessed the effects of omega-3 FA in women with polycystic ovary syndrome (PCOS), nine trials involving 591 patients were included. Compared with the control group, omega-3 FA increased adiponectin level (weighted mean difference (WMD) 1.34; 95% CI 0.51 to 2.17; p = 0. 002) [144]. In the meta-analysis of RCTs in patients with type 2 diabetes, omega-3 FA increased adiponectin by 0.57 µg/mL (95% CI 0.15 to 1.31; p = 0.01) [145]. Another meta-analysis in patients with type 2 diabetes showed a nonsignificant increase (MD = 0.17 µg/mL (95% CI 0.11 to 0.44)) of adiponectin [146].

5.4. Anti-Diabetic Drugs

5.4.1. Thiazolidinediones

A systematic review which summarizes the evidence of the effect of thiazolidinediones (pioglitazone and rosiglitazone) on circulating adiponectin levels was performed through a systematic search in PubMed, Scopus, and Cochrane Library. A significant increase in adiponectin (80-178%) after thiazolidinediones treatment was observed in all included studies [147]. Our systematic review also reported that pioglitazone increased serum adiponectin levels [148]. Further, stopping pioglitazone was associated with a subsequent decrease in adiponectin (from 9.7 ± 9.1 to 5.1 ± 4.5 µg/ml) [149].

5.4.2. Metformin

To provide high-quality evidence about the effect of metformin on adipocytokines in patients with PCOS, relevant studies that assessed the levels of adiponectin in patients with PCOS treated with metformin were reviewed and analyzed [150]. A total of 34 data sets were included, with four different outcomes, involving 744 women with PCOS. Metformin treatment was associated with significantly elevated serum adiponectin concentrations [standard mean difference (SMD) −0.43; 95%CI −0.75 to −0.11]. In a meta-analysis to investigate and determine the role of metformin on serum adiponectin levels in patients with type 2 diabetes, 18 cohort studies conducted among Asians and Caucasians from 2004 to 2013 were examined [151]. Post-treatment serum adiponectin levels were higher than pre-treatment levels in patients with type 2 diabetes (SMD = 0.19, 95% CI 0.09 to 0.30, $p < 0.001$).

5.4.3. α-Glycosidase Inhibitors

Miglitol, one of α-glycosidase inhibitors, has been reported to increase serum adiponectin levels [152]. Adiponectin levels were significantly increased by miglitol ($p < 0.01$), and the significant increase in adiponectin by miglitol was inversely correlated with the ratio between the 60 minute change in blood glucose at three months and the change at baseline ($r = −0.59$, $p = 0.02$), which was independent of age, sex, changes in hemoglobin A1c and BMI, and the baseline concentration of adiponectin [153]. Another α-glycosidase inhibitor, acarbose, has been also reported to lead to a significant increase of adiponectin [154–156].

5.4.4. Dipeptidyl peptidase-4 inhibitors (DPP4i)

The PubMed, Embase, and Cochrane library databases were searched from inception to February 2016. RCTs evaluating DPP4i (sitagliptin and vildagliptin) versus placebo or an active control drug in type 2 diabetic patients, lasting ≥12 weeks, were identified [157]. Weighted mean differences in adiponectin levels were calculated by using a fixed- or random-effects model. Ten RCTs, including 1495 subjects, were identified. Compared with the placebo, DPP4i (sitagliptin and vildagliptin) treatment significantly elevated adiponectin levels by 0.74 µg/mL (95%CI, 0.45 to 1.03), whereas, the difference was 0.00 µg/mL (95% CI, −0.57 to 0.56) when using an active-comparison.

5.4.5. Glucagon-like peptide-1 (GLP-1) analogues

The GLP-1 receptor agonist liraglutide did not change adiponectin levels in women with PCOS [158]. Liraglutide reduced HbA1c and adiponectin (all $p < 0.05$) in patients with non-alcoholic steatohepatitis [159]. An eight-week liraglutide therapy was associated with an increase in the levels of adiponectin (4480 vs. 6290 pg/mL, $p < 0.002$) in patients with type 2 diabetes [160]. However, liraglutide reduced serum adiponectin levels in Japanese patients with type 2 diabetes [161,162]. Exenatide significantly increased adiponectin levels after three months compared with baseline in patients with obesity and type 2 diabetes ($p < 0.05$) [163]. The adiponectin level was significantly increased by the addition of exenatide (0.39 ± 0.32 vs. −1.62 ± 0.97 µg/mL in exenatide and placebo groups, respectively, $p = 0.045$) in patients with poorly controlled type 2 diabetes [164].

5.4.6. Sodium–glucose cotransporter 2 inhibitors (SGLT-2i)

The new drugs for type 2 diabetes SGLT-2i are reversible inhibitor of SGLT-2, leading to a reduction of renal glucose reabsorption and a decrease of plasma glucose, in an insulin-independent manner. Since SGLT-2i are proved to be significantly associated with weight loss, we have predicted that SGLT-2 inhibitors may increase adiponectin [165]. Dapagliflozin, ipragliflozin, and canagliflozin showed a significant increase of adiponectin [166–172].

5.4.7. Sulfonyl Urea

In RCTs which investigated the effects of new anti-diabetic drugs (pioglitazone, DPP4i, and SGLT-2i) on adiponectin, glimepiride, a sulfonyl urea, has been used as a comparator [168,173–178]. Glimepiride is less likely to increase adiponectin than other oral anti-diabetic drugs. To observe the efficacy and safety of adding glimepiride to an established insulin therapy in poorly controlled type 2 diabetes and to assess the resulting changes in the HMW adiponectin serum levels and glycemia after glimepiride treatment, 56 subjects with poorly controlled insulin-treated type 2 diabetes were randomly assigned to either the glimepiride-treated group (n = 29) or the insulin-increasing group (n = 27) [179]. HMW adiponectin serum levels were significantly increased in the glimepiride-treated group compared with the insulin-increasing group. Changes in HbA1c were inversely correlated with changes in serum HMW adiponectin in the glimepiride-treated group (r = −0.452, p = 0.02).

5.5. Hypolipidemia Drugs

5.5.1. Statin

A meta-analysis of 12 RCTs with 16 comparisons and 1042 patients showed that serum adiponectin was not significantly affected by simvastatin (WMD: 0.42 µg/mL; 95% CI, −0.66 to 1.50 µg/mL) [180]. In a systematic review and meta-analysis of 43 studies, a significant increase in plasma adiponectin levels was observed after statin therapy (WMD: 0.57 µg/mL, 95% CI: 0.18 to 0.95, p = 0.004) [181]. In subgroup analysis, atorvastatin, simvastatin, rosuvastatin, pravastatin, and pitavastatin were found to change plasma adiponectin concentrations by 0.70 µg/mL (95% CI: −0.26 to 1.65), 0.50 µg/mL (95% CI: −0.44 to 1.45), −0.70 µg/mL (95% CI: −1.08 to −0.33), 0.62 µg/mL (95% CI: −0.12 to 1.35), and 0.51 µg/mL (95% CI: 0.30 to 0.72), respectively.

5.5.2. Ezetimibe

A meta-analysis of 23 RCTs did not suggest any significant effect of adding ezetimibe to statin therapy on plasma concentrations of adiponectin (SMD 0.34, 95% CI −0.28 to 0.96; p = 0.288) [182].

5.5.3. Fibrate

Out of 12 RCTs comprising 443 cases and 437 controls met the selection criteria for systematic review, 9 RCTs (399 cases and 401 controls) were included in the meta-analysis. Quantitative data synthesis revealed a significant effect of fibrate therapy in increasing circulating adiponectin levels (WMD: 0.38 µg/mL; 95%CI: 0.13 to 0.63 µg/mL; p = 0.003) [183]. In the head-to-head comparison of fibrates versus statins for the elevation of circulating adiponectin concentrations by a systematic review and meta-analysis, monotherapies with either fibrates or statins had comparable effects on circulating concentrations of adiponectin [184].

5.6. Anti-Hypertensive Drugs

Angiotensin II receptor blocker (ARB)

Telmisartan has been proposed to be a promising cardiometabolic ARB due to its unique PPAR-γ-inducing property. In a meta-analysis of RCTs, the pooled analysis suggested a significant increase in % changes of adiponectin (0.75; 95% CI, 0.40 to 1.09; p < 0.0001) among patients with metabolic syndrome randomized to receive telmisartan or control therapy [185]. The pooled analysis of the 11 trials (1088 patients) demonstrated a statistically significant increase in the percent changes of adiponectin levels (MD, 15.74%; 95% CI, 4.95% to 26.52%; p = 0.004) with telmisartan relative to other ARB therapies [186]. A systematic review of the effect of telmisartan on insulin sensitivity in hypertensive patients with insulin resistance or diabetes was performed [187]. Eight trials involving a total of 763 patients met the inclusion criteria. Telmisartan was superior to other ARBs in increasing adiponectin level (MD, 0.93 µg/dL; 95% CI, 0.28 to 1.59 µg/dL; p = 0.005).

5.7. Summary of Possible Factors Which Increase Circulating Adiponectin Levels

The summary of possible factors which increase circulating adiponectin levels are shown in Table 1.

Table 1. Possible factors which increase circulating adiponectin levels.

1. Weight Loss
Bariatric Surgery
Sibutramine
Low Calorie Diet
2. Exercise
3. Nutritional Factors
Resveratrol
Astaxanthin
Mixed-Carotenoid Supplementation (β-carotene, α-carotene, Lutein, Zeaxanthin, Lycopene, Astaxanthin, γ-tocopherol)
Tomato Juice
β-carotene
β-cryptoxanthin
Antioxidant Supplementation (Vitamin E, Vitamin C, β-carotene)
Omega-3 Fatty Acids
4. Anti-Diabetic Drugs
Thiazolidinediones
Metformin
α-Glycosidase Inhibitors (Miglitol, Acarbose)
Dipeptidyl Peptidase-4 Inhibitors
Glucagon-Like Peptide-1Analugues (Liraglutide < Exenatide)
Sodium-Glucose Cotransporter 2 Inhibitors
5. Hypolipidemia Drugs
Statin
Fibrate
6. Anti-Hypertensive Drugs
Angiotensin II Receptor blockers (Telmisartan)

6. Conclusions

Adiponectin reduces inflammatory cytokines and oxidative stress, which lead to an improvement of insulin resistance. Adiponectin-induced improvement of insulin resistance and adiponectin itself reduce hepatic gluconeogenesis and glycogenolysis and increase the utilization of glucose and FA by skeletal muscles, resulting in lower glucose levels. Adiponectin has also β-cell protective effect. A great number of previous studies demonstrated that adiponectin increases HDL and decreases TG. Adiponectin increases ABCA1 and LPL and decreases hepatic lipase, which may elevate HDL. Increased mass and activity of LPL and VLDL-receptor and reduced apo-CIII may increase VLDL catabolism and result in the reduction of serum TG. Further, adiponectin has various anti-atherosclerotic properties such as reduction of scavenger receptor in macrophages and increase of cholesterol efflux. These findings suggest that high circulating adiponectin levels can protect against atherosclerosis. Weight loss, exercise, nutritional factors, anti-diabetic drugs, hypolipidemic drugs, and anti-hypertensive drugs have been associated with an increase of serum adiponectin levels.

Author Contributions: H.Y. (Hidekatsu Yanai) and H.Y. (Hiroshi Yoshida) conceived the review; H.Y. (Hidekatsu Yanai) wrote the paper; H.Y. (Hiroshi Yoshida) edited the paper and provided critical guidance. Both authors read and approved the final version of this paper.

Funding: This review research received no external funding.

Conflicts of Interest: The authors declare no conflict of interest in relation to the present review paper.

Abbreviations

ABCA1	ATP-binding cassette transporter A1
AMPK	adenosine monophosphate-activated protein kinase
AOX	antioxidant
ARB	angiotensin II receptor blockers
BMI	body mass index
CAD	coronary artery disease
CI	confidence intervals
CRP	C-reactive protein
CVD	cardiovascular diseases
DPP4i	dipeptidyl peptidase-4 inhibitors
GLUT-4	glucose transporter-4
G6Pase	glucose-6-phosphatase
eNOS	endothelial nitric oxide synthase
FA	fatty acid
FFA	free fatty acids
GLP-1	glucagon-like peptide-1
HDL	high-density lipoprotein
HMW	high-molecular weight
HL	hepatic lipase
HOMA-IR	homeostasis model assessment of insulin resistance
HR	hazard ratio
HSL	hormone-sensitive lipase
IDL	intermediate-density lipoprotein
IL	interleukin
iNOS	inducible nitric oxide synthase
LDL	low-density lipoprotein
LPL	lipoprotein lipase
MCS	mixed-carotenoid supplementation
NADPH	nicotinamide adenine dinucleotide phosphate
NF-κB	nuclear factor-κB
NO	nitric oxide
PCOS	polycystic ovary syndrome
PPAR	peroxisome proliferator-activated receptor
PEPCK	phosphoenolpyruvate carboxy kinase
RCTs	randomized controlled trials
S1P	sphingosine 1-phosphate
Sd-LDL	small dense LDL
SGLT-2i	sodium–glucose cotransporter 2 inhibitors
SMCs	smooth muscle cells
SMD	standard mean difference
SR	scavenger receptor
TNF-α	tumor necrosis factor-alpha
TG	triglycerides
VLDL	very low density lipoprotein
VLDL-R	very low density lipoprotein receptor
WMD	weighted mean difference

Int. J. Mol. Sci. **2019**, *20*, 1190

References

1. Maeda, K.; Okubo, K.; Shimomura, I.; Funahashi, T.; Matsuzawa, Y.; Matsubara, K. cDNA cloning and expression of a novel adipose specific collagen-like factor, apM1 (AdiPose Most abundant Gene transcript 1). *Biochem. Biophys. Res. Commun.* **1996**, *221*, 286–289. [CrossRef]

2. Yokota, T.; Oritani, K.; Takahashi, I.; Ishikawa, J.; Matsuyama, A.; Ouchi, N.; Kihara, S.; Funahashi, T.; Tenner, A.J.; Tomiyama, Y.; et al. Adiponectin, a new member of the family of soluble defense collagens, negatively regulates the growth of myelomonocytic progenitors and the functions of macrophages. *Blood* **2000**, *96*, 1723–1732.

3. Ouchi, N.; Kihara, S.; Arita, Y.; Nishida, M.; Matsuyama, A.; Okamoto, Y.; Ishigami, M.; Kuriyama, H.; Kishida, K.; Nishizawa, H.; et al. Adipocyte-derived plasma protein, adiponectin, suppresses lipid accumulation and class A scavenger receptor expression in human monocyte-derived macrophages. *Circulation* **2001**, *103*, 1057–1063. [CrossRef] [PubMed]

4. Waki, H.; Yamauchi, T.; Kamon, J.; Ito, Y.; Uchida, S.; Kita, S.; Hara, K.; Hada, Y.; Vasseur, F.; Froguel, P.; et al. Impaired multimerization of human adiponectin mutants associated with diabetes. Molecular structure and multimer formation of adiponectin. *J. Biol. Chem.* **2003**, *278*, 40352–40363. [CrossRef] [PubMed]

5. Pajvani, U.B.; Du, X.; Combs, T.P.; Berg, A.H.; Rajala, M.W.; Schulthess, T.; Engel, J.; Brownlee, M.; Scherer, P.E. Structure-function studies of the adipocyte-secreted hormone Acrp30/adiponectin. Implications for metabolic regulation and bioactivity. *J. Biol. Chem.* **2003**, *278*, 9073–9085. [CrossRef] [PubMed]

6. Yamauchi, T.; Kamon, J.; Ito, Y.; Tsuchida, A.; Yokomizo, T.; Kita, S.; Sugiyama, T.; Miyagishi, M.; Hara, K.; Tsunoda, M.; et al. Cloning of adiponectin receptors that mediate antidiabetic metabolic effects. *Nature* **2003**, *423*, 762–769. [CrossRef] [PubMed]

7. Hug, C.; Wang, J.; Ahmad, N.S.; Bogan, J.S.; Tsao, T.S.; Lodish, H.F. T-cadherin is a receptor for hexameric and high-molecular-weight forms of Acrp30/adiponectin. *Proc. Natl. Acad. Sci. USA* **2004**, *101*, 10308–10313. [CrossRef] [PubMed]

8. Achari, A.E.; Jain, S.K. Adiponectin, a Therapeutic Target for Obesity, Diabetes, and Endothelial Dysfunction. *Int. J. Mol. Sci.* **2017**, *18*, 1321. [CrossRef]

9. Rosen, E.D.; Spiegelman, B.M. Adipocytes as regulators of energy balance and glucose homeostasis. *Nature* **2006**, *444*, 847–853. [CrossRef] [PubMed]

10. Ghadge, A.A.; Diwan, A.G.; Harsulkar, A.M.; Kuvalekar, A.A. Gender dependent effects of fasting blood glucose levels and disease duration on biochemical markers in type 2 diabetics: A pilot study. *Diabetes Metab. Syndr.* **2017**, *11*, S481–S489. [CrossRef] [PubMed]

11. Arita, Y.; Kihara, S.; Ouchi, N.; Takahashi, M.; Maeda, K.; Miyagawa, J.; Hotta, K.; Shimomura, I.; Nakamura, T.; Miyaoka, K.; et al. Paradoxical decrease of an adipose-specific protein, adiponectin, in obesity. *Biochem. Biophys. Res. Commun.* **1999**, *257*, 79–83. [CrossRef] [PubMed]

12. Funahashi, T.; Nakamura, T.; Shimomura, I.; Maeda, K.; Kuriyama, H.; Takahashi, M.; Arita, Y.; Kihara, S.; Matsuzawa, Y. Role of adipocytokines on the pathogenesis of atherosclerosis in visceral obesity. *Intern. Med.* **1999**, *38*, 202–206. [CrossRef] [PubMed]

13. Matsuzawa, Y.; Funahashi, T.; Nakamura, T. Molecular mechanism of metabolic syndrome X: Contribution of adipocytokines adipocyte-derived bioactive substances. *Ann. N. Y. Acad. Sci.* **1999**, *892*, 146–154. [CrossRef] [PubMed]

14. Okamoto, Y.; Arita, Y.; Nishida, M.; Muraguchi, M.; Ouchi, N.; Takahashi, M.; Igura, T.; Inui, Y.; Kihara, S.; Nakamura, T.; et al. An adipocyte-derived plasma protein, adiponectin, adheres to injured vascular walls. *Horm. Metab. Res.* **2000**, *32*, 47–50. [CrossRef] [PubMed]

15. Tilg, H.; Moschen, A.R. Adipocytokines: Mediators linking adipose tissue, inflammation and immunity. *Nat. Rev. Immunol.* **2006**, *6*, 772–783. [CrossRef] [PubMed]

16. Zhang, P.; Wang, Y.; Fan, Y.; Tang, Z.; Wang, N. Overexpression of adiponectin receptors potentiates the antiinflammatory action of sub-effective dose of globular adiponectin in vascular endothelial cells. *Arterioscler. Thromb. Vasc. Biol.* **2009**, *29*, 67–74. [CrossRef] [PubMed]

17. Weisberg, S.P.; McCann, D.; Desai, M.; Rosenbaum, M.; Leibel, R.L.; Ferrante, A.W., Jr. Obesity is associated with macrophage accumulation in adipose tissue. *J. Clin. Investig.* **2003**, *112*, 1796–1808. [CrossRef] [PubMed]

18. Xu, H.; Barnes, G.T.; Yang, Q.; Tan, G.; Yang, D.; Chou, C.J.; Sole, J.; Nichols, A.; Ross, J.S.; Tartaglia, L.A.; et al. Chronic inflammation in fat plays a crucial role in the development of obesity-related insulin resistance. *J. Clin. Investig.* **2003**, *112*, 1821–1830. [CrossRef] [PubMed]

19. Guha, M.; Bai, W.; Nadler, J.L.; Natarajan, R. Molecular mechanisms of tumor necrosis factor alpha gene expression in monocytic cells via hyperglycemia-induced oxidant stress-dependent and -independent pathways. *J. Biol. Chem.* **2000**, *275*, 17728–17739. [CrossRef] [PubMed]

20. Morohoshi, M.; Fujisawa, K.; Uchimura, I.; Numano, F. Glucose-dependent interleukin 6 and tumor necrosis factor production by human peripheral blood monocytes in vitro. *Diabetes* **1996**, *45*, 954–959. [CrossRef] [PubMed]

21. Barzilay, J.I.; Abraham, L.; Heckbert, S.R.; Cushman, M.; Kuller, L.H.; Resnick, H.E.; Tracy, R.P. The relation of markers of inflammation to the development of glucose disorders in the elderly: The Cardiovascular Health Study. *Diabetes* **2001**, *50*, 2384–2389. [CrossRef] [PubMed]

22. Freeman, D.J.; Norrie, J.; Caslake, M.J.; Gaw, A.; Ford, I.; Lowe, G.D.; O'Reilly, D.S.; Packard, C.J.; Sattar, N. C-reactive protein is an independent predictor of risk for the development of diabetes in the West of Scotland Coronary Prevention Study. *Diabetes* **2002**, *51*, 1596–1600. [CrossRef] [PubMed]

23. Mirza, S.; Hossain, M.; Mathews, C.; Martinez, P.; Pino, P.; Gay, J.L.; Rentfro, A.; McCormick, J.B.; Fisher-Hoch, S.P. Type 2-diabetes is associated with elevated levels of TNF-alpha, IL-6 and adiponectin and low levels of leptin in a population of Mexican Americans: A cross-sectional study. *Cytokine* **2012**, *57*, 136–142. [CrossRef] [PubMed]

24. Bertoni, A.G.; Burke, G.L.; Owusu, J.A.; Carnethon, M.R.; Vaidya, D.; Barr, R.G.; Jenny, N.S.; Ouyang, P.; Rotter, J.I. Inflammation and the incidence of type 2 diabetes: The Multi-Ethnic Study of Atherosclerosis (MESA). *Diabetes Care* **2010**, *33*, 804–810. [CrossRef] [PubMed]

25. Marques-Vidal, P.; Schmid, R.; Bochud, M.; Bastardot, F.; von Känel, R.; Paccaud, F.; Glaus, J.; Preisig, M.; Waeber, G.; Vollenweider, P. Adipocytokines, hepatic and inflammatory biomarkers and incidence of type 2 diabetes. The CoLaus study. *PLoS ONE* **2012**, *7*, e51768. [CrossRef] [PubMed]

26. Ebrahimi-Mamaeghani, M.; Mohammadi, S.; Arefhosseini, S.R.; Fallah, P.; Bazi, Z. Adiponectin as a potential biomarker of vascular disease. *Vasc. Health Risk Manag.* **2015**, *11*, 55–70. [PubMed]

27. Ouchi, N.; Kihara, S.; Arita, Y.; Okamoto, Y.; Maeda, K.; Kuriyama, H.; Hotta, K.; Nishida, M.; Takahashi, M.; Muraguchi, M.; et al. Adiponectin, an adipocyte-derived plasma protein, inhibits endothelial NF-κB signaling through a cAMP-dependent pathway. *Circulation* **2000**, *102*, 1296–1301. [CrossRef] [PubMed]

28. Ouchi, N.; Walsh, K. Adiponectin as an anti-inflammatory factor. *Clin. Chim. Acta* **2007**, *380*, 24–30. [CrossRef] [PubMed]

29. Ouchi, N.; Kihara, S.; Arita, Y.; Maeda, K.; Kuriyama, H.; Okamoto, Y.; Hotta, K.; Nishida, M.; Takahashi, M.; Nakamura, T.; et al. Novel modulator for endothelial adhesion molecules adipocyte-derived plasma protein adiponectin. *Circulation* **1999**, *100*, 2473–2476. [CrossRef] [PubMed]

30. Kobashi, C.; Urakaze, M.; Kishida, M.; Kibayashi, E.; Kobayashi, H.; Kihara, S.; Funahashi, T.; Takata, M.; Temaru, R.; Sato, A.; et al. Adiponectin inhibits endothelial synthesis of interleukin-8. *Circ. Res.* **2005**, *97*, 1245–1252. [CrossRef] [PubMed]

31. Libby, P.; Ridker, P.M.; Maseri, A. Inflammation and atherosclerosis. *Circulation* **2002**, *105*, 1135–1143. [CrossRef] [PubMed]

32. Wolf, A.M.; Wolf, D.; Rumpold, H.; Enrich, B.; Tilg, H. Adiponectin induces the anti-inflammatory cytokines IL-10 and IL-1RA in human leukocytes. *Biochem. Biophys. Res. Commun.* **2004**, *323*, 630–635. [CrossRef] [PubMed]

33. Tao, L.; Gao, E.; Jiao, X.; Yuan, Y.; Li, S.; Christopher, T.A.; Lopez, B.L.; Koch, W.; Chan, L.; Goldstein, B.J.; et al. Adiponectin cardioprotection after myocardial ischemia/reperfusion involves the reduction of oxidative/nitrative stress. *Circulation* **2007**, *115*, 1408–1416. [CrossRef] [PubMed]

34. Matsuda, M.; Shimomura, I. Roles of adiponectin and oxidative stress in obesity-associated metabolic and cardiovascular diseases. *Rev. Endocr. Metab. Disord.* **2014**, *15*, 1–10. [CrossRef] [PubMed]

35. Holland, W.L.; Miller, R.A.; Wang, Z.V.; Sun, K.; Barth, B.M.; Bui, H.H.; Davis, K.E.; Bikman, B.T.; Halberg, N.; Rutkowski, J.M.; et al. Receptor-mediated activation of ceramidase activity initiates the pleiotropic actions of adiponectin. *Nat. Med.* **2011**, *17*, 55–63. [CrossRef]

36. Rakatzi, I.; Mueller, H.; Ritzeler, O.; Tennagels, N.; Eckel, J. Adiponectin counteracts cytokine- and fatty acid-induced apoptosis in the pancreatic beta-cell line INS-1. *Diabetologia* **2004**, *47*, 249–258. [CrossRef] [PubMed]

37. Kim, J.Y.; van de Wall, E.; Laplante, M.; Azzara, A.; Trujillo, M.E.; Hofmann, S.M.; Schraw, T.; Durand, J.L.; Li, H.; Li, G.; et al. Obesity-associated improvements in metabolic profile through expansion of adipose tissue. *J. Clin. Investig.* **2007**, *117*, 2621–2637. [CrossRef] [PubMed]

38. Tao, C.; Sifuentes, A.; Holland, W.L. Regulation of glucose and lipid homeostasis by adiponectin: Effects on hepatocytes, pancreatic β cells and adipocytes. *Best Pract. Res. Clin. Endocrinol. Metab.* **2014**, *28*, 43–58. [CrossRef]

39. Yamauchi, T.; Kamon, J.; Minokoshi, Y.A.; Ito, Y.; Waki, H.; Uchida, S.; Yamashita, S.; Noda, M.; Kita, S.; Ueki, K. Adiponectin stimulates glucose utilization and fatty-acid oxidation by activating amp-activated protein kinase. *Nat. Med.* **2002**, *8*, 1288–1295. [CrossRef]

40. Fruebis, J.; Tsao, T.S.; Javorschi, S.; Ebbets-Reed, D.; Erickson, M.R.S.; Yen, F.T.; Bihain, B.E.; Lodish, H.F. Proteolytic cleavage product of 30-kDa adipocyte complement-related protein increases fatty acid oxidation in muscle and causes weight loss in mice. *Proc. Natl. Acad. Sci. USA* **2001**, *98*, 2005–2010. [CrossRef]

41. Ceddia, R.B.; Somwar, R.; Maida, A.; Fang, X.; Bikopoulos, G.; Sweeney, G. Globular adiponectin increases glut4 translocation and glucose uptake but reduces glycogen synthesis in rat skeletal muscle cells. *Diabetologia* **2005**, *48*, 132–139. [CrossRef] [PubMed]

42. Combs, T.P.; Berg, A.H.; Obici, S.; Scherer, P.E.; Rossetti, L. Endogenous glucose production is inhibited by the adipose-derived protein Acrp30. *J. Clin. InvestIG.* **2001**, *108*, 1875–1881. [CrossRef] [PubMed]

43. Yamauchi, T.; Kamon, J.; Waki, H.; Terauchi, Y.; Kubota, N.; Hara, K.; Mori, Y.; Ide, T.; Murakami, K.; Tsuboyama-Kasaoka, N. The fat-derived hormone adiponectin reverses insulin resistance associated with both lipoatrophy and obesity. *Nat. Med.* **2001**, *7*, 941–946. [CrossRef]

44. Shklyaev, S.; Aslanidi, G.; Tennant, M.; Prima, V.; Kohlbrenner, E.; Kroutov, V.; Campbell-Thompson, M.; Crawford, J.; Shek, E.W.; Scarpace, P.J.; et al. Sustained peripheral expression of transgene adiponectin offsets the development of diet-induced obesity in rats. *Proc. Natl. Acad. Sci. USA* **2003**, *100*, 14217–14222. [CrossRef] [PubMed]

45. Miller, R.A.; Chu, Q.; Le Lay, J.; Scherer, P.E.; Ahima, R.S.; Kaestner, K.H.; Foretz, M.; Viollet, B.; Birnbaum, M.J. Adiponectin suppresses gluconeogenic gene expression in mouse hepatocytes independent of LKB1-AMPK signaling. *J. Clin. Investig.* **2011**, *121*, 2518–2528. [CrossRef] [PubMed]

46. Ma, Y.; Liu, D. Hydrodynamic delivery of adiponectin and adiponectin receptor 2 gene blocks high-fat diet-induced obesity and insulin resistance. *Gene Ther.* **2013**, *20*, 846–852. [CrossRef] [PubMed]

47. Combs, T.P.; Marliss, E.B. Adiponectin signaling in the liver. *Rev. Endocr. Metab. Disord.* **2014**, *15*, 137–147. [CrossRef] [PubMed]

48. Wu, X.; Motoshima, H.; Mahadev, K.; Stalker, T.J.; Scalia, R.; Goldstein, B.J. Involvement of AMP-activated protein kinase in glucose uptake stimulated by the globular domain of adiponectin in primary rat adipocytes. *Diabetes* **2003**, *52*, 1355–1363. [CrossRef]

49. Wang, C.; Mao, X.; Wang, L.; Liu, M.; Wetzel, M.D.; Guan, K.L.; Dong, L.Q.; Liu, F. Adiponectin sensitizes insulin signaling by reducing p70 S6 kinase-mediated serine phosphorylation of IRS-1. *J. Biol. Chem.* **2007**, *282*, 7991–7996. [CrossRef]

50. Saltiel, A.R.; Pessin, J.E. Insulin signaling pathways in time and space. *Trends Cell Biol.* **2002**, *12*, 65–71. [CrossRef]

51. Danielsson, A.; Ost, A.; Lystedt, E.; Kjolhede, P.; Gustavsson, J.; Nystrom, F.H.; Strålfors, P. Insulin resistance in human adipocytes occurs downstream of IRS1 after surgical cell isolation but at the level of phosphorylation of IRS1 in type 2 diabetes. *FEBS J.* **2005**, *272*, 141–151. [CrossRef] [PubMed]

52. Kovacs, P.; Hanson, R.L.; Lee, Y.H.; Yang, X.; Kobes, S.; Permana, P.A.; Bogardus, C.; Baier, L.J. The role of insulin receptor substrate-1 gene (IRS1) in type 2 diabetes in Pima Indians. *Diabetes* **2003**, *52*, 3005–3009. [CrossRef]

53. Lindsay, R.S.; Funahashi, T.; Hanson, R.L.; Matsuzawa, Y.; Tanaka, S.; Tataranni, P.A.; Knowler, W.C.; Krakoff, J. Adiponectin and development of type 2 diabetes in the Pima Indian population. *Lancet* **2002**, *360*, 57–58. [CrossRef]

54. Thorand, B.; Zierer, A.; Baumert, J.; Meisinger, C.; Herder, C.; Koenig, W. Associations between leptin and the leptin/adiponectin ratio and incident Type 2 diabetes in middle-aged men and women: Results from the MONICA/KORA Augsburg study 1984–2002. *Diabet. Med.* **2010**, *27*, 1004–1011. [CrossRef]
55. Liu, C.; Feng, X.; Li, Q.; Wang, Y.; Li, Q.; Hua, M. Adiponectin, TNF-α and inflammatory cytokines and risk of type 2 diabetes: A systematic review and meta-analysis. *Cytokine* **2016**, *86*, 100–109. [CrossRef] [PubMed]
56. Zhang, M.; Chen, P.; Chen, S.; Sun, Q.; Zeng, Q.C.; Chen, J.Y.; Liu, Y.X.; Cao, X.H.; Ren, M.; Wang, J.K. The association of new inflammatory markers with type 2 diabetes mellitus and macrovascular complications: A preliminary study. *Eur. Rev. Med. Pharmacol. Sci.* **2014**, *18*, 1567–1572. [PubMed]
57. Wannamethee, S.G.; Lowe, G.D.; Rumley, A.; Cherry, L.; Whincup, P.H.; Sattar, N. Adipokines and risk of type 2 diabetes in older men. *Diabetes Care* **2007**, *30*, 1200–1205. [CrossRef] [PubMed]
58. Ley, S.H.; Harris, S.B.; Connelly, P.W.; Mamakeesick, M.; Gittelsohn, J.; Hegele, R.A.; Retnakaran, R.; Zinman, B.; Hanley, A.J. Adipokines and incident type 2 diabetes in an Aboriginal Canadian [corrected] population: The Sandy Lake Health and Diabetes Project. *Diabetes Care* **2008**, *31*, 1410–1415. [CrossRef] [PubMed]
59. Christou, G.A.; Kiortsis, D.N. Adiponectin and lipoprotein metabolism. *Obes. Rev.* **2013**, *14*, 939–949. [CrossRef]
60. Yamamoto, Y.; Hirose, H.; Saito, I.; Tomita, M.; Taniyama, M.; Matsubara, K.; Okazaki, Y.; Ishii, T.; Nishikai, K.; Saruta, T. Correlation of the adipocyte-derived protein adiponectin with insulin resistance index and serum high-density lipoprotein-cholesterol, independent of body mass index, in the Japanese population. *Clin. Sci.* **2002**, *103*, 137–142. [CrossRef]
61. Matsubara, M.; Maruoka, S.; Katayose, S. Decreased plasma adiponectin concentrations in women with dyslipidemia. *J. Clin. Endocrinol. Metab.* **2002**, *87*, 2764–2769. [CrossRef] [PubMed]
62. Christou, G.A.; Tellis, K.C.; Elisaf, M.C.; Tselepis, A.D.; Kiortsis, D.N. High density lipoprotein is positively correlated with the changes in circulating total adiponectin and high molecular weight adiponectin during dietary and fenofibrate treatment. *Hormones* **2012**, *11*, 178–188. [CrossRef] [PubMed]
63. Ezenwaka, C.E.; Kalloo, R.; Uhlig, M.; Eckel, J. Relationship between adiponectin and metabolic variables in Caribbean offspring of patients with type 2 diabetes mellitus. *Horm. Metab. Res.* **2004**, *36*, 238–242. [PubMed]
64. Kazumi, T.; Kawaguchi, A.; Hirano, T.; Yoshino, G. Serum adiponectin is associated with high-density lipoprotein cholesterol, triglycerides, and low-density lipoprotein particle size in young healthy men. *Metabolism* **2004**, *53*, 589–593. [CrossRef] [PubMed]
65. Shetty, G.K.; Economides, P.A.; Horton, E.S.; Mantzoros, C.S.; Veves, A. Circulating adiponectin and resistin levels in relation to metabolic factors, inflammatory markers, and vascular reactivity in diabetic patients and subjects at risk for diabetes. *Diabetes Care* **2004**, *27*, 2450–2457. [CrossRef] [PubMed]
66. Kangas-Kontio, T.; Huotari, A.; Ruotsalainen, H.; Herzig, K.H.; Tamminen, M.; Ala-Korpela, M.; Savolainen, M.J.; Kakko, S. Genetic and environmental determinants of total and high-molecular weight adiponectin in families with low HDL-cholesterol and early onset coronary heart disease. *Atherosclerosis* **2010**, *210*, 479–485. [CrossRef]
67. Shim, C.Y.; Park, S.; Kim, J.S.; Shin, D.J.; Ko, Y.G.; Kang, S.M.; Choi, D.; Ha, J.W.; Jang, Y.; Chung, N. Association of plasma retinol-binding protein 4, adiponectin, and high molecular weight adiponectin with insulin resistance in non-diabetic hypertensive patients. *Yonsei Med. J.* **2010**, *51*, 375–384. [CrossRef] [PubMed]
68. Kwon, K.; Jung, S.H.; Choi, C.; Park, S.H. Reciprocal association between visceral obesity and adiponectin: In healthy premenopausal women. *Int. J. Cardiol.* **2005**, *101*, 385–390. [CrossRef]
69. Im, J.A.; Kim, S.H.; Lee, J.W.; Shim, J.Y.; Lee, H.R.; Lee, D.C. Association between hypoadiponectinemia and cardiovascular risk factors in nonobese healthy adults. *Metabolism* **2006**, *55*, 1546–1550. [CrossRef]
70. Tomono, Y.; Hiraishi, C.; Yoshida, H. Age and sex differences in serum adiponectin and its association with lipoprotein fractions. *Ann. Clin. Biochem.* **2018**, *55*, 165–171. [CrossRef]
71. Van Linthout, S.; Foryst-Ludwig, A.; Spillmann, F.; Peng, J.; Feng, Y.; Meloni, M.; Van Craeyveld, E.; Kintscher, U.; Schultheiss, H.P.; De Geest, B.; et al. Impact of HDL on adipose tissue metabolism and adiponectin expression. *Atherosclerosis* **2010**, *210*, 438–444. [CrossRef] [PubMed]
72. Oku, H.; Matsuura, F.; Koseki, M.; Sandoval, J.C.; Yuasa-Kawase, M.; Tsubakio-Yamamoto, K.; Masuda, D.; Maeda, N.; Ohama, T.; Ishigami, M.; et al. Adiponectin deficiency suppresses ABCA1 expression and ApoA-I synthesis in the liver. *FEBS. Lett.* **2007**, *581*, 5029–5033. [CrossRef] [PubMed]

73. Matsuura, F.; Oku, H.; Koseki, M.; Sandoval, J.C.; Yuasa-Kawase, M.; Tsubakio-Yamamoto, K.; Masuda, D.; Maeda, N.; Tsujii, K.; Ishigami, M.; et al. Adiponectin accelerates reverse cholesterol transport by increasing high density lipoprotein assembly in the liver. *Biochem. Biophys. Res. Commun.* **2007**, *358*, 1091–1095. [CrossRef] [PubMed]

74. Qiao, L.; Zou, C.; van der Westhuyzen, D.R.; Shao, J. Adiponectin reduces plasma triglyceride by increasing VLDL triglyceride catabolism. *Diabetes* **2008**, *57*, 1824–1833. [CrossRef] [PubMed]

75. Tsubakio-Yamamoto, K.; Matsuura, F.; Koseki, M.; Oku, H.; Sandoval, J.C.; Inagaki, M.; Nakatani, K.; Nakaoka, H.; Kawase, R.; Yuasa-Kawase, M.; et al. Adiponectin prevents atherosclerosis by increasing cholesterol efflux from macrophages. *Biochem. Biophys. Res. Commun.* **2008**, *375*, 390–394. [CrossRef] [PubMed]

76. Kitajima, K.; Miura, S.; Yamauchi, T.; Uehara, Y.; Kiya, Y.; Rye, K.A.; Kadowaki, T.; Saku, K. Possibility of increasing cholesterol efflux by adiponectin and its receptors through the ATP binding cassette transporter A1 in HEK293T cells. *Biochem. Biophys. Res. Commun.* **2011**, *411*, 305–311. [CrossRef] [PubMed]

77. Schneider, J.G.; von Eynatten, M.; Schiekofer, S.; Nawroth, P.P.; Dugi, K.A. Low plasma adiponectin levels are associated with increased hepatic lipase activity in vivo. *Diabetes Care* **2005**, *28*, 2181–2186. [CrossRef]

78. Clarenbach, J.J.; Vega, G.L.; Adams-Huet, B.; Considine, R.V.; Ricks, M.; Sumner, A.E. Variability in postheparin hepatic lipase activity is associated with plasma adiponectin levels in African Americans. *J. Investig. Med.* **2007**, *55*, 187–194. [CrossRef]

79. Ng, T.W.; Watts, G.F.; Farvid, M.S.; Chan, D.C.; Barrett, P.H. Adipocytokines and VLDL metabolism: Independent regulatory effects of adiponectin, insulin resistance, and fat compartments on VLDL apolipoprotein B-100 kinetics? *Diabetes* **2005**, *54*, 795–802. [CrossRef]

80. Okada, T.; Saito, E.; Kuromori, Y.; Miyashita, M.; Iwata, F.; Hara, M.; Harada, K. Relationship between serum adiponectin level and lipid composition in each lipoprotein fraction in adolescent children. *Atherosclerosis* **2006**, *188*, 179–183. [CrossRef]

81. Vanhala, M.; Kumpula, L.S.; Soininen, P.; Kangas, A.J.; Ala-Korpela, M.; Kautiainen, H.; Mäntyselkä, P.; Saltevo, J. High serum adiponectin is associated with favorable lipoprotein subclass profile in 6.4-year follow-up. *Eur. J. Endocrinol.* **2011**, *164*, 549–552. [CrossRef] [PubMed]

82. Yoshida, H.; Hirowatari, Y.; Kurosawa, H.; Tada, N. Implications of decreased serum adiponectin for type IIb hyperlipidaemia and increased cholesterol levels of very-low-density lipoprotein in type II diabetic patients. *Clin. Sci.* **2005**, *109*, 297–302. [CrossRef] [PubMed]

83. Chan, D.C.; Barrett, P.H.; Ooi, E.M.; Ji, J.; Chan, D.T.; Watts, G.F. Very low density lipoprotein metabolism and plasma adiponectin as predictors of high-density lipoprotein apolipoprotein A-I kinetics in obese and nonobese men. *J. Clin. Endocrinol. Metab.* **2009**, *94*, 989–997. [CrossRef] [PubMed]

84. Lapointe, A.; Tchernof, A.; Lamarche, B.; Piché, M.E.; Weisnagel, J.; Bergeron, J.; Lemieux, S. Plasma adiponectin concentration is strongly associated with VLDL-TG catabolism in postmenopausal women. *Nutr. Metab. Cardiovasc. Dis.* **2011**, *21*, 254–260. [CrossRef] [PubMed]

85. Mead, J.R.; Irvine, S.A.; Ramji, D.P. Lipoprotein lipase: Structure, function, regulation, and role in disease. *J. Mol. Med.* **2002**, *80*, 753–769. [CrossRef] [PubMed]

86. von Eynatten, M.; Schneider, J.G.; Humpert, P.M.; Rudofsky, G.; Schmidt, N.; Barosch, P.; Hamann, A.; Morcos, M.; Kreuzer, J.; Bierhaus, A.; et al. Decreased plasma lipoprotein lipase in hypoadiponectinemia: An association independent of systemic inflammation and insulin resistance. *Diabetes Care* **2004**, *27*, 2925–2929. [CrossRef] [PubMed]

87. Kobayashi, J.; Kusunoki, M.; Murase, Y.; Kawashiri, M.; Higashikata, T.; Miwa, K.; Katsuda, S.; Takata, M.; Asano, A.; Nohara, A.; et al. Relationship of lipoprotein lipase and hepatic triacylglycerol lipase activity to serum adiponectin levels in Japanese hyperlipidemic men. *Horm. Metab. Res.* **2005**, *37*, 505–509. [CrossRef]

88. Combs, T.P.; Pajvani, U.B.; Berg, A.H.; Lin, Y.; Jelicks, L.A.; Laplante, M.; Nawrocki, A.R.; Rajala, M.W.; Parlow, A.F.; Cheeseboro, L.; et al. A transgenic mouse with a deletion in the collagenous domain of adiponectin displays elevated circulating adiponectin and improved insulin sensitivity. *Endocrinology* **2004**, *145*, 367–383. [CrossRef]

89. Tsubakio-Yamamoto, K.; Sugimoto, T.; Nishida, M.; Okano, R.; Monden, Y.; Kitazume-Taneike, R.; Yamashita, T.; Nakaoka, H.; Kawase, R.; Yuasa-Kawase, M.; et al. Serum adiponectin level is correlated with the size of HDL and LDL particles determined by high performance liquid chromatography. *Metabolism* **2012**, *61*, 1763–1770. [CrossRef]

90. Chan, D.C.; Watts, G.F.; Ng, T.W.; Uchida, Y.; Sakai, N.; Yamashita, S.; Barrett, P.H. Adiponectin and other adipocytokines as predictors of markers of triglyceride-rich lipoprotein metabolism. *Clin. Chem.* **2005**, *51*, 578–585. [CrossRef]

91. Sztalryd, C.; Kraemer, F.B. Regulation of hormone-sensitive lipase in streptozotocin-induced diabetic rats. *Metabolism* **1995**, *44*, 1391–1396. [CrossRef]

92. Pilz, S.; Horejsi, R.; Möller, R.; Almer, G.; Scharnagl, H.; Stojakovic, T.; Dimitrova, R.; Weihrauch, G.; Borkenstein, M.; Maerz, W.; et al. Early atherosclerosis in obese juveniles is associated with low serum levels of adiponectin. *J. Clin. Endocrinol. Metab.* **2005**, *90*, 4792–4796. [CrossRef] [PubMed]

93. Kantartzis, K.; Rittig, K.; Balletshofer, B.; Machann, J.; Schick, F.; Porubska, K.; Fritsche, A.; Häring, H.U.; Stefan, N. The relationships of plasma adiponectin with a favorable lipid profile, decreased inflammation, and less ectopic fat accumulation depend on adiposity. *Clin. Chem.* **2006**, *52*, 1934–1942. [CrossRef] [PubMed]

94. Staiger, H.; Kaltenbach, S.; Staiger, K.; Stefan, N.; Fritsche, A.; Guirguis, A.; Péterfi, C.; Weisser, M.; Machicao, F.; Stumvoll, M.; et al. Expression of adiponectin receptor mRNA in human skeletal muscle cells is related to in vivo parameters of glucose and lipid metabolism. *Diabetes* **2004**, *53*, 2195–2201. [CrossRef] [PubMed]

95. Eckel, R.H.; Grundy, S.M.; Zimmet, P.Z. The metabolic syndrome. *Lancet* **2005**, *365*, 1415–1428. [CrossRef]

96. Rizzo, M.; Kotur-Stevuljevic, J.; Berneis, K.; Spinas, G.; Rini, G.B.; Jelic-Ivanovic, Z.; Spasojevic-Kalimanovska, V.; Vekic, J. Atherogenic dyslipidemia and oxidative stress: A new look. *Transl. Res.* **2009**, *153*, 217–223. [CrossRef] [PubMed]

97. Nakamura, T.; Kugiyama, K. Triglycerides and remnant particles as risk factors for coronary artery disease. *Curr. Atheroscler. Rep.* **2006**, *8*, 107–110. [CrossRef]

98. Masuda, D.; Yamashita, S. Postprandial Hyperlipidemia and Remnant Lipoproteins. *J. Atheroscler. Thromb.* **2017**, *24*, 95–109. [CrossRef]

99. Ouchi, N.; Ohishi, M.; Kihara, S.; Funahashi, T.; Nakamura, T.; Nagaretani, H.; Kumada, M.; Ohashi, K.; Okamoto, Y.; Nishizawa, H.; et al. Association of hypoadiponectinemia with impaired vasoreactivity. *Hypertension* **2003**, *42*, 231–234. [CrossRef]

100. Shimabukuro, M.; Higa, N.; Asahi, T.; Oshiro, Y.; Takasu, N.; Tagawa, T.; Ueda, S.; Shimomura, I.; Funahashi, T.; Matsuzawa, Y. Hypoadiponectinemia is closely linked to endothelial dysfunction in man. *J. Clin. Endocrinol. Metab.* **2003**, *88*, 3236–3240. [CrossRef]

101. Kumada, M.; Kihara, S.; Sumitsuji, S.; Kawamoto, T.; Matsumoto, S.; Ouchi, N.; Arita, Y.; Okamoto, Y.; Shimomura, I.; Hiraoka, H.; et al. Coronary artery disease. Association of hypoadiponectinemia with coronary artery disease in men. *Arterioscler. Thromb. Vasc. Biol.* **2003**, *23*, 85–89. [CrossRef] [PubMed]

102. Matsuda, M.; Shimomura, I.; Sata, M.; Arita, Y.; Nishida, M.; Maeda, N.; Kumada, M.; Okamoto, Y.; Nagaretani, H.; Nishizawa, H.; et al. Role of adiponectin in preventing vascular stenosis. The missing link of adipo-vascular axis. *J. Biol. Chem.* **2002**, *277*, 37487–37491. [CrossRef] [PubMed]

103. Kubota, N.; Terauchi, Y.; Kubota, T.; Kumagai, H.; Itoh, S.; Satoh, H.; Yano, W.; Ogata, H.; Tokuyama, K.; Takamoto, I.; et al. Pioglitazone ameliorates insulin resistance and diabetes by both adiponectin-dependent and -independent pathways. *J. Biol. Chem.* **2006**, *281*, 8748–8755. [CrossRef] [PubMed]

104. Torigoe, M.; Matsui, H.; Ogawa, Y.; Murakami, H.; Murakami, R.; Cheng, X.W.; Numaguchi, Y.; Murohara, T.; Okumura, K. Impact of the high-molecular-weight form of adiponectin on endothelial function in healthy young men. *Clin. Endocrinol.* **2007**, *67*, 276–281. [CrossRef] [PubMed]

105. Ouedraogo, R.; Wu, X.; Xu, S.Q.; Fuchsel, L.; Motoshima, H.; Mahadev, K.; Hough, K.; Scalia, R.; Goldstein, B.J. Adiponectin suppression of high-glucose-induced reactive oxygen species in vascular endothelial cells: Evidence for involvement of a cAMP signaling pathway. *Diabetes* **2006**, *55*, 1840–1846. [CrossRef] [PubMed]

106. Miyatani, Y.; Yasui, T.; Uemura, H.; Yamada, M.; Matsuzaki, T.; Kuwahara, A.; Tsuchiya, N.; Yuzurihara, M.; Kase, Y.; Irahara, M. Associations of circulating adiponectin with estradiol and monocyte chemotactic protein-1 in postmenopausal women. *Menopause* **2008**, *15*, 536–541. [CrossRef] [PubMed]

107. Xiao, X.; Dong, Y.; Zhong, J.; Cao, R.; Zhao, X.; Wen, G.; Liu, J. Adiponectin protects endothelial cells from the damages induced by the intermittent high level of glucose. *Endocrine* **2011**, *40*, 386–393. [CrossRef]

108. Kajikawa, M.; Maruhashi, T.; Matsumoto, T.; Iwamoto, Y.; Iwamoto, A.; Oda, N.; Kishimoto, S.; Matsui, S.; Aibara, Y.; Hidaka, T.; et al. Relationship between serum triglyceride levels and endothelial function in a large community-based study. *Atherosclerosis* **2016**, *249*, 70–75. [CrossRef]

109. Jamwal, S.; Sharma, S. Vascular endothelium dysfunction: A conservative target in metabolic disorders. *Inflamm. Res.* **2018**, *67*, 391–405. [CrossRef]

110. Shi, Y.; Vanhoutte, P.M. Macro- and microvascular endothelial dysfunction in diabetes. *J. Diabetes.* **2017**, *9*, 434–449. [CrossRef]

111. Wang, Y.; Lam, K.S.; Xu, J.Y.; Lu, G.; Xu, L.Y.; Cooper, G.J.; Xu, A. Adiponectin inhibits cell proliferation by interacting with several growth factors in an oligomerization-dependent manner. *J. Biol. Chem.* **2005**, *280*, 18341–18347. [CrossRef] [PubMed]

112. Arita, Y.; Kihara, S.; Ouchi, N.; Maeda, K.; Kuriyama, H.; Okamoto, Y.; Kumada, M.; Hotta, K.; Nishida, M.; Takahashi, M.; et al. Adipocyte-derived plasma protein adiponectin acts as a platelet-derived growth factor-BB-binding protein and regulates growth factor-induced common postreceptor signal in vascular smooth muscle cell. *Circulation* **2002**, *105*, 2893–2898. [CrossRef] [PubMed]

113. Marsche, G.; Zelzer, S.; Meinitzer, A.; Kern, S.; Meissl, S.; Pregartner, G.; Weghuber, D.; Almer, G.; Mangge, H. Adiponectin Predicts High-Density Lipoprotein Cholesterol Efflux Capacity in Adults Irrespective of Body Mass Index and Fat Distribution. *J. Clin. Endocrinol. Metab.* **2017**, *102*, 4117–4123. [CrossRef] [PubMed]

114. Wang, M.; Wang, D.; Zhang, Y.; Wang, X.; Liu, Y.; Xia, M. Adiponectin increases macrophages cholesterol efflux and suppresses foam cell formation in patients with type 2 diabetes mellitus. *Atherosclerosis* **2013**, *229*, 62–70. [CrossRef] [PubMed]

115. Kubota, M.; Nakanishi, S.; Hirano, M.; Maeda, S.; Yoneda, M.; Awaya, T.; Yamane, K.; Kohno, N. Relationship between serum cholesterol efflux capacity and glucose intolerance in Japanese-Americans. *J. Atheroscler. Thromb.* **2014**, *21*, 1087–1097. [CrossRef] [PubMed]

116. Yassine, H.N.; Belopolskaya, A.; Schall, C.; Stump, C.S.; Lau, S.S.; Reaven, P.D. Enhanced cholesterol efflux to HDL through the ABCA1 transporter in hypertriglyceridemia of type 2 diabetes. *Metabolism* **2014**, *63*, 727–734. [CrossRef] [PubMed]

117. de Vries, R.; Groen, A.K.; Perton, F.G.; Dallinga-Thie, G.M.; van Wijland, M.J.; Dikkeschei, L.D.; Wolffenbuttel, B.H.; van Tol, A.; Dullaart, R.P. Increased cholesterol efflux from cultured fibroblasts to plasma from hypertriglyceridemic type 2 diabetic patients: Roles of pre beta-HDL, phospholipid transfer protein and cholesterol esterification. *Atherosclerosis* **2008**, *196*, 733–741. [CrossRef]

118. Fournier, N.; Francone, O.; Rothblat, G.; Goudouneche, D.; Cambillau, M.; Kellner-Weibel, G.; Robinet, P.; Royer, L.; Moatti, N.; Simon, A.; et al. Enhanced efflux of cholesterol from ABCA1-expressing macrophages to serum from type IV hypertriglyceridemic subjects. *Atherosclerosis* **2003**, *171*, 287–293. [CrossRef]

119. Khosravi-Largani, M.; Nojomi, M.; Aghili, R.; Otaghvar, H.A.; Tanha, K.; Seyedi, S.H.S.; Mottaghi, A. Evaluation of all Types of Metabolic Bariatric Surgery and its Consequences: A Systematic Review and Meta-Analysis. *Obes. Surg.* **2018**. [CrossRef]

120. De Vincentis, A.; Pedone, C.; Vespasiani-Gentilucci, U.; Picardi, A.; Derosa, G.; Maffioli, P.; Sahebkar, A. Effect of Sibutramine on Plasma C-Reactive Protein, Leptin and Adiponectin Concentrations: A Systematic Review and Meta-Analysis of Randomized Controlled Trials. *Curr. Pharm. Des.* **2017**, *23*, 870–878. [CrossRef]

121. Salehi-Abargouei, A.; Izadi, V.; Azadbakht, L. The effect of low calorie diet on adiponectin concentration: A systematic review and meta-analysis. *Horm. Metab. Res.* **2015**, *47*, 549–555. [CrossRef] [PubMed]

122. Yoshida, H.; Ishikawa, T.; Suto, M.; Kurosawa, H.; Hirowatari, Y.; Ito, K.; Yanai, H.; Tada, N.; Suzuki, M. Effects of supervised aerobic exercise training on serum adiponectin and parameters of lipid and glucose metabolism in subjects with moderate dyslipidemia. *J. Atheroscler. Thromb.* **2010**, *17*, 1160–1166. [CrossRef] [PubMed]

123. Dinca, M.; Serban, M.C.; Sahebkar, A.; Mikhailidis, D.P.; Toth, P.P.; Martin, S.S.; Blaha, M.J.; Blüher, M.; Gurban, C.; Penson, P.; et al. Does vitamin D supplementation alter plasma adipokines concentrations? A systematic review and meta-analysis of randomized controlled trials. *Pharmacol. Res.* **2016**, *107*, 360–371. [CrossRef] [PubMed]

124. Sirico, F.; Bianco, A.; D'Alicandro, G.; Castaldo, C.; Montagnani, S.; Spera, R.; Di Meglio, F.; Nurzynska, D. Effects of Physical Exercise on Adiponectin, Leptin, and Inflammatory Markers in Childhood Obesity: Systematic Review and Meta-Analysis. *Child. Obes.* **2018**, *14*, 207–217. [CrossRef] [PubMed]

125. Yu, N.; Ruan, Y.; Gao, X.; Sun, J. Systematic Review and Meta-Analysis of Randomized, Controlled Trials on the Effect of Exercise on Serum Leptin and Adiponectin in Overweight and Obese Individuals. *Horm. Metab. Res.* **2017**, *49*, 164–173. [CrossRef] [PubMed]

126. García-Hermoso, A.; Ceballos-Ceballos, R.J.; Poblete-Aro, C.E.; Hackney, A.C.; Mota, J.; Ramírez-Vélez, R. Exercise, adipokines and pediatric obesity: A meta-analysis of randomized controlled trials. *Int. J. Obes.* **2017**, *41*, 475–482. [CrossRef] [PubMed]

127. García-Hermoso, A.; Ramírez-Vélez, R.; Ramírez-Campillo, R.; Peterson, M.D.; Martínez-Vizcaíno, V. Concurrent aerobic plus resistance exercise versus aerobic exercise alone to improve health outcomes in paediatric obesity: A systematic review and meta-analysis. *Br. J. Sports Med.* **2018**, *52*, 161–166. [CrossRef] [PubMed]

128. Mousa, A.; Naderpoor, N.; Teede, H.; Scragg, R.; de Courten, B. Vitamin D supplementation for improvement of chronic low-grade inflammation in patients with type 2 diabetes: A systematic review and meta-analysis of randomized controlled trials. *Nutr. Rev.* **2018**, *76*, 380–394. [CrossRef]

129. Suksomboon, N.; Poolsup, N.; Darli Ko Ko, H. Effect of vitamin K supplementation on insulin sensitivity: A meta-analysis. *Diabetes Metab. Syndr. Obes.* **2017**, *10*, 169–177. [CrossRef]

130. Öztürk, E.; Arslan, A.K.K.; Yerer, M.B.; Bishayee, A. Resveratrol and diabetes: A critical review of clinical studies. *Biomed. Pharmacother.* **2017**, *95*, 230–234. [CrossRef]

131. Mohammadi-Sartang, M.; Mazloom, Z.; Sohrabi, Z.; Sherafatmanesh, S.; Barati-Boldaji, R. Resveratrol supplementation and plasma adipokines concentrations? A systematic review and meta-analysis of randomized controlled trials. *Pharmacol. Res.* **2017**, *117*, 394–405. [CrossRef] [PubMed]

132. Kishimoto, Y.; Yoshida, H.; Kondo, K. Potential Anti-Atherosclerotic Properties of Astaxanthin. *Mar. Drugs* **2016**, *14*, 35. [CrossRef] [PubMed]

133. Yoshida, H.; Yanai, H.; Ito, K.; Tomono, Y.; Koikeda, T.; Tsukahara, H.; Tada, N. Administration of natural astaxanthin increases serum HDL-cholesterol and adiponectin in subjects with mild hyperlipidemia. *Atherosclerosis* **2010**, *209*, 520–523. [CrossRef] [PubMed]

134. Canas, J.A.; Lochrie, A.; McGowan, A.G.; Hossain, J.; Schettino, C.; Balagopal, P.B. Effects of Mixed Carotenoids on Adipokines and Abdominal Adiposity in Children: A Pilot Study. *J. Clin. Endocrinol. Metab.* **2017**, *102*, 1983–1990. [CrossRef] [PubMed]

135. Li, Y.F.; Chang, Y.Y.; Huang, H.C.; Wu, Y.C.; Yang, M.D.; Chao, P.M. Tomato juice supplementation in young women reduces inflammatory adipokine levels independently of body fat reduction. *Nutrition* **2015**, *31*, 691–696. [CrossRef] [PubMed]

136. Llanos, A.A.; Peng, J.; Pennell, M.L.; Krok, J.L.; Vitolins, M.Z.; Degraffinreid, C.R.; Paskett, E.D. Effects of tomato and soy on serum adipokine concentrations in postmenopausal women at increased breast cancer risk: A cross-over dietary intervention trial. *J. Clin. Endocrinol. Metab.* **2014**, *99*, 625–632. [CrossRef] [PubMed]

137. Ben Amara, N.; Tourniaire, F.; Maraninchi, M.; Attia, N.; Amiot-Carlin, M.J.; Raccah, D.; Valéro, R.; Landrier, J.F.; Darmon, P. Independent positive association of plasma β-carotene concentrations with adiponectin among non-diabetic obese subjects. *Eur. J. Nutr.* **2015**, *54*, 447–454. [CrossRef] [PubMed]

138. Suzuki, K.; Inoue, T.; Hashimoto, S.; Ochiai, J.; Kusuhara, Y.; Ito, Y.; Hamajima, N. Association of serum carotenoids with high molecular weight adiponectin and inflammation markers among Japanese subjects. *Clin. Chim. Acta* **2010**, *411*, 1330–1334. [CrossRef]

139. Iwamoto, M.; Imai, K.; Ohta, H.; Shirouchi, B.; Sato, M. Supplementation of highly concentrated β-cryptoxanthin in a satsuma mandarin beverage improves adipocytokine profiles in obese Japanese women. *Lipids Health Dis.* **2012**, *11*, 52. [CrossRef]

140. Vincent, H.K.; Bourguignon, C.M.; Weltman, A.L.; Vincent, K.R.; Barrett, E.; Innes, K.E.; Taylor, A.G. Effects of antioxidant supplementation on insulin sensitivity, endothelial adhesion molecules, and oxidative stress in normal-weight and overweight young adults. *Metabolism* **2009**, *58*, 254–262. [CrossRef]

141. Vincent, H.K.; Bourguignon, C.M.; Vincent, K.R.; Weltman, A.L.; Bryant, M.; Taylor, A.G. Antioxidant supplementation lowers exercise-induced oxidative stress in young overweight adults. *Obesity* **2006**, *14*, 2224–2235. [CrossRef] [PubMed]

142. Wu, J.H.; Cahill, L.E.; Mozaffarian, D. Effect of fish oil on circulating adiponectin: A systematic review and meta-analysis of randomized controlled trials. *J. Clin. Endocrinol. Metab.* **2013**, *98*, 2451–2459. [CrossRef] [PubMed]

143. Becic, T.; Studenik, C. Effects of Omega-3 Supplementation on Adipocytokines in Prediabetes and Type 2 Diabetes Mellitus: Systematic Review and Meta-Analysis of Randomized Controlled Trials. *Diabetes Metab. J.* **2018**, *42*, 101–116. [CrossRef] [PubMed]

144. Yang, K.; Zeng, L.; Bao, T.; Ge, J. Effectiveness of Omega-3 fatty acid for polycystic ovary syndrome: A systematic review and meta-analysis. *Reprod. Biol. Endocrinol.* **2018**, *16*, 27. [CrossRef] [PubMed]

145. Bahreini, M.; Ramezani, A.H.; Shishehbor, F.; Mansoori, A. The Effect of Omega-3 on Circulating Adiponectin in Adults with Type 2 Diabetes Mellitus: A Systematic Review and Meta-Analysis of Randomized Controlled Trials. *Can. J. Diabetes* **2018**, *42*, 553–559. [CrossRef] [PubMed]

146. Farimani, A.R.; Hariri, M.; Azimi-Nezhad, M.; Borji, A.; Zarei, S.; Hooshmand, E. The effect of n-3 PUFAs on circulating adiponectin and leptin in patients with type 2 diabetes mellitus: A systematic review and meta-analysis of randomized controlled trials. *Acta Diabetol.* **2018**, *55*, 641–652. [CrossRef]

147. Polyzos, S.A.; Mantzoros, C.S. Adiponectin as a target for the treatment of nonalcoholic steatohepatitis with thiazolidinediones: A systematic review. *Metabolism* **2016**, *65*, 1297–1306. [CrossRef]

148. Yanai, H.; Adachi, H. The Low-Dose (7.5 mg/day) Pioglitazone Therapy. *J. Clin. Med. Res.* **2017**, *9*, 821–825. [CrossRef]

149. Lutchman, G.; Modi, A.; Kleiner, D.E.; Promrat, K.; Heller, T.; Ghany, M.; Borg, B.; Loomba, R.; Liang, T.J.; Premkumar, A.; et al. The effects of discontinuing pioglitazone in patients with nonalcoholic steatohepatitis. *Hepatology* **2007**, *46*, 424–429. [CrossRef]

150. Kong, W.; Niu, X.; Zeng, T.; Lu, M.; Chen, L. Impact of Treatment with Metformin on Adipocytokines in Patients with Polycystic Ovary Syndrome: A Meta-Analysis. *PLoS ONE* **2015**, *10*, e0140565. [CrossRef]

151. Su, J.R.; Lu, Z.H.; Su, Y.; Zhao, N.; Dong, C.L.; Sun, L.; Zhao, S.F.; Li, Y. Relationship of Serum Adiponectin Levels and Metformin Therapy in Patients with Type 2 Diabetes. *Horm. Metab. Res.* **2016**, *48*, 92–98. [CrossRef] [PubMed]

152. Shimabukuro, M.; Higa, M.; Yamakawa, K.; Masuzaki, H.; Sata, M. Miglitol, α-glycosidase inhibitor, reduces visceral fat accumulation and cardiovascular risk factors in subjects with the metabolic syndrome: A randomized comparable study. *Int. J. Cardiol.* **2013**, *167*, 2108–2113. [CrossRef] [PubMed]

153. Yokoyama, H.; Kannno, S.; Ishimura, I.; Node, K. Miglitol increases the adiponectin level and decreases urinary albumin excretion in patients with type 2 diabetes mellitus. *Metabolism* **2007**, *56*, 1458–1463. [CrossRef] [PubMed]

154. Wang, J.S.; Lin, S.D.; Lee, W.J.; Su, S.L.; Lee, I.T.; Tu, S.T.; Tseng, Y.H.; Lin, S.Y.; Sheu, W.H. Effects of acarbose versus glibenclamide on glycemic excursion and oxidative stress in type 2 diabetic patients inadequately controlled by metformin: A 24-week, randomized, open-label, parallel-group comparison. *Clin. Ther.* **2011**, *33*, 1932–1942. [CrossRef] [PubMed]

155. Shimazu, T.; Inami, N.; Satoh, D.; Kajiura, T.; Yamada, K.; Iwasaka, T.; Nomura, S. Effect of acarbose on platelet-derived microparticles, soluble selectins, and adiponectin in diabetic patients. *J. Thromb. Thrombolysis* **2009**, *28*, 429–435. [CrossRef] [PubMed]

156. Ochiai, H.; Ooka, H.; Shida, C.; Ishikawa, T.; Inoue, D.; Okazaki, R. Acarbose treatment increases serum total adiponectin levels in patients with type 2 diabetes. *Endocr. J.* **2008**, *55*, 549–556. [CrossRef] [PubMed]

157. Liu, X.; Men, P.; Wang, Y.; Zhai, S.; Liu, G. Impact of dipeptidyl peptidase-4 inhibitors on serum adiponectin: A meta-analysis. *Lipids Health Dis.* **2016**, *15*, 204. [CrossRef]

158. Frøssing, S.; Nylander, M.; Chabanova, E.; Frystyk, J.; Holst, J.J.; Kistorp, C.; Skouby, S.O.; Faber, J. Effect of liraglutide on ectopic fat in polycystic ovary syndrome: A randomized clinical trial. *Diabetes Obes. Metab.* **2018**, *20*, 215–218. [CrossRef]

159. Armstrong, M.J.; Hull, D.; Guo, K.; Barton, D.; Hazlehurst, J.M.; Gathercole, L.L.; Nasiri, M.; Yu, J.; Gough, S.C.; Newsome, P.N.; et al. Glucagon-like peptide 1 decreases lipotoxicity in non-alcoholic steatohepatitis. *J. Hepatol.* **2016**, *64*, 399–408. [CrossRef]

160. Hogan, A.E.; Gaoatswe, G.; Lynch, L.; Corrigan, M.A.; Woods, C.; O'Connell, J.; O'Shea, D. Glucagon-like peptide 1 analogue therapy directly modulates innate immune-mediated inflammation in individuals with type 2 diabetes mellitus. *Diabetologia* **2014**, *57*, 781–784. [CrossRef]

161. Suzuki, D.; Toyoda, M.; Kimura, M.; Miyauchi, M.; Yamamoto, N.; Sato, H.; Tanaka, E.; Kuriyama, Y.; Miyatake, H.; Abe, M.; et al. Effects of liraglutide, a human glucagon-like peptide-1 analogue, on body weight, body fat area and body fat-related markers in patients with type 2 diabetes mellitus. *Intern. Med.* **2013**, *52*, 1029–1034. [CrossRef] [PubMed]

162. Yanai, H.; Hamasaki, H.; Adachi, H.; Moriyama, S.; Hirowatari, Y. Effects of Liraglutide, a Human Glucagon-Like Peptide-1 Analog, on Glucose/Lipid Metabolism, and Adipocytokines in Patients With Type 2 Diabetes. *J. Endocrinol. Metab.* **2011**, *1*, 149–151. [CrossRef]

163. Shi, L.; Zhu, J.; Yang, P.; Tang, X.; Yu, W.; Pan, C.; Shen, M.; Zhu, D.; Cheng, J.; Ye, X. Comparison of exenatide and acarbose on intra-abdominal fat content in patients with obesity and type-2 diabetes: A randomized controlled trial. *Obes. Res. Clin. Pract.* **2017**, *11*, 607–615. [CrossRef] [PubMed]

164. Lin, C.H.; Hsieh, S.H.; Sun, J.H.; Tsai, J.S.; Huang, Y.Y. Glucose Variability and β- Cell Response by GLP-1 Analogue added-on CSII for Patients with Poorly Controlled Type 2 Diabetes. *Sci. Rep.* **2015**, *5*, 16968. [CrossRef] [PubMed]

165. Yanai, H.; Katsuyama, H.; Hamasaki, H.; Adachi, H.; Moriyama, S.; Yoshikawa, R.; Sako, A. Sodium-Glucose Cotransporter 2 Inhibitors: Possible Anti-Atherosclerotic Effects Beyond Glucose Lowering. *J. Clin. Med. Res.* **2016**, *8*, 10–14. [CrossRef] [PubMed]

166. Nomiyama, T.; Shimono, D.; Horikawa, T.; Fujimura, Y.; Ohsako, T.; Terawaki, Y.; Fukuda, T.; Motonaga, R.; Tanabe, M.; Yanase, T. Efficacy and safety of sodium-glucose cotransporter 2 inhibitor ipragliflozin on glycemic control and cardiovascular parameters in Japanese patients with type 2 diabetes mellitus; Fukuoka Study of Ipragliflozin (FUSION). *Endocr. J.* **2018**, *65*, 859–867. [CrossRef] [PubMed]

167. Sugiyama, S.; Jinnouchi, H.; Kurinami, N.; Hieshima, K.; Yoshida, A.; Jinnouchi, K.; Nishimura, H.; Suzuki, T.; Miyamoto, F.; Kajiwara, K.; et al. The SGLT2 Inhibitor Dapagliflozin Significantly Improves the Peripheral Microvascular Endothelial Function in Patients with Uncontrolled Type 2 Diabetes Mellitus. *Intern. Med.* **2018**, *57*, 2147–2156. [CrossRef]

168. Garvey, W.T.; Van Gaal, L.; Leiter, L.A.; Vijapurkar, U.; List, J.; Cuddihy, R.; Ren, J.; Davies, M.J. Effects of canagliflozin versus glimepiride on adipokines and inflammatory biomarkers in type 2 diabetes. *Metabolism* **2018**, *85*, 32–37. [CrossRef]

169. Tobita, H.; Sato, S.; Miyake, T.; Ishihara, S.; Kinoshita, Y. Effects of Dapagliflozin on Body Composition and Liver Tests in Patients with Nonalcoholic Steatohepatitis Associated with Type 2 Diabetes Mellitus: A Prospective, Open-label, Uncontrolled Study. *Curr. Ther. Res. Clin. Exp.* **2017**, *87*, 13–19. [CrossRef]

170. Hayashi, T.; Fukui, T.; Nakanishi, N.; Yamamoto, S.; Tomoyasu, M.; Osamura, A.; Ohara, M.; Yamamoto, T.; Ito, Y.; Hirano, T. Dapagliflozin decreases small dense low-density lipoprotein-cholesterol and increases high-density lipoprotein 2-cholesterol in patients with type 2 diabetes: Comparison with sitagliptin. *Cardiovasc. Diabetol.* **2017**, *16*, 8. [CrossRef]

171. Ishihara, H.; Yamaguchi, S.; Nakao, I.; Okitsu, A.; Asahina, S. Efficacy and safety of ipragliflozin as add-on therapy to insulin in Japanese patients with type 2 diabetes mellitus (IOLITE): A multi-centre, randomized, placebo-controlled, double-blind study. *Diabetes Obes. Metab.* **2016**, *18*, 1207–1216. [CrossRef] [PubMed]

172. Okamoto, A.; Yokokawa, H.; Sanada, H.; Naito, T. Changes in Levels of Biomarkers Associated with Adipocyte Function and Insulin and Glucagon Kinetics during Treatment with Dapagliflozin among Obese Type 2 Diabetes Mellitus Patients. *Drugs R D* **2016**, *16*, 255–261. [CrossRef] [PubMed]

173. Nomoto, H.; Miyoshi, H.; Furumoto, T.; Oba, K.; Tsutsui, H.; Inoue, A.; Atsumi, T.; Manda, N.; Kurihara, Y.; Aoki, S. A Randomized Controlled Trial Comparing the Effects of Sitagliptin and Glimepiride on Endothelial Function and Metabolic Parameters: Sapporo Athero-Incretin Study 1 (SAIS1). *PLoS ONE* **2016**, *11*, e0164255. [CrossRef] [PubMed]

174. Ohira, M.; Yamaguchi, T.; Saiki, A.; Ban, N.; Kawana, H.; Nagumo, A.; Murano, T.; Shirai, K.; Tatsuno, I. Pioglitazone improves the cardio-ankle vascular index in patients with type 2 diabetes mellitus treated with metformin. *Diabetes Metab. Syndr. Obes.* **2014**, *7*, 313–319. [CrossRef] [PubMed]

175. Sam, S.; Haffner, S.; Davidson, M.H.; D'Agostino, R., Sr.; Perez, A.; Mazzone, T. Pioglitazone-mediated changes in lipoprotein particle composition are predicted by changes in adiponectin level in type 2 diabetes. *J. Clin. Endocrinol. Metab.* **2012**, *97*, E110–E114. [CrossRef] [PubMed]

176. Pfützner, A.; Schöndorf, T.; Tschöpe, D.; Lobmann, R.; Merke, J.; Müller, J.; Lehmann, U.; Fuchs, W.; Forst, T. PIOfix-study: Effects of pioglitazone/metformin fixed combination in comparison with a combination of metformin with glimepiride on diabetic dyslipidemia. *Diabetes Technol. Ther.* **2011**, *13*, 637–643. [CrossRef] [PubMed]

177. Derosa, G.; Maffioli, P.; Ferrari, I.; Mereu, R.; Ragonesi, P.D.; Querci, F.; Franzetti, I.G.; Gadaleta, G.; Ciccarelli, L.; Piccinni, M.N.; et al. Effects of one year treatment of vildagliptin added to pioglitazone or glimepiride in poorly controlled type 2 diabetic patients. *Horm. Metab. Res.* **2010**, *42*, 663–669. [CrossRef] [PubMed]

178. Forst, T.; Weber, M.M.; Löbig, M.; Lehmann, U.; Müller, J.; Hohberg, C.; Friedrich, C.; Fuchs, W.; Pfützner, A. Pioglitazone in addition to metformin improves erythrocyte deformability in patients with Type 2 diabetes mellitus. *Clin. Sci.* **2010**, *119*, 345–351. [CrossRef] [PubMed]

179. Li, C.J.; Zhang, J.Y.; Yu, D.M.; Zhang, Q.M. Adding glimepiride to current insulin therapy increases high-molecular weight adiponectin levels to improve glycemic control in poorly controlled type 2 diabetes. *Diabetol. Metab. Syndr.* **2014**, *6*, 41. [CrossRef] [PubMed]

180. Chen, W.; Huang, Z.; Bi, M.; Xu, X.; Zhao, N. Effects of simvastatin on serum adiponectin: A meta-analysis of randomized controlled trials. *Lipids Health Dis.* **2017**, *16*, 53. [CrossRef]

181. Chruściel, P.; Sahebkar, A.; Rembek-Wieliczko, M.; Serban, M.C.; Ursoniu, S.; Mikhailidis, D.P.; Jones, S.R.; Mosteoru, S.; Blaha, M.J.; Martin, S.S.; et al. Impact of statin therapy on plasma adiponectin concentrations: A systematic review and meta-analysis of 43 randomized controlled trial arms. *Atherosclerosis* **2016**, *253*, 194–208. [CrossRef] [PubMed]

182. Dolezelova, E.; Stein, E.; Derosa, G.; Maffioli, P.; Nachtigal, P.; Sahebkar, A. Effect of ezetimibe on plasma adipokines: A systematic review and meta-analysis. *Br. J. Clin. Pharmacol.* **2017**, *83*, 1380–1396. [CrossRef] [PubMed]

183. Sahebkar, A.; Watts, G.F. Fibrate therapy and circulating adiponectin concentrations: A systematic review and meta-analysis of randomized placebo-controlled trials. *Atherosclerosis* **2013**, *230*, 110–120. [CrossRef] [PubMed]

184. Sahebkar, A. Head-to-head comparison of fibrates versus statins for elevation of circulating adiponectin concentrations: A systematic review and meta-analysis. *Metabolism* **2013**, *62*, 1876–1885. [CrossRef] [PubMed]

185. Takagi, H.; Niwa, M.; Mizuno, Y.; Goto, S.N.; Umemoto, T. Telmisartan as a metabolic sartan: The first meta-analysis of randomized controlled trials in metabolic syndrome. *J. Am. Soc. Hypertens.* **2013**, *7*, 229–235. [CrossRef]

186. Takagi, H.; Umemoto, T. Telmisartan increases adiponectin levels: A meta-analysis and meta-regression of randomized head-to-head trials. *Int. J. Cardiol.* **2012**, *155*, 448–451. [CrossRef]

187. Suksomboon, N.; Poolsup, N.; Prasit, T. Systematic review of the effect of telmisartan on insulin sensitivity in hypertensive patients with insulin resistance or diabetes. *Clin. Pharm. Ther.* **2012**, *37*, 319–327. [CrossRef]

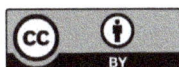

International Journal of
Molecular Sciences

MDPI

Review

Mechanisms of Adiponectin Action: Implication of Adiponectin Receptor Agonism in Diabetic Kidney Disease

Yaeni Kim [1] and Cheol Whee Park [1,2,*]

[1] Division of Nephrology, Department of Internal Medicine, College of Medicine, The Catholic University of Korea, 222, Banpo-daero, Seocho-gu, Seoul 06591, Korea; yaenikim82@gmail.com
[2] Institute for Aging and Metabolic Diseases, College of Medicine, The Catholic University of Korea, Seoul 06591, Korea
*   Correspondence: cheolwhee@hanmail.net; Tel.: +82-2-2258-6038; Fax: +82-2-599-3589

Received: 26 February 2019; Accepted: 8 April 2019; Published: 10 April 2019

Abstract: Adiponectin, an adipokine secreted by adipocytes, exerts favorable effects in the milieu of diabetes and metabolic syndrome through its anti-inflammatory, antifibrotic, and antioxidant effects. It mediates fatty acid metabolism by inducing AMP-activated protein kinase (AMPK) phosphorylation and increasing peroxisome proliferative-activated receptor (PPAR)-α expression through adiponectin receptor (AdipoR)1 and AdipoR2, respectively, which in turn activate PPAR gamma coactivator 1 alpha (PGC-1α), increase the phosphorylation of acyl CoA oxidase, and upregulate the uncoupling proteins involved in energy consumption. Moreover, adiponectin potently stimulates ceramidase activity associated with its two receptors and enhances ceramide catabolism and the formation of its anti-apoptotic metabolite, sphingosine 1 phosphate (S1P), independently of AMPK. Low circulating adiponectin levels in obese patients with a risk of insulin resistance, type 2 diabetes, and cardiovascular diseases, and increased adiponectin expression in the state of albuminuria suggest a protective and compensatory role for adiponectin in mitigating further renal injury during the development of overt diabetic kidney disease (DKD). We propose AdipoRon, an orally active synthetic adiponectin receptor agonist as a promising drug for restoration of DKD without inducing systemic adverse effects. Its renoprotective role against lipotoxicity and oxidative stress by enhancing the AMPK/PPARα pathway and ceramidase activity through AdipoRs is revealed here.

Keywords: adiponectin; metabolism; AdipoRon; lipotoxicity

1. Introduction

With the advent of modern conveniences promoting increased dietary ingestion and a sedentary lifestyle, it is inevitable that a higher proportion of the population is exposed to a state of energy excess that contributes to the exponential growth of diabetes and obesity-related diseases [1]. White adipose tissue stores energy in the form of triglycerides during nutritional affluence, but as its storage capacity becomes saturated, excess fat is redirected to non-adipose tissues, entering alternative non-oxidative pathways and promoting the organ-specific production of toxic lipid metabolites [2].

Derangements in lipid metabolism play a crucial role in the development and progression of diabetic kidney disease (DKD). The accumulation of free fatty acids, which are otherwise used as an energy source, in glomerular and tubular epithelial cells of diabetic kidneys indicates a state of energy surplus. This altered energy balance leads to lipotoxicity in the kidney, which is characterized by the deposition of fatty acid metabolites such as triglycerides, diacylglycerols, and ceramides, leading to intrarenal toxicity and cell death [3].

The role of adipose tissue or adipocytes as an endocrine organ secreting various adipokines, in particular adiponectin, has come to the forefront in the fight against diabetes and metabolic syndrome because it has been demonstrated to exert pro-metabolic effects through the modulation of glucose and lipid homeostasis both directly, in an organ-specific manner, and indirectly, by systemic amelioration of insulin sensitivity [4]. Indeed, the increased circulating adiponectin levels in patients with end-stage renal disease [5] and the increased expression of adiponectin receptors that positively correlates with serum and urinary adiponectin levels in rats with chronic renal failure [6] indicate that there might be an intriguing link between adiponectin and the kidney in the setting of renal injury. In this review, we deal with the molecular signaling pathways involved in adiponectin and its receptor binding, placing an emphasis on the recent progress in research on the role of the adiponectin receptor agonist, AdipoRon, in DKD.

2. Adiponectin in Renal Physiology: Its Association with Albuminuria and Glomerular Filtration Rate

Adiponectin circulates in a combination of three forms: (1) low-molecular-weight trimers that oligomerize to form (2) middle-molecular-weight hexamers that in turn agglomerate to form (3) high-order structures of oligomers of up to 800 kDa that potentiate the strongest insulin-sensitizing activity in hepatocytes [7]. Circulating adiponectin is primarily eliminated by the liver, and secondarily by the kidneys [8]. Since adiponectin monomers (28 kDa) and dimers are small enough to cross the glomerular filtration barrier, they can be detected in the urine of healthy individuals [9], whereas high-molecular-weight adiponectin has been reported to be excreted to a considerable extent in the urine of albuminuric and proteinuric patients, possibly as a result of leakage through a dysfunctional glomerular filtration barrier [10].

The association between plasma adiponectin concentration and urinary adiponectin excretion rate in proteinuric patients with or without diabetes is unclear. In those with low-grade microalbuminuria, a study involving subjects mainly of obese and metabolic syndrome backgrounds with a preserved glomerular filtration rate (GFR) found that urinary adiponectin and albumin excretion rates were negatively correlated with the plasma adiponectin level [11–13]. In contrast, a study population consisting of diabetics with reduced GFR and macroalbuminuria demonstrated a positive relationship between circulating adiponectin levels and urinary adiponectin and albumin excretion rates [5,14]. In a subpopulation analysis, an inverse relationship between the serum adiponectin level and urinary protein excretion rate in patients with type 2 diabetes with preserved GFR was attributed to the decrease in serum adiponectin associated with increased insulin resistance [15], whereas an increase in serum adiponectin levels has been established in patients with type 1 diabetes [16]. This increase in urinary or serum adiponectin concentration is not in its receptor-bound form and thus it is not metabolically active. Markedly increased adiponectin has been consistently reported in patients with both chronic kidney disease (CKD) and end-stage renal disease (ESRD), and this upregulation of circulating adiponectin has been deemed a compensatory mechanism to relieve further renal injury and subsequent unbound form adiponectin in excess may have been filtered through loosened and defective glomerular filtration barrier and excreted in the urine [17,18].

Several contradictory observations have been reported in the literature to date. It is hard to interpret the adiponectin-albuminuria association in the setting of DKD since impaired GFR frequently coexists that tends to increase circulating adiponectin level, and its impact cannot be investigated separately from the presence of albuminuria. Moreover, the effect of antidiabetic regimen that patients might have been following could also influence circulating adiponectin levels, further hindering the identification of a causal relationship. Collectively, an increase in serum adiponectin together with decreased urinary adiponectin and albumin excretion rates and decreased GFR point towards a renoprotective role for adiponectin in decreasing its urinary loss and preserving renal function. Nevertheless, it is important to balance these strong clinical correlations with consideration of whether alterations in adiponectin are always a cause or a consequence of disease states, and thus, it is likely that the timing of targeted adiponectin therapy will be vital to its success in this metabolic milieu.

3. Expression of Adiponectin and Its Receptors and Their Implication for Renoprotection

In the kidney, adiponectin is found on the endothelium of the glomerular and peritubular capillaries, on the smooth muscle cells of intrarenal arteries/arterioles, and proximal and distal tubular epithelial cells [19,20]. It has been reported that a fair amount of AdipoR1 is expressed in the cells constituting the glomerulus: endothelial cells, podocytes, mesangial cells, and Bowman's capsule epithelial cells, as well as in proximal tubular cells, whereas AdipoR2 is expressed to a lesser degree on glomeruli and proximal tubular cells [20,21].

The renoprotective properties of adiponectin through binding to its receptors have been implicated in several rodent models. Sharma et al. demonstrated that adiponectin knockout mice exhibited increased albuminuria and segmentally fused podocyte foot processes that were restored by adiponectin administration. In addition, albumin permeability across a differentiated podocyte cell monolayer was reduced by the addition of adiponectin in vitro. 5-aminoimidazole-4-carboxamide-1-β-D-ribonucleoside (AICAR), a specific activator of AMPK, reduced the permeability of podocytes to albumin, whereas adenine 9-β-D-arabinofuranoside, a specific inhibitor of AMPK, increased the permeability of podocytes to albumin, suggesting a protective role of adiponectin against the development of albuminuria, at least in part, through the direct action of adiponectin-induced activation of the AMPK pathway in podocytes. This was independent of adiponectin's systemic effect, since AMPK activation in podocytes was induced specifically by restoring the localization of zona occludens-1 along the plasma membrane of podocytes, which contributed to the podocytes' structural and functional integrity associated with tight junction adherence and the narrowing of the slit diaphragm [21].

Rutkowski et al. generated a mouse model that allowed the induction of caspase-8-mediated apoptosis specifically in podocytes (POD-ATTAC mice). POD-ATTAC mice lacking adiponectin developed significant albuminuria and ablated podocytes; however, adiponectin-overexpressing POD-ATTAC mice recovered renal function and ameliorated podocyte injury and interstitial fibrosis, suggesting that adiponectin helped to reverse podocyte injury and restore renal function [22].

Fang et al. confirmed the hypothesis that adiponectin may attenuate the deleterious effects of angiotensin II in renal tubular cells by showing that angiotensin II-induced nicotinamide adenine dinucleotide phosphate (NADPH) oxidase activation and oxidative stress were attenuated by AdipoR1 activation. Activation of AMPK with AICAR mimicked the effect of adiponectin on angiotensin II-induced activation of NADPH oxidase. Angiotensin II-induced activation of NADPH oxidase was abrogated by coincubation with the AMPK inhibitor compound C, indicating that the renoprotective effect of adiponectin binding to AdipoR1 was achieved through the subsequent activation of AMPK [23].

Yu et al. created a chronic renal failure rat model by adenine administration that exhibited increased serum and urinary adiponectin levels that positively correlated with the intrarenal expression of both AdipoR1 and AdipoR2. Significant upregulation of the expression of adiponectin and its receptors might be reflective of an adaptive renal response to compensate for ongoing renal injury [6]. These data suggest that adiponectin's effect on its specific target organ might be achieved by binding to its receptors in the relevant tissues, independently of its systemic effect. The above-mentioned studies investigating the renoprotective effects of adiponectin concerning podocyte recovery were carried out exclusively in rodent experimental settings. Therefore, the relevance of these studies to the human situation in different pathological backgrounds should be interpreted with caution.

Our study investigating the expression of adiponectin receptors in human diabetic kidneys demonstrated significantly decreased expression of AdipoR1 and AdipoR2, even at an early stage of CKD, that was maintained throughout the progression of CKD stages compared to that of non-diabetic kidneys, and this down-regulation of adiponectin receptors might be in part due to the increased insulin resistance in diabetes [24,25]. This is in keeping with the evidence that obesity decreases not only plasma adiponectin levels but also AdipoR1/R2 expression, thereby reducing adiponectin sensitivity and leading to insulin resistance, which in turn aggravates hyperinsulinemia [26]. This suggests that both upregulation of AdipoR1 and AdipoR2 expression and agonism of AdipoRs could be potential targets for novel treatments for insulin resistance and type 2 diabetes.

4. Signaling Pathways Associated with Adiponectin and Its Receptor Binding

Adiponectin exerts its effects via binding to three receptors: AdipoR1, AdipoR2, and T-cadherin. AdipoR1 and AdipoR2 have seven transmembrane domains and are significantly homologous, sharing 67 % amino acid identity [27], whereas T-cadherin is considered to be an adiponectin-binding protein but its functional significance has not been completely determined. It is thought that the latter receptor has no effect on adiponectin's cellular signaling or function, since it does not have an intracellular domain [28]. The binding of adiponectin to its receptors can regulate glucose and lipid homeostasis by promoting a strong insulin-sensitizing effect, fatty acid oxidation, mitochondrial biogenesis, and mediating anti-oxidative and anti-inflammatory effects. AMPK and PPARα are primary targets activated by AdipoR1 and AdipoR2, respectively [29,30].

AMPK is a metabolic master switch that regulates downstream signals based on shifts in the surrounding energy reservoir [31]. AMPK activation can be triggered as a result of the conformational change incurred by an adenosine monophosphate (AMP) binding to its γ subunit and phosphorylation of the α subunit by upstream kinases, including a compound consisting of three proteins: STE-related adaptor (STRAD), mouse protein 25, and the tumor-suppressor liver kinase B1 (LKB1) [32]. LKB1 activation and calcium influx-induced activation of Ca^{2+}/calmodulin-dependent protein kinase kinase β (CaMKKβ) are triggered upon AdipoR1 activation that primarily potentiates AMPK stimulation [33]. Upon activation, AMPK signals through its downstream substrates to achieve energy homeostasis by stimulating processes that generate ATP through actions such as glucose transport, mitochondrial biogenesis, and fatty acid oxidation, while inhibiting those that use ATP through the opposing actions of fatty acid, protein, and glycogen synthesis [31].

AMPK modulates glucose transport in a similar way to insulin. AMPK promotes glucose uptake in peripheral tissues by promoting GLUT4 translocation to the cell membrane and upregulating the expression of hexokinase II [34]. Hyperglycemia-induced oxidative stress upregulates vascular endothelial growth factor expression in podocytes that increases vascular permeability and activates classical pathways associated with the production of advanced glycosylation end products and the activation of protein kinase C and aldose reductase that contribute to the development of DKD through its characteristic pathological changes in mesangial cell proliferation and hypertrophy, exacerbated matrix production, and basement membrane thickening [35,36]. Therefore, targeting AMPK could ameliorate these adverse effects by enhancing insulin sensitivity at the systemic level and regulating glucotoxicity-induced oxidative stress in the target organ as well.

AMPK is also known to mediate the intracellular signaling pathway of class O forkhead box (FoxO) proteins. FoxO proteins are transcription factors that regulate the expression of antioxidant enzymes; promote mitochondrial biogenesis, cell survival, and longevity in several tissues; and participate in tumor suppression [37]. The transcriptional activity of the subfamily member FoxO3a is modulated by AMPK in response to metabolic stress to shield quiescent cells from reactive oxygen species (ROS) by antagonizing apoptosis, which reduces oxidative stress by directly increasing the quantity of antioxidant enzymes such as thioredoxin, peroxiredoxin, manganese superoxide dismutase (SOD), and catalase [38]. Therefore, when activated upon ROS exposure, the AMPK-FoxO3a signaling pathway upregulates the expression of silent information regulator T1 (SIRT1), a well-known FoxO3a coactivator, that is thought to mediate apoptotic and autophagy crosstalk [39]. Our previous study investigating the effect of resveratrol suggested that resveratrol can ameliorate renal cell apoptosis and oxidative stress via activation of the AMPK-SIRT1-PGC1α axis and its consequent effects on the phosphatidylinositol-3 kinase (PI3K)-Akt (protein kinase B)-FoxO3a pathway, which induces mitochondrial biogenesis and enhances its capacity to alleviate oxidative stress in DKD [40]. The renoprotective role of human recombinant extracellular superoxide dismutase (EC-SOD) on DKD—amelioration of hyperglycemia-induced oxidative stress, inflammation, and apoptosis through the activation AMPK-PGC1α-nuclear factor erythroid 2-related factor 2 (Nrf2) and AMPK-FoxOs pathways—was also demonstrated in our recent study [41].

The AMPK dependent phosphorylation of downstream target substrates involved in regulating protein translation, cell growth, and autophagy includes tuberous sclerosis complex protein-2 (TSC2) and mammalian target of rapamycin (mTOR) complex 1 that repress protein synthesis and deliver their renoprotective effect by inhibiting the accumulation of extracellular matrix in DKD [42].

AMPK modulates changes in lipid metabolism via the regulation of fatty acid oxidation and cholesterol synthesis in the target organ. AMPK phosphorylation decreases the activity of the lipogenesis-associated enzymes sterol regulatory element-binding protein-1 (SREBP-1), acetyl CoA carboxylase-1 (ACC-1), and hydroxymethylglutaryl CoA reductase (HMGCR), which in turn limit malonyl CoA production, attenuating the inhibition of carnitine palmitoyl transferase-1 (CPT-1) activity that potentiates the transport of fatty acids into the mitochondria for beta oxidation and interrupts fatty acid synthesis [43].

Moreover, AdipoR2-induced activation of PPARα promotes fatty acid catabolism by upregulating genes involved in fatty acid transport, binding and activation, and peroxisomal and mitochondrial fatty acid β-oxidation. PPARα-mediated gene transcription upregulates the PGC1α and ERR1α axis that enhances mitochondrial oxidative capacity to reduce oxidative stress and further contributes to decreased lipid accumulation in the target organ [44]. As a result, the increased endothelial nitric oxide synthase (eNOS) level is expected to neutralize ROS, reduce adhesion molecule synthesis, and suppress cell proliferation, which collectively help to confer protective effects on endothelial cells against albuminuria development in the kidney [24]. We recently unraveled a causal relationship between lipotoxicity and lymphangiogenesis using the PPARα agonist fenofibrate that improved intrarenal lipotoxicity and secondary lymphatic proliferation through PPARα-AMPK-pACC signaling in DKD [45].

Adiponectin modifies the effects of toxic ceramide accumulation by binding to AdipoR1/2, which increases ceramidase activity, catalyzing the conversion of ceramide to sphingosine and subsequently sphingosine-1 phosphate (S1P), independently of AMPK [46]. Ceramides consist of sphinosines and fatty acids that make up sphingomyelin, one of the major lipids in the bilayer of the cell membrane. In addition to its original role as a structural element, sphingomyelin acts as a cellular signaling molecule and regulates the differentiation, proliferation, programmed cell death, and apoptosis of cells [47]. Among its different subtypes, ceramide (C)16, C18, and C24 are associated with adverse clinical outcomes with their fatty acid components accumulating in the target organ promoting cell apoptosis and insulin resistance [48]. Surplus fatty acids in target organ cells stimulate the transcription of enzymes involved in ceramide biosynthesis that disrupt the association between inhibitor 2 of protein phosphatase 2A (I2PP2A) and protein phosphatase 2A (PP2A) [49]. PP2A impairs NO bioavailability by promoting the dephosphorylation and inactivation of Akt and B-cell lymphoma 2 (Bcl-2), leading to endothelial dysfunction and apoptosis, respectively [50,51]. Consequently, increased ceramidase activity results in a net increase in the S1P to ceramide ratio that promotes three key metabolic effects: it provides sphingosine and free fatty acids as ligands for PPARα, promotes the formation of the pro-survival factor S1P, and decreases ceramide accumulation that further increases insulin sensitivity and NO production. This is in line with our recent finding that AdipoR activation may ameliorate intrarenal triglyceride accumulation and endothelial dysfunction through increased ceramidase activity and the subsequent normalized ceramide to S1P ratio in DKD [25].

The studies discussed above are only a handful of many that describe the activation of AMPK, PPARα, and enhanced ceramidase activity through AdipoR binding. Highlighting the concept of lipotoxicity as a main contributor to the development of DKD, it is noteworthy that AdipoR1 and AdipoR2 serve as receptors for globular and full-length adiponectin that are primarily involved in cellular signaling pathways promoting mitochondrial oxidative capacity and fatty acid oxidation. This raises the potential for AdipoR activation via adiponectin binding as a therapeutic target for optimizing lipid metabolism in DKD.

5. Adiponectin and Adiponectin Receptors as Therapeutic Targets for DKD

5.1. Strategy for Upregulation of Adiponectin and Its Receptors

The general consensus based on the available literature indicates that adiponectin is renoprotective and, therefore, it seems a logical approach that antidiabetic therapy should be aimed at enhancing adiponectin effects by increasing the plasma level of adiponectin itself or by activating adiponectin receptors to increase adiponectin sensitivity, which subsequently would render pleiotropic metabolic effects via their downstream signaling pathways.

Pravastatin therapy significantly improves insulin sensitivity and increases plasma adiponectin levels in patients with hypercholesterolemia and in those with coronary heart disease with impaired glucose tolerance. The mechanism involving HMG-CoA reductase inhibition may account for the reported increased plasma adiponectin level via which this particular statin delivers its therapeutic effect [52]. Blocking the renin-angiotensin-aldosterone system (RAAS) by either physiologic or pharmacologic modulation of RAAS activity, e.g., by using enalapril or valsartan, increased adiponectin production and upregulated circulating adiponectin. Valsartan blocks the constitutive angiotensin II type 1 receptor activity involving the nuclear factor κB (NF-κB) pathway that limits PPARγ activity in mature adipocytes, thus attenuating the proinflammatory response and enhancing the insulin-sensitizing activities of mature adipocytes, which may underlie the beneficial metabolic impact of angiotensin II receptor blockers (ARBs) [53]. Increasing the level of adiponectin using RAAS blockers might improve the anti-inflammatory response in DKD by activating the AMPK and cyclooxygenase-2 pathways, and decreasing tumor necrosis factor-α (TNF-α) activity. Adiponectin has also been shown to inhibit angiotensin II–induced activation of NADPH oxidase via the AdipoR1-mediated activation of both AMPK and cAMP-Epac pathways [54]. Tesaglitazar is a PPARα/γ dual agonist that exerts its favorable effect by increasing plasma adiponectin levels. It not only improved insulin resistance and lipid metabolism at the systemic level, but also prevented albuminuria and renal glomerular fibrosis in a diabetic mouse model, proving its potential as a promising antidiabetic agent for DKD [55]. Fenofibrate has been reported to increase adiponectin expression in adipose tissue and serum adiponectin levels through PPARα activation and the elevation of high-density lipoprotein levels [56]. Salsalate treatment demonstrated metabolic improvements in terms of increased insulin sensitivity and lipid profiles in obese Hispanics by significantly increasing serum adiponectin levels, which occurred without alterations in adiposity [57]. Thiazolidinediones (TZD), e.g., pioglitazone and rosiglitazone, have been shown to directly upregulate adiponectin gene transcription via activation of PPARγ in adipose tissue, thereby promoting adipocyte differentiation and/or increasing the number of small adipocytes that are more sensitive to insulin [58,59]. However, whether the TZD-induced increase in the plasma adiponectin level is causally involved in the TZD-mediated insulin-sensitizing effects has not been addressed experimentally. Rosiglitazone, a PPARγ agonist, not only improved metabolic parameters encompassing plasma adiponectin, fasting glucose, glucose metabolic clearance rate, and TNF-α, but also alleviated albuminuria, suggesting its potency as a renoprotective agent for T2D patients [60]. It has also become clear that a fasted/starved state, caloric restriction, and/or weight loss lead to increases in circulating levels of adiponectin, and that SIRT1 increases adiponectin or inhibits inflammatory cytokines by deacetylating PPARγ [61].

However, there are significant side-effects associated with chronic adiponectin upregulation. Notably, mice genetically engineered to overexpress adiponectin and those treated with molecules that stimulate adiponectin secretion, such as thiazolidinediones and fibroblast growth factor 21, showed reduced bone density [62]. Heart damage—left ventricular hypertrophy in particular—was one of the other adverse effects that has been observed in rodents upon chronic increase in adiponectin production [63,64]. Adiponectin may also promote adipogenesis and angiogenesis associated with weight gain and the growth of tumors, respectively [65]. Lastly, infertility can be triggered by chronically elevated adiponectin concentrations [66]. The mechanism by which chronic adiponectin exposure mediates detrimental effects on various tissues is unclear. However, experimental evidences indicate that its innate properties to self-associate into higher-order structures with high turn-over rate and sexual dimorphism may attribute to the yet unraveled defaults associated with chronic adiponectin exposure [8]. Moreover, in case of its association with reduced bone mass, it is implicated that circulating adiponectin especially in its full-length form, rather than globular form, indirectly inhibits bone mass by increasing insulin sensitivity and inhibiting the action of insulin in tissues [67,68]. These potential pitfalls will need to be addressed with deliberation when establishing a strategy exploiting the upregulation of adiponectin and its receptors.

5.2. Development of an AdipoR Agonist, AdipoRon

Okada-Iwabu et al. identified several molecules that activate adiponectin receptors and focused their in-depth analysis on devising an orally active synthetic compound called "AdipoRon." AdipoRon binds, at a low micromolar concentration, to both AdipoR1 and AdipoR2. It is capable of producing the pro-metabolic effects of adiponectin by binding to both AdipoR1/2 and subsequently activating AMPK, PPARα, and the transcriptional coactivator PGC1α, which boost mitochondrial proliferation and energy metabolism [69]. When diabetic mice fed a high-fat diet were treated with AdipoRon, the metabolic improvements, including enhanced glucose and lipid metabolism and insulin sensitivity, were conferred in the liver and skeletal muscle, which ultimately increased their exercise endurance capacity and extended their life span [69]. Overexpression of the oxidative stress-relieving genes catalase and SOD might have led to the increase in lifespan [70]. Despite the aforementioned concerns, AdipoRon did not promote weight gain in mice, and the reported observation of a prolonged life span in diabetic mice helps to obviate some of these concerns, even though many of these effects require a more chronic exposure to be manifested. Although the studies described focused on the endocrine effects of AdipoRon, it is again important to consider the potential local effects of AdipoRon in the target organ that is the diabetic kidney.

5.3. Role of AdipoRon in DKD

In human diabetic kidneys, the expression of AdipoR1, AdipoR2, and CaMKKβ, and the number of phosphorylated LKB1- and AMPK-positive cells significantly decreased when compared to those of controls and the extent of glomerulosclerosis and tubulointerstitial fibrosis correlated with renal functional deterioration. In a diabetic mouse model, AdipoRon directly activated intrarenal AdipoR1 and AdipoR2, which increased CaMKKβ, phosphorylated Ser^{431}LKB1, phosphorylated Thr^{172}AMPK, and PPARα expression independently of the systemic effects of adiponectin. AdipoRon also decreased intrarenal ceramide species and restored the activity of acid ceramidase, the concentration of S1P, and the ratio of ceramide to S1P. In vitro studies confirmed that AdipoRon increased the intracellular Ca^{2+} influx that activated the CaMKKβ/phosphorylated Ser^{431}LKB1/phosphorylated Thr^{172}AMPK/PPARα pathway and downstream signaling, thus decreasing oxidative stress and apoptosis and improving endothelial dysfunction in human glomerular endothelial cells and murine podocytes treated with high-glucose- and palmitate-media. Adiponectin receptor agonism recovered podocytes' structural integrity as demonstrated by increased slit-diaphragm diameter and decreased foot process width, and glomerular basement membrane (GBM) thickness in electron microscope (EM) findings. We also confirmed favorable impact of AdipoRon on renal phenotype; it ameliorated features of DKD through decreased intrarenal fibrosis, inflammation and apoptosis as shown by decreased mesangial fraction area and expression of collagen IV, TGF-β, and F4/80 on PAS and immunohistochemical staining. Collectively, AdipoRon treatment exerted renoprotective effects by improving diabetes-induced oxidative stress and apoptosis by ameliorating relevant intracellular pathways associated with lipid accumulation and endothelial dysfunction. Our study results suggest that AdipoRon may be a promising drug for the restoration of diabetic nephropathy by reducing lipotoxicity through the activation of adiponectin receptors and downstream targets through stimulation of the intracellular Ca^{2+}/AMPK-LKB1/PPARα pathway and also by increasing ceramidase activity [24,25].

6. Conclusions and Future Perspectives

The rationale for targeting adiponectin is based on the well-documented beneficial physiological actions of adiponectin spanning diabetes, inflammation, and metabolic diseases, and it is expected that studies in animal models will translate well to human physiology in the case of adiponectin. An excess intake of fatty acids can promote lipotoxicity and lipoapopotosis in several target organs, including diabetic kidneys. The binding of adiponectin to AdipoRs exerts renoprotective effects by regulating fatty acid metabolism; it enhances beta oxidation and ceramidase activity. AdipoRon can activate AdipoRs without affecting the systemic adiponectin level. It ameliorates lipotoxicity in DKD by increasing intrarenal AdipoRs that promote ceramidase activity and activates their downstream signaling, including the intracellular Ca^{2+}-CaMKKβ/LKB1-AMPK/PPARα pathway (Figure 1). The discovery of the small molecular compound AdipoRon is an attractive therapeutic option that would mimic or enhance the established pro-metabolic actions of adiponectin but without the detrimental side effects due to chronic adiponectin exposure. Our recent studies highlight that targeting adiponectin receptors with low molecular weight agonists is a viable strategy, and that developing higher-affinity agonists with improved pharmacokinetics with a tissue- or cell-specific delivery approach should be pursued in the future.

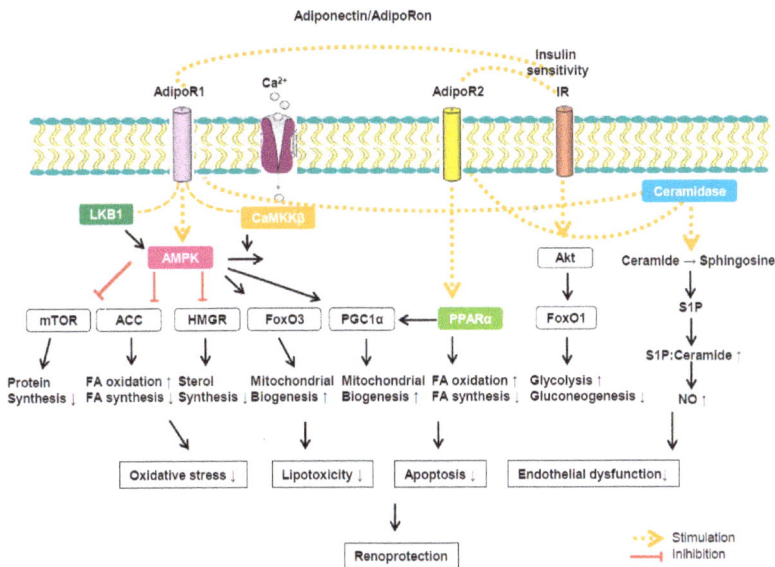

Figure 1. Signaling pathways associated with adiponectin and its receptor binding. AdipoR1 increases calcium influx to activate Ca^{2+}/calmodulin-dependent protein kinase kinase β (CaMKKβ) and subsequent downstream kinases. AdipoR1 also activates liver kinase B1 (LKB1) and AMPK that can increase peroxisome proliferator-activated receptor (PPAR) gamma coactivator 1 alpha (PGC-1) expression. Activation of associated downstream pathways exert prometabolic effects by enhancing fatty acid oxidation and mitochondrial biogenesis. AdipoR2 activate PPARα to increase fatty acid oxidation and insulin sensitivity. AdipopR1/2 has ceramidase activity and can catalyze the conversion of ceramide to sphingosine, which produces sphingosine-1-phosphate (S1P), subsequently increasing S1P to ceramide ratio that further ameliorates endothelial dysfunction through increased NO level. Insulin-stimulated FoxO1 phosphorylation through PI3K and AKT can reduce hepatic gluconeogenesis.

Int. J. Mol. Sci. **2019**, *20*, 1782

Author Contributions: Y.K. and C.W.P. designed and wrote the manuscript. The authors critically analyzed the manuscript and approved its final version for publication.

Acknowledgments: This study was supported by grants from the Basic Science Research Program through the National Research Foundation of Korea (NRF) funded by the Ministry of Education, Science and Technology (CWP: 2016R1A2B2015980).

Conflicts of Interest: The authors declare no conflict of interest.

References

1. Park, C.W. Diabetic kidney disease: From epidemiology to clinical perspectives. *Diabetes Metab. J.* **2014**, *38*, 252–260. [CrossRef]
2. Martinez de Morentin, P.B.; Varela, L.; Ferno, J.; Nogueiras, R.; Dieguez, C.; Lopez, M. Hypothalamic lipotoxicity and the metabolic syndrome. *Biochim. Biophys. Acta* **2010**, *1801*, 350–361. [CrossRef]
3. Stadler, K.; Goldberg, I.J.; Susztak, K. The evolving understanding of the contribution of lipid metabolism to diabetic kidney disease. *Curr. Diabetes Rep.* **2015**, *15*, 40. [CrossRef]
4. Ruan, H.; Dong, L.Q. Adiponectin signaling and function in insulin target tissues. *J. Mol. Cell Biol.* **2016**, *8*, 101–109. [CrossRef]
5. Martinez Cantarin, M.P.; Waldman, S.A.; Doria, C.; Frank, A.M.; Maley, W.R.; Ramirez, C.B.; Keith, S.W.; Falkner, B. The adipose tissue production of adiponectin is increased in end-stage renal disease. *Kidney Int.* **2013**, *83*, 487–494. [CrossRef] [PubMed]
6. Yu, Y.; Bao, B.J.; Fan, Y.P.; Shi, L.; Li, S.Q. Changes of adiponectin and its receptors in rats following chronic renal failure. *Ren. Fail.* **2014**, *36*, 92–97. [CrossRef] [PubMed]
7. Esmaili, S.; Xu, A.; George, J. The multifaceted and controversial immunometabolic actions of adiponectin. *TEM* **2014**, *25*, 444–451. [CrossRef]
8. Halberg, N.; Schraw, T.D.; Wang, Z.V.; Kim, J.Y.; Yi, J.; Hamilton, M.P.; Luby-Phelps, K.; Scherer, P.E. Systemic fate of the adipocyte-derived factor adiponectin. *Diabetes* **2009**, *58*, 1961–1970. [CrossRef] [PubMed]
9. Shimotomai, T.; Kakei, M.; Narita, T.; Koshimura, J.; Hosoba, M.; Kato, M.; Komatsuda, A.; Ito, S. Enhanced urinary adiponectin excretion in IgA-nephropathy patients with proteinuria. *Ren. Fail.* **2005**, *27*, 323–328. [CrossRef] [PubMed]
10. Shen, Y.Y.; Hughes, J.T.; Charlesworth, J.A.; Kelly, J.J.; Peake, P.W. Adiponectin is present in the urine in its native conformation, and specifically reduces the secretion of MCP-1 by proximal tubular cells. *Nephrology* **2008**, *13*, 405–410. [CrossRef] [PubMed]
11. Barlovic, D.P.; Zaletel, J.; Prezelj, J. Adipocytokines are associated with renal function in patients with normal range glomerular filtration rate and type 2 diabetes. *Cytokine* **2009**, *46*, 142–145. [CrossRef] [PubMed]
12. Barlovic, D.P.; Zaletel, J.; Prezelj, J. Association between adiponectin and low-grade albuminuria is BMI-dependent in type 2 diabetes. *Kidney Blood Press. Res.* **2010**, *33*, 405–410. [CrossRef]
13. Tamba, S.; Nakatsuji, H.; Kishida, K.; Noguchi, M.; Ogawa, T.; Okauchi, Y.; Nishizawa, H.; Imagawa, A.; Nakamura, T.; Matsuzawa, Y.; et al. Relationship between visceral fat accumulation and urinary albumin-creatinine ratio in middle-aged Japanese men. *Atherosclerosis* **2010**, *211*, 601–605. [CrossRef] [PubMed]
14. Jorsal, A.; Petersen, E.H.; Tarnow, L.; Hess, G.; Zdunek, D.; Frystyk, J.; Flyvbjerg, A.; Lajer, M.; Rossing, P. Urinary adiponectin excretion rises with increasing albuminuria in type 1 diabetes. *J. Diabetes Complicat.* **2013**, *27*, 604–608. [CrossRef]
15. Kacso, I.M.; Bondor, C.I.; Kacso, G. Plasma adiponectin is related to the progression of kidney disease in type 2 diabetes patients. *Scand. J. Clin. Lab. Investig.* **2012**, *72*, 333–339. [CrossRef]
16. Bjornstad, P.; Pyle, L.; Kinney, G.L.; Rewers, M.; Johnson, R.J.; Maahs, D.M.; Snell-Bergeon, J.K. Adiponectin is associated with early diabetic kidney disease in adults with type 1 diabetes: A Coronary Artery Calcification in Type 1 Diabetes (CACTI) Study. *J. Diabetes Complicat.* **2017**, *31*, 369–374. [CrossRef]
17. Lim, C.C.; Teo, B.W.; Tai, E.S.; Lim, S.C.; Chan, C.M.; Sethi, S.; Wong, T.Y.; Sabanayagam, C. Elevated serum leptin, adiponectin and leptin to adiponectin ratio is associated with chronic kidney disease in Asian adults. *PLoS ONE* **2015**, *10*, e0122009. [CrossRef]

18. Park, J.T.; Yoo, T.H.; Kim, J.K.; Oh, H.J.; Kim, S.J.; Yoo, D.E.; Lee, M.J.; Shin, D.H.; Han, S.H.; Han, D.S.; et al. Leptin/adiponectin ratio is an independent predictor of mortality in nondiabetic peritoneal dialysis patients. *Perit. Dial. Int.* **2013**, *33*, 67–74. [CrossRef] [PubMed]

19. Von Eynatten, M.; Liu, D.; Hock, C.; Oikonomou, D.; Baumann, M.; Allolio, B.; Korosoglou, G.; Morcos, M.; Campean, V.; Amann, K.; et al. Urinary adiponectin excretion: A novel marker for vascular damage in type 2 diabetes. *Diabetes* **2009**, *58*, 2093–2099. [CrossRef] [PubMed]

20. Perri, A.; Vizza, D.; Lofaro, D.; Gigliotti, P.; Leone, F.; Brunelli, E.; Malivindi, R.; De Amicis, F.; Romeo, F.; De Stefano, R.; et al. Adiponectin is expressed and secreted by renal tubular epithelial cells. *J. Nephrol.* **2013**, *26*, 1049–1054. [CrossRef] [PubMed]

21. Sharma, K.; Ramachandrarao, S.; Qiu, G.; Usui, H.K.; Zhu, Y.; Dunn, S.R.; Ouedraogo, R.; Hough, K.; McCue, P.; Chan, L.; et al. Adiponectin regulates albuminuria and podocyte function in mice. *J. Clin. Investig.* **2008**, *118*, 1645–1656. [CrossRef]

22. Rutkowski, J.M.; Wang, Z.V.; Park, A.S.; Zhang, J.; Zhang, D.; Hu, M.C.; Moe, O.W.; Susztak, K.; Scherer, P.E. Adiponectin promotes functional recovery after podocyte ablation. *JASN* **2013**, *24*, 268–282. [CrossRef]

23. Fang, F.; Liu, G.C.; Kim, C.; Yassa, R.; Zhou, J.; Scholey, J.W. Adiponectin attenuates angiotensin II-induced oxidative stress in renal tubular cells through AMPK and cAMP-Epac signal transduction pathways. *Am. J. Physiol. Ren. Physiol.* **2013**, *304*, F1366–F1374. [CrossRef]

24. Kim, Y.; Lim, J.H.; Kim, M.Y.; Kim, E.N.; Yoon, H.E.; Shin, S.J.; Choi, B.S.; Kim, Y.S.; Chang, Y.S.; Park, C.W. The Adiponectin Receptor Agonist AdipoRon Ameliorates Diabetic Nephropathy in a Model of Type 2 Diabetes. *JASN* **2018**, *29*, 1108–1127. [CrossRef]

25. Choi, S.R.; Lim, J.H.; Kim, M.Y.; Kim, E.N.; Kim, Y.; Choi, B.S.; Kim, Y.S.; Kim, H.W.; Lim, K.M.; Kim, M.J.; et al. Adiponectin receptor agonist AdipoRon decreased ceramide, and lipotoxicity, and ameliorated diabetic nephropathy. *Metab. Clin. Exp.* **2018**, *85*, 348–360. [CrossRef]

26. Tsuchida, A.; Yamauchi, T.; Ito, Y.; Hada, Y.; Maki, T.; Takekawa, S.; Kamon, J.; Kobayashi, M.; Suzuki, R.; Hara, K.; et al. Insulin/Foxo1 pathway regulates expression levels of adiponectin receptors and adiponectin sensitivity. *J. Biol. Chem.* **2004**, *279*, 30817–30822. [CrossRef]

27. Yamauchi, T.; Kamon, J.; Ito, Y.; Tsuchida, A.; Yokomizo, T.; Kita, S.; Sugiyama, T.; Miyagishi, M.; Hara, K.; Tsunoda, M.; et al. Cloning of adiponectin receptors that mediate antidiabetic metabolic effects. *Nature* **2003**, *423*, 762–769. [CrossRef]

28. Hug, C.; Wang, J.; Ahmad, N.S.; Bogan, J.S.; Tsao, T.S.; Lodish, H.F. T-cadherin is a receptor for hexameric and high-molecular-weight forms of Acrp30/adiponectin. *Proc. Natl. Acad. Sci. USA* **2004**, *101*, 10308–10313. [CrossRef]

29. Yamauchi, T.; Kamon, J.; Minokoshi, Y.; Ito, Y.; Waki, H.; Uchida, S.; Yamashita, S.; Noda, M.; Kita, S.; Ueki, K.; et al. Adiponectin stimulates glucose utilization and fatty-acid oxidation by activating AMP-activated protein kinase. *Nat. Med.* **2002**, *8*, 1288–1295. [CrossRef]

30. Mao, X.; Kikani, C.K.; Riojas, R.A.; Langlais, P.; Wang, L.; Ramos, F.J.; Fang, Q.; Christ-Roberts, C.Y.; Hong, J.Y.; Kim, R.Y.; et al. APPL1 binds to adiponectin receptors and mediates adiponectin signalling and function. *Nat. Cell Biol.* **2006**, *8*, 516–523. [CrossRef]

31. Kim, Y.; Park, C.W. Adenosine monophosphate-activated protein kinase in diabetic nephropathy. *Kidney Res. Clin. Pract.* **2016**, *35*, 69–77. [CrossRef]

32. Hawley, S.A.; Boudeau, J.; Reid, J.L.; Mustard, K.J.; Udd, L.; Makela, T.P.; Alessi, D.R.; Hardie, D.G. Complexes between the LKB1 tumor suppressor, STRAD alpha/beta and MO25 alpha/beta are upstream kinases in the AMP-activated protein kinase cascade. *J. Biol.* **2003**, *2*, 28. [CrossRef]

33. Hawley, S.A.; Selbert, M.A.; Goldstein, E.G.; Edelman, A.M.; Carling, D.; Hardie, D.G. 5′-AMP activates the AMP-activated protein kinase cascade, and Ca^{2+}/calmodulin activates the calmodulin-dependent protein kinase I cascade, via three independent mechanisms. *J. Biol. Chem.* **1995**, *270*, 27186–27191. [CrossRef]

34. Jensen, T.E.; Sylow, L.; Rose, A.J.; Madsen, A.B.; Angin, Y.; Maarbjerg, S.J.; Richter, E.A. Contraction-stimulated glucose transport in muscle is controlled by AMPK and mechanical stress but not sarcoplasmatic reticulum Ca^{2+} release. *Mol. Metab.* **2014**, *3*, 742–753. [CrossRef] [PubMed]

35. Fioretto, P.; Mauer, M. Histopathology of diabetic nephropathy. *Semin. Nephrol.* **2007**, *27*, 195–207. [CrossRef]

36. Kim, Y.; Park, C.W. New therapeutic agents in diabetic nephropathy. *Korean J. Intern. Med.* **2017**, *32*, 11–25. [CrossRef] [PubMed]

37. Sanchez, A.M.; Csibi, A.; Raibon, A.; Cornille, K.; Gay, S.; Bernardi, H.; Candau, R. AMPK promotes skeletal muscle autophagy through activation of forkhead FoxO3a and interaction with Ulk1. *J. Cell. Biochem.* **2012**, *113*, 695–710. [CrossRef]

38. Chiribau, C.B.; Cheng, L.; Cucoranu, I.C.; Yu, Y.S.; Clempus, R.E.; Sorescu, D. FOXO3A regulates peroxiredoxin III expression in human cardiac fibroblasts. *J. Biol. Chem.* **2008**, *283*, 8211–8217. [CrossRef]

39. Canto, C.; Gerhart-Hines, Z.; Feige, J.N.; Lagouge, M.; Noriega, L.; Milne, J.C.; Elliott, P.J.; Puigserver, P.; Auwerx, J. AMPK regulates energy expenditure by modulating NAD+ metabolism and SIRT1 activity. *Nature* **2009**, *458*, 1056–1060. [CrossRef] [PubMed]

40. Kim, M.Y.; Lim, J.H.; Youn, H.H.; Hong, Y.A.; Yang, K.S.; Park, H.S.; Chung, S.; Ko, S.H.; Shin, S.J.; Choi, B.S.; et al. Resveratrol prevents renal lipotoxicity and inhibits mesangial cell glucotoxicity in a manner dependent on the AMPK-SIRT1-PGC1alpha axis in db/db mice. *Diabetologia* **2013**, *56*, 204–217. [CrossRef]

41. Hong, Y.A.; Lim, J.H.; Kim, M.Y.; Kim, Y.; Park, H.S.; Kim, H.W.; Choi, B.S.; Chang, Y.S.; Kim, H.W.; Kim, T.Y.; et al. Extracellular Superoxide Dismutase Attenuates Renal Oxidative Stress through the Activation of Adenosine Monophosphate-Activated Protein Kinase in Diabetic Nephropathy. *Antioxid. Redox Signal.* **2018**, *28*, 1543–1561. [CrossRef]

42. Luo, X.; Deng, L.; Lamsal, L.P.; Xu, W.; Xiang, C.; Cheng, L. AMP-activated protein kinase alleviates extracellular matrix accumulation in high glucose-induced renal fibroblasts through mTOR signaling pathway. *Cell. Physiol. Biochem.* **2015**, *35*, 191–200. [CrossRef]

43. Li, Y.; Xu, S.; Mihaylova, M.M.; Zheng, B.; Hou, X.; Jiang, B.; Park, O.; Luo, Z.; Lefai, E.; Shyy, J.Y.; et al. AMPK phosphorylates and inhibits SREBP activity to attenuate hepatic steatosis and atherosclerosis in diet-induced insulin-resistant mice. *Cell Metab.* **2011**, *13*, 376–388. [CrossRef]

44. Kersten, S. Integrated physiology and systems biology of PPARalpha. *Mol. Metab.* **2014**, *3*, 354–371. [CrossRef]

45. Kim, Y.; Hwang, S.D.; Lim, J.H.; Kim, M.Y.; Kim, E.N.; Choi, B.S.; Kim, Y.S.; Kim, H.W.; Park, C.W. Attenuated Lymphatic Proliferation Ameliorates Diabetic Nephropathy and High-Fat Diet-Induced Renal Lipotoxicity. *Sci. Rep.* **2019**, *9*, 1994. [CrossRef]

46. Holland, W.L.; Miller, R.A.; Wang, Z.V.; Sun, K.; Barth, B.M.; Bui, H.H.; Davis, K.E.; Bikman, B.T.; Halberg, N.; Rutkowski, J.M.; et al. Receptor-mediated activation of ceramidase activity initiates the pleiotropic actions of adiponectin. *Nat. Med.* **2011**, *17*, 55–63. [CrossRef]

47. Kuzmenko, D.I.; Klimentyeva, T.K. Role of Ceramide in Apoptosis and Development of Insulin Resistance. *Biochem. Biokhimiia* **2016**, *81*, 913–927. [CrossRef]

48. Summers, S.A. The ART of Lowering Ceramides. *Cell Metab.* **2015**, *22*, 195–196. [CrossRef]

49. Symons, J.D.; Abel, E.D. Lipotoxicity contributes to endothelial dysfunction: A focus on the contribution from ceramide. *Rev. Endocr. Metab. Dis.* **2013**, *14*, 59–68. [CrossRef]

50. Ruvolo, P.P.; Deng, X.; Ito, T.; Carr, B.K.; May, W.S. Ceramide induces Bcl2 dephosphorylation via a mechanism involving mitochondrial PP2A. *J. Biol. Chem.* **1999**, *274*, 20296–20300. [CrossRef]

51. Zhang, Q.J.; Holland, W.L.; Wilson, L.; Tanner, J.M.; Kearns, D.; Cahoon, J.M.; Pettey, D.; Losee, J.; Duncan, B.; Gale, D.; et al. Ceramide mediates vascular dysfunction in diet-induced obesity by PP2A-mediated dephosphorylation of the eNOS-Akt complex. *Diabetes* **2012**, *61*, 1848–1859. [CrossRef]

52. Sugiyama, S.; Fukushima, H.; Kugiyama, K.; Maruyoshi, H.; Kojima, S.; Funahashi, T.; Sakamoto, T.; Horibata, Y.; Watanabe, K.; Koga, H.; et al. Pravastatin improved glucose metabolism associated with increasing plasma adiponectin in patients with impaired glucose tolerance and coronary artery disease. *Atherosclerosis* **2007**, *194*, e43–e51. [CrossRef]

53. Hasan, A.U.; Ohmori, K.; Hashimoto, T.; Kamitori, K.; Yamaguchi, F.; Ishihara, Y.; Ishihara, N.; Noma, T.; Tokuda, M.; Kohno, M. Valsartan ameliorates the constitutive adipokine expression pattern in mature adipocytes: A role for inverse agonism of the angiotensin II type 1 receptor in obesity. *Hypertens. Res.* **2014**, *37*, 621–628. [CrossRef] [PubMed]

54. Kintscher, U.; Unger, T. Vascular protection in diabetes: A pharmacological view of angiotensin II type 1 receptor blockers. *Acta Diabetol.* **2005**, *42*, S26–S32. [CrossRef] [PubMed]

55. Yang, J.; Zhang, D.; Li, J.; Zhang, X.; Fan, F.; Guan, Y. Role of PPARgamma in renoprotection in Type 2 diabetes: Molecular mechanisms and therapeutic potential. *Clin. Sci.* **2009**, *116*, 17–26. [CrossRef] [PubMed]

56. Tsunoda, F.; Asztalos, I.B.; Horvath, K.V.; Steiner, G.; Schaefer, E.J.; Asztalos, B.F. Fenofibrate, HDL, and cardiovascular disease in Type-2 diabetes: The DAIS trial. *Atherosclerosis* **2016**, *247*, 35–39. [CrossRef]

57. Alderete, T.L.; Sattler, F.R.; Richey, J.M.; Allayee, H.; Mittelman, S.D.; Sheng, X.; Tucci, J.; Gyllenhammer, L.E.; Grant, E.G.; Goran, M.I. Salsalate treatment improves glycemia without altering adipose tissue in nondiabetic obese hispanics. *Obesity* **2015**, *23*, 543–551. [CrossRef] [PubMed]

58. Iwaki, M.; Matsuda, M.; Maeda, N.; Funahashi, T.; Matsuzawa, Y.; Makishima, M.; Shimomura, I. Induction of adiponectin, a fat-derived antidiabetic and antiatherogenic factor, by nuclear receptors. *Diabetes* **2003**, *52*, 1655–1663. [CrossRef]

59. Yu, J.G.; Javorschi, S.; Hevener, A.L.; Kruszynska, Y.T.; Norman, R.A.; Sinha, M.; Olefsky, J.M. The effect of thiazolidinediones on plasma adiponectin levels in normal, obese, and type 2 diabetic subjects. *Diabetes* **2002**, *51*, 2968–2974. [CrossRef]

60. Miyazaki, Y.; Cersosimo, E.; Triplitt, C.; DeFronzo, R.A. Rosiglitazone decreases albuminuria in type 2 diabetic patients. *Kidney Int.* **2007**, *72*, 1367–1373. [CrossRef]

61. Guarente, L. Sirtuins as potential targets for metabolic syndrome. *Nature* **2006**, *444*, 868–874. [CrossRef]

62. Wei, W.; Dutchak, P.A.; Wang, X.; Ding, X.; Wang, X.; Bookout, A.L.; Goetz, R.; Mohammadi, M.; Gerard, R.D.; Dechow, P.C.; et al. Fibroblast growth factor 21 promotes bone loss by potentiating the effects of peroxisome proliferator-activated receptor gamma. *Proc. Natl. Acad. Sci. USA* **2012**, *109*, 3143–3148. [CrossRef] [PubMed]

63. Ayerden Ebinc, F.; Ebinc, H.; Derici, U.; Aral, A.; Aybay, C.; Tacoy, G.; Koc, E.; Mutluay, R.; Altok Reis, K.; Erten, Y.; et al. The relationship between adiponectin levels and proinflammatory cytokines and left ventricular mass in dialysis patients. *J. Nephrol.* **2009**, *22*, 216–223.

64. Durand, J.L.; Nawrocki, A.R.; Scherer, P.E.; Jelicks, L.A. Gender differences in adiponectin modulation of cardiac remodeling in mice deficient in endothelial nitric oxide synthase. *J. Cell. Biochem.* **2012**, *113*, 3276–3287. [CrossRef]

65. Yamauchi, T.; Kamon, J.; Waki, H.; Terauchi, Y.; Kubota, N.; Hara, K.; Mori, Y.; Ide, T.; Murakami, K.; Tsuboyama-Kasaoka, N.; et al. The fat-derived hormone adiponectin reverses insulin resistance associated with both lipoatrophy and obesity. *Nat. Med.* **2001**, *7*, 941–946. [CrossRef] [PubMed]

66. Combs, T.P.; Pajvani, U.B.; Berg, A.H.; Lin, Y.; Jelicks, L.A.; Laplante, M.; Nawrocki, A.R.; Rajala, M.W.; Parlow, A.F.; Cheeseboro, L.; et al. A transgenic mouse with a deletion in the collagenous domain of adiponectin displays elevated circulating adiponectin and improved insulin sensitivity. *Endocrinology* **2004**, *145*, 367–383. [CrossRef]

67. Reid, I.R.; Cornish, J.; Baldock, P.A. Nutrition-related peptides and bone homeostasis. *J. Bone Miner. Res.* **2006**, *21*, 495–500. [CrossRef]

68. Ealey, K.N.; Kaludjerovic, J.; Archer, M.C.; Ward, W.E. Adiponectin is a negative regulator of bone mineral and bone strength in growing mice. *Exp. Biol. Med.* **2008**, *233*, 1546–1553. [CrossRef]

69. Okada-Iwabu, M.; Yamauchi, T.; Iwabu, M.; Honma, T.; Hamagami, K.; Matsuda, K.; Yamaguchi, M.; Tanabe, H.; Kimura-Someya, T.; Shirouzu, M.; et al. A small-molecule AdipoR agonist for type 2 diabetes and short life in obesity. *Nature* **2013**, *503*, 493–499. [CrossRef]

70. Okada-Iwabu, M.; Iwabu, M.; Ueki, K.; Yamauchi, T.; Kadowaki, T. Perspective of Small-Molecule AdipoR Agonist for Type 2 Diabetes and Short Life in Obesity. *Diabetes Metab. J.* **2015**, *39*, 363–372. [CrossRef]

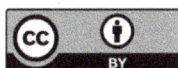

International Journal of
Molecular Sciences

MDPI

Article

Kojyl Cinnamate Ester Derivatives Increase Adiponectin Expression and Stimulate Adiponectin-Induced Hair Growth Factors in Human Dermal Papilla Cells

Phil June Park and Eun-Gyung Cho *

Basic Research & Innovation Division, R&D Unit, Amorepacific Corporation, 1920 Yonggu-daero, Giheung-gu, Yongin-si, Gyeonggi-do 17074, Korea; mosme@amorepacific.com
* Correspondence: egcho@amorepacific.com; Tel.: +82-31-280-5961

Received: 11 March 2019; Accepted: 12 April 2019; Published: 15 April 2019

Abstract: Adiponectin (APN), released mainly from adipose tissue, is a well-known homeostatic factor for regulating glucose levels, lipid metabolism, and insulin sensitivity. A recent study showed that human hair follicles express APN receptors and the presence of APN-mediated hair growth signaling, thereby suggesting that APN is a potent hair growth-promoting adipokine. Previously, kojyl cinnamate ester derivatives (KCEDs) were synthesized in our institute as new anti-aging or adiponectin-/adipogenesis-inducing compounds. Here, we tested the activity of these derivatives to induce endogenous APN secretion. Among the derivatives, KCED-1 and KCED-2 showed improved activity in inducing APN mRNA expression, secretion of APN protein, and adipogenesis in human subcutaneous fat cells (hSCFs) when compared with the effects of Seletinoid G, a verified APN inducer. When human follicular dermal papilla cells were treated with the culture supernatant of KCED-1- or KCED-2-treated hSCFs, the mRNA expression of APN-induced hair growth factors such as insulin-like growth factor, hepatocyte growth factor, and vascular endothelial growth factor was upregulated compared with that in the control. Taken together, our study shows that among kojyl cinnamate ester derivatives, KCED-1, KCED-2, as well as Seletinoid G are effective inducers of endogenous APN production in subcutaneous fat tissues, which may in turn contribute to the promotion of hair growth in the human scalp.

Keywords: adiponectin; adiponectin inducer; kojyl cinnamate ester derivative; adipogenesis; hair growth-related factor; human follicular dermal papilla cell

1. Introduction

Adipose tissue, an active metabolic and endocrine organ, plays important roles in physiological and pathological processes by secreting a variety of soluble factors [1]. Particularly, subcutaneous fat, a white adipose tissue beneath the skin dermis and the largest adipose tissue in the body, is involved in regulating body temperature and skin elasticity in normal states. However, its dysregulation is associated with abnormal states including obesity, which has impacts on skin physiology, skin manifestations, dermatologic diseases, and lipodystrophy [2–4], indicating the important functions of adipocytes or adipocyte-derived factors in skin pathophysiology.

Adiponectin (APN), along with leptin, is a key hormone that is exclusively released from white adipocytes including those in subcutaneous adipose tissue and is involved in regulating glucose levels, lipid metabolism, and insulin sensitivity [5,6]. Three types of receptor for APN have been verified: adiponectin receptor 1 (AdipoR1), AdipoR2, and T-cadherin. AdipoR1 and AdipoR2 are integral membrane proteins possessing seven-transmembrane domains; the N- and C-termini are internal and external, respectively. Both receptors bind to APNs, which exist in a trimer, a hexamer, and high-molecular weight 12- to 18-mer by combining via collagen domain at the N-terminus, and activate p38 MAPK, AMPK, and PPARα, thereby mediating APN-induced biological functions such as increased fatty acid oxidation, increased glucose uptake, and decreased gluconeogenesis [5,7]. T-cadherin is suggested to be important for APN-mediated cardioprotection [7]. Besides its roles in regulating energy metabolism, APN was recently reported to decrease ceramide and increase sphingosine-1 phosphate, thereby protecting from apoptosis [7,8], and to display in vitro hair growth-promoting effects on human hair follicles that express three types of APN receptors [9]. APN promotes hair shaft elongation in organ culture, and this effect is comparable to that of minoxidil, a representative drug for promoting hair growth. Although the stimulation of APN-associated hair growth signals via APN receptors has been suggested as a potential clinical strategy, synthetic APNs are expensive, thereby necessitating alternative methods.

Previously, we synthesized kojyl cinnamate ester derivatives (KCEDs) via the sequential reaction of kojic acid (KA) with thionyl chloride and then with 3,4-(methylenedioxy) cinnamic acid (CA), generating Seletinoid G (SG; Compound 4b) [10,11], which shows anti-aging activity and promotes APN production in adipose tissue-derived stem cells (ADSCs) [11,12]. Similar to SG, two derivatives (Compounds 4a and 4c) were verified to show improved activity for APN production during adipogenesis, importantly indicating that an α,β-unsaturated carbonyl ester structure and intact KA moiety in the derivatives are essential for promoting adipogenesis. Because of the insoluble nature of the three verified derivatives, we further screened new KCEDs that harbor an α,β-unsaturated carbonyl structure with KA moiety but were estimated to show high solubility. Finally, we selected two derivatives, KCED-1 and KCED-2, and in this study examined their potential to induce APN expression and adipogenesis using human subcutaneous fat cells (hSCFs). Furthermore, we investigated whether these two compounds could be used to promote APN-associated hair-growth signals in human follicular dermal papilla cells (hDPCs).

2. Results and Discussion

2.1. Selected Kojyl Cinnamate Ester Derivatives Show No Significant Effect On hSCF Viability

To determine the appropriate non-cytotoxic concentration of various compounds including SG and newly selected derivatives (KCED-1 and KCED-2) (Figure 1), hSCFs were treated with each compound and cell viability was measured at 24 and 72 h. KA and cinnamic acid (CA), which are structural moieties for KCEDs [10], and glibenclamide (GC), a well-known adiponectin inducer [13], were used as negative or positive controls. These control compounds did not cause severe changes in cell viability at tested concentrations (Figure 2). SG increased cell viability at concentrations ≤ 10 µM when treated for 24 h but decreased significantly at concentrations ≥ 5 µM at 72 h (Figure 2A). Compared with SG, KCED-1 and -2 increased cell viability at concentrations ≥ 10 µM at 24 h (Figure 2B,C). In particular, KCED-1 increased cell viability at concentrations of 25 µM and 50 µM even at 72 h, whereas SG and KCED-2 did not increase or decrease cell viability (Figure 2B,C), suggesting that KCED-1 and -2, and particularly KCED-1, are less toxic to the cells than SG. Although SG and KCED-2 showed significant cytotoxicity at some concentrations, according to ISO 10993-5, substances eliciting a cell viability above 80% are considered to be non-cytotoxic. Therefore, various concentrations (10 µM, 25 µM, and 50 µM) of these three compounds were applied for examining cellular effects.

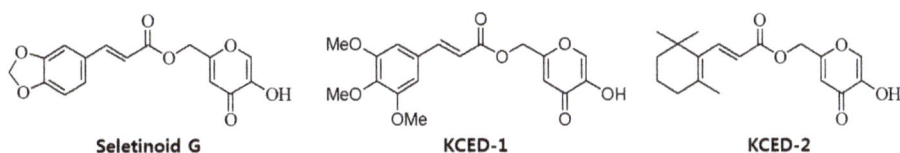

Figure 1. The structures of the kojyl cinnamate ester derivatives Seletinoid G, KCED-1, and KCED-2.

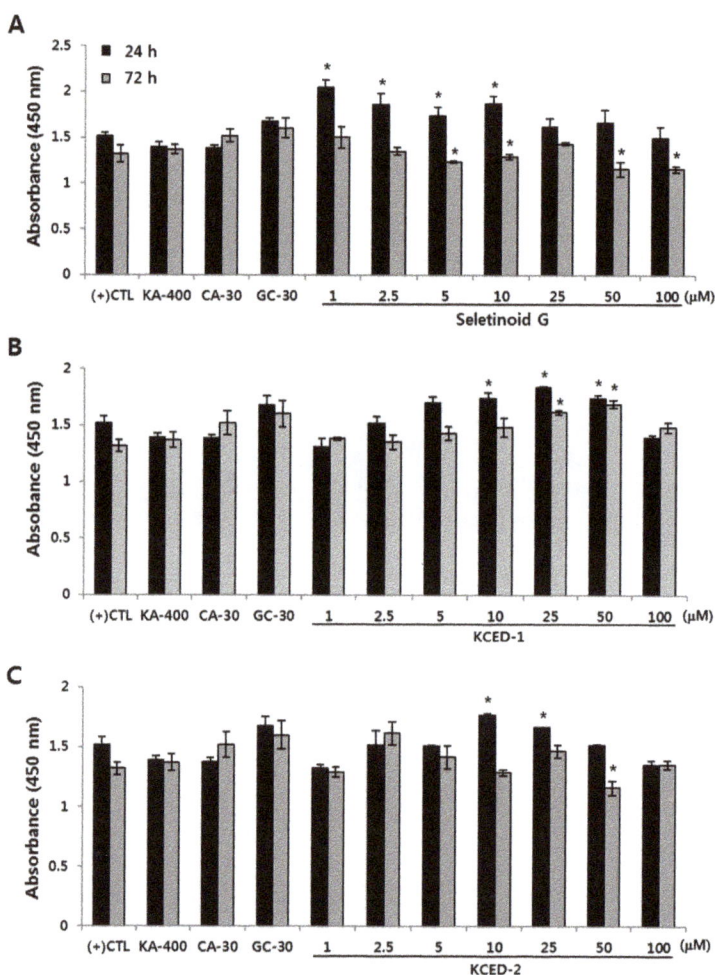

Figure 2. The effect of SG, KCED-1, and KCED-2 on cell viability of human subcutaneous fat cells (hSCFs). The hSCFs were treated with (**A**) SG, (**B**) KCED-1, and (**C**) KCED-2 for 24 or 72 h, after which the cell viability was analyzed. The data are presented as the mean ± SD (* $p < 0.05$). KA-400, kojic acid-400 μM; CA-30, cinnamic acid-30 μM; GC-30, glibenclamide-30 μM; CTL, control.

2.2. Selected Kojyl Cinnamate Ester Derivatives Induce mRNA Expression of APN

It is known that APN is released into the medium when adipocytes mature by forming lipid droplets in the cytosol [11,14]. To validate whether newly selected KCED-1 and -2 are effective in APN production and secretion, we treated the differentiated hSCFs with the compounds and examined the mRNA expression levels of APN. SG has the ability to differentiate adipocytes and promote APN production [11]; therefore, we compared the activities of the selected compounds with that of SG. The mRNA expression of APN gene (*ADIPOQ*) in hSCFs was greatly upregulated by treatments with SG, KCED-1, or KCED-2 in a dose-dependent manner compared with that of GC, the positive control for APN induction (Figure 3). KA and CA did not induce the mRNA expression of *ADIPOQ* significantly, and KCED-2 showed the strongest effect on increasing *ADIPOQ* levels at concentrations of 25 μM and 50 μM.

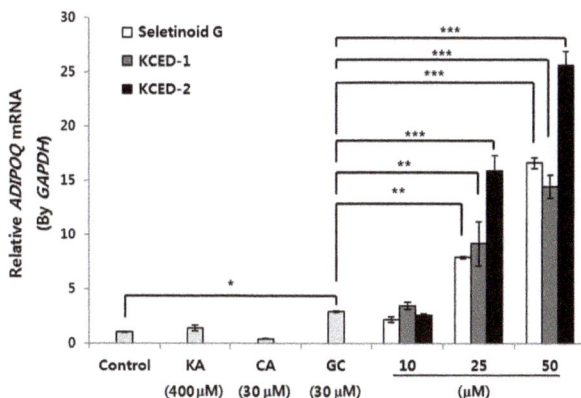

Figure 3. Upregulation of *ADIPOQ* mRNA expression by SG, KCED-1, and KCED-2 in hSCFs. The hSCFs were treated with the indicated concentration of each compound for 14 days, and the mRNA expression of *ADIPOQ* was analyzed by qRT-PCR. The data are presented as the mean ± SD (n = 3; $* p < 0.05$, $** p < 0.01$, and $*** p < 0.001$). KA, kojic acid; CA, cinnamic acid; GC, glibenclamide.

2.3. Selected Kojyl Cinnamate Ester Derivatives Promote APN Secretion and Stimulate Adipogenesis in hSCFs

Inspired by the dramatic increase in *ADIPOQ* mRNA levels, we determined the secreted protein levels of APN after treatments with SG, KCED-1, and KCED-2 during differentiation of hSCFs. Compared with the non-treated control, treatments with KA and GC, but not CA, increased the secretion of APN weakly but significantly (Figure 4A). Compared with GC, SG, KCED-1, and KCED-2 dramatically increased the APN secretion at concentrations of 25 μM and 50 μM. Consistent with the result in mRNA expression, KCED-2 treatment increased the APN secretion significantly at concentrations as low as 10 μM, which is one-third of the GC concentration, and showed the strongest effect on APN induction. APN is an essential factor in regulating lipid metabolism by inducing adipogenesis, fatty acid oxidation, and mitochondria biogenesis, thereby protecting obesity, insulin resistance, and type 2 diabetes [15–17]. We examined the degree of adipocyte differentiation by staining the lipid droplets formed after treatment with each compound. Compared with the non-treated control cells, where the lipid droplets were barely formed and stained, hSCFs treated with KA, CA, or GC showed weak but increased signals in Oil Red O staining, with GC showing the strongest signal among the three (Figure 4B). Compared with the effects of these compounds, hSCFs treated with SG, KCED-1, or KCED-2 showed remarkably increased signals in lipid staining in dose-dependent manners, indicating the increased formation of lipid droplets and strong adipogenesis by the KCEDs. Consistent with the results observed with induction of APN mRNA and protein levels, KCED-2 showed the stronger effect in inducing adipogenesis than SG and KCED-1, when considering the signal intensity at identical concentrations.

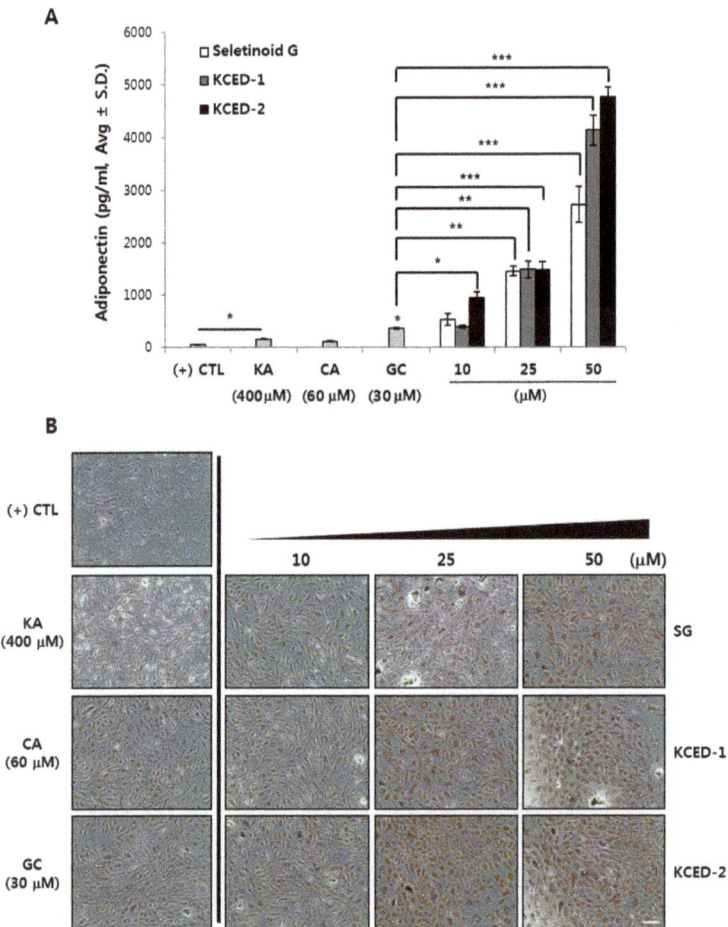

Figure 4. SG, KCED-1, and KCED-2 promote adiponectin secretion and stimulate adipogenesis in hSCFs. The hSCFs were pre-cultured for two days and differentiated for another 14 days using the differentiation medium supplemented with each compound. (**A**) The secreted APN levels were quantitatively determined using ELISA assay kit. The data are presented as the mean ± SD ($n = 3$; * $p < 0.05$, ** $p < 0.01$, and *** $p < 0.001$). (**B**) Lipids droplets were stained with Oil Red O dye. Scale bar, 200 μm.

2.4. APN-Containing Culture Supernatants Induce the Expression of Hair Growth-related Factors in Human Follicular Dermal Papilla Cells

Based on the previous report that APN shows hair growth-promoting effect on human hair follicles in vitro and ex vivo organ culture [9], APN has been suggested as a potential hair growth-promoting adipokine. Therefore, we investigated whether the hSCF-derived, APN-enriched conditioned media after treatments of SG, KCED-1, or KCED-2 could influence the expression of hair growth-related factors in hDPCs, which are known to express APN receptors [9]. Synthetic APN peptides were used as positive control and the treatment of these peptides significantly upregulated the mRNA expression of insulin-like growth factor 1 (*IGF-1*), vascular endothelial growth factor (*VEGF*), and hepatocyte growth factor (*HGF*), which were previously verified to be increased by APN in cultured hDPCs [9], compared with that seen in non-treated control (Figure 5). In contrast to these growth factors, transforming growth factor beta-1 (*TGF-β1*) was not significantly affected by APN peptides in our culture system, although it was reduced by APN treatment in hDPCs in previous study [9]. We treated hDPCs with various concentrations (5%, 10%, and 50%) of SG-, KCED-1-, or KCED-2-treated hSCF conditioned media for 48 h and examined the mRNA expression of hair growth-related factors. As expected, hDPCs showed increased mRNA levels of *IGF-1*, *VEGF*, and *HGF* in a concentration-dependent manner and the effects were comparable to those seen after APN peptide-treatment (Figure 5). *TGF-β1* mRNA levels were prone to be decreased weakly but relatively by the treatments of KCED-1-, KCED-2-treated, or 50% of SG-treated hSCF conditioned media compared with control treatment. These results suggest that SG-, KCED-1-, or KCED-2-treated hSCF media could contribute to hair growth promotion in vitro by stimulating hDPCs similar to treatment with APN.

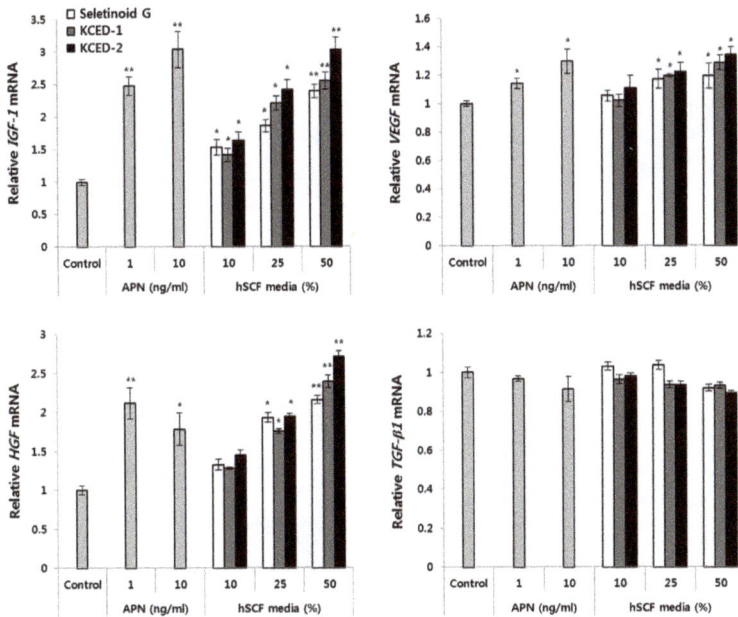

Figure 5. The SG-, KCED-1-, or KCED-2-treated hSCF media increase the mRNA levels of hair growth-related growth factors in hDPCs. The hDPCs were treated with different volumes of 50 μM SG-, KCED-1-, or KCED-2-treated hSCFs media for 48 h. The mRNA expression of hair growth-related growth factors was analyzed by RT-qPCR using respective Taqman probes. The data are presented as the mean ± SD ($n = 3$; * $p < 0.05$, ** $p < 0.01$).

Based on the APN amounts released by treatment of hSCFs with 50 μM SG, KCED-1, or KCED-2 (Figure 4A), the APN concentration in hDPC culture medium treated with 50% hSCF-conditioned medium was estimated to be in the range of about 1.5 to 2.5 ng/mL, which was comparable to those of APN peptides effectively upregulating the expression of hair growth-related factors (Figure 5). Besides APN, other secretory factors might be induced by SG, KCED-1, or KCED-2 treatments in hSCFs and contribute to hair growth promotion in hDPCs. Whether the enriched APNs in SG-, KCED-1-, or KCED-2-treated hSCF media are mainly involved in inducing mRNA expression of hair growth-related factors in hSCFs remains to be addressed using neutralizing antibodies or siRNAs against APN receptors. At least, SG, KCED-1, and KCED-2 did not seem to affect hair growth-related factors by themselves in hDPCs based on our preliminary examination.

There are several items of literature claiming that hair follicles (HFs) interact strongly with adipocytes in dermal white adipose tissue (dWAT) located in the superficial layer of the subcutaneous adipose tissue (sWAT) and that HF cycling correlates with spatiotemporal behavior of these adipocytes, i.e., it has different ratio of proliferation (preadipocyte) and differentiation (mature adipocyte) states [18–21], suggesting close interaction between HFs and dermal and subcutaneous WAT. Therefore, dermal adipocytes have been suggested as a potential target not only for counteracting skin aging but also for hair growth [21,22]. Interactions between HFs and adipocytes are expected to involve various soluble factors including microRNAs and possibly APN secreted from adipocytes from dermal and subcutaneous WAT. Extracellular vesicles containing exosome derived from skin adipocytes are also considered to be potent mediators reflecting local WAT contents, i.e., immature and mature states of adipocyte during the hair cycle [21]. Considering the three-dimensional structure of HF, which is surrounded by the epidermis, dermis, vessels, sebaceous gland, hair erector muscle, and dermal and subcutaneous WAT, the effects of APN and APN-enriched conditioned media derived from hSCFs on hair growth may be worthy of being evaluated via human HF organ culture. A schematic diagram for the roles of the kojyl cinnamate ester derivatives SG, KCED-1, and KCED-2 in adipogenesis and hair growth is illustrated in Figure 6. Given that intrinsic or extrinsic aging is known to correlate with a continuous reduction of WAT [22], we expect that kojyl cinnamate ester derivatives, as well as APN, could be also used as anti-aging agents by promoting adipogenesis of dermal and subcutaneous WAT.

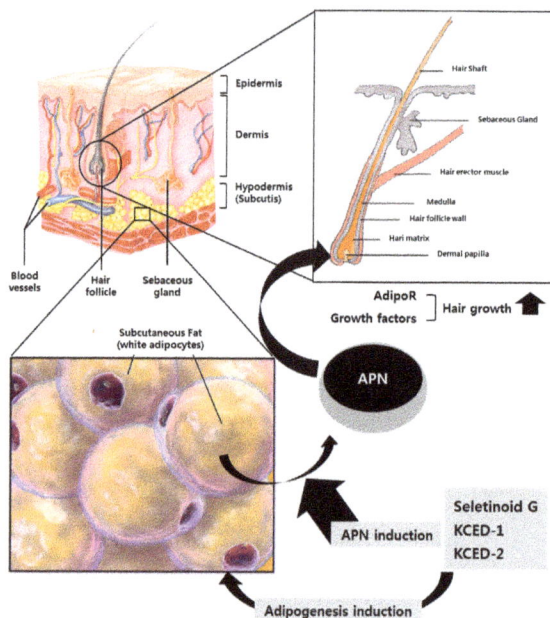

Figure 6. Schematic diagram illustrating the roles of kojyl cinnamate ester derivatives in adipogenesis and hair growth. Kojyl cinnamate ester derivatives including SG, KCED-1, and KCED-2 can promote adipogenesis and induction of *APN* mRNA levels and secretion of APN protein from human subcutaneous fat tissue. The secreted APN can promote hair growth via APN receptors.

3. Materials and Methods

3.1. Compounds

Seletinoid G [IUPAC name: (5-hydroxy-4-oxo-4H-pyran-2-yl)methyl (2E)-3-(2H-1,3-benzodioxol-5-yl)prop-2-enoate; Patent #, KR2016-0116831], kojyl cinnamate ester derivative-1 (KCED-1) [IUPAC name: 3-(3,4,5-Trimethoxy-phenyl)-acrylic acid 5-hydroxy-4-oxo-4*H*-pyran-2-ylmethyl ester] and KCED-2 [IUPAC name: 3-(2,6,6-Trimethyl-cyclohex-1-enyl)-acrylic acid 5-hydroxy-4-oxo-4Hpyran-2-ylmethyl ester] were synthesized and supplied by R&D Unit, Amorepacific Corp. (Yongin, South Korea). The structure of each compound is described in Figure 1. KA, CA, and GC were purchased from Sigma-Aldrich (St. Louis, MO, USA). Human adiponectin was purchased from ProSpec (Rehobot, Israel).

3.2. Cell Culture, Differentiation, and Compound Treatment

Human subcutaneous fat cells (hSCFs) representing subcutaneous preadipocytes (#SP-F-2) and Subcutaneous Preadipocyte Media were purchased from ZenBio Inc. (Research Triangle Park, NC, USA) and cultured in a humidified 5% CO_2 incubator. To induce differentiation, hSCFs in a confluency ≥95% were cultured in Dulbecco's modified Eagle's medium (DMEM; Lonza, Walkersville, MD, USA) supplemented with 10% fetal bovine serum (FBS; PAA, Pasching, Austria), 10 µg/mL insulin (Sigma-Aldrich, St. Louis, MO, USA), 0.5 mM 3-isobutyl-1-methylxanthine (IBMX; Sigma-Aldrich, St. Louis, MO, USA), 1 µM dexamethasone (DEX; Sigma-Aldrich, St. Louis, MO, USA), and 1 µM troglitazone (Sigma-Aldrich, St. Louis, MO, USA) for two days. The cells were further incubated in DMEM supplemented with 10% FBS and 10 µg/mL insulin with or without compounds for additional 14 days. The medium containing compounds was replaced every other day. Human follicular dermal papilla cells (hDPCs) and the culture medium were purchased from Cefobio Co. (Seoul, Korea). The hDPCs were cultured in a humidified 5% CO_2 incubator according to the manufacturer's instruction.

3.3. Cell Viability Assay

The hSCF viability was measured using EZ-Cytox Cell viability assay kit (MTT assay, Daeil lab Service, South Korea) according to the manufacturer's instructions. In brief, hSCFs were cultured for seven days and treated with various concentrations of each chemical (SG, KCED-1, KCED-2) for 24 and 72 h. EZ-Cytox solution (10 µL) was added to each well and incubated at 37 °C for 2 h. Absorbance at 450 nm was measured using a spectrophotometer (Synergy H2, BioTek., Winooski, VT, USA). All experiments were triplicated and the data are presented as the absorbance.

3.4. Quantitative Real-time PCR (RT-qPCR)

Total RNA was extracted using TRIzol reagent (Life Technologies, Carlsbad, CA, USA) according to the manufacturer's instructions. One µg of total RNA was utilized to synthesize cDNAs using the RevertAid First Strand cDNA Synthesis kit (Thermo Scientific, Waltham, MA, USA). One µg of cDNA sample was subjected to PCR analysis using each TaqMan® probe (Life Technologies, Carlsbad, CA, USA), Quantitect Probe PCR kit (Qiagen, Valencia, CA, USA), and the 7500 fast real-time PCR system (Life Technologies, Carlsbad, CA, USA). Each TaqMan® probe was as follows: Adiponectin (*ADIPOQ*; #Hs00605917_m1), insulin-like growth factor 1 (*IGF-1*; #Hs01547656_m1), vascular endothelial growth factor (*VEGF*; #Hs00900055_m1), hepatocyte growth factor (*HGF*; #Hs00300159_m1), transforming growth factor β-1 (*TGF-β1*; #Hs00998133_m1), and glyceraldehyde-3-phosphate dehydrogenase (*GAPDH*; #4352339E). All data were acquired from three independent experiments and are presented as a fold change relative to the *GAPDH* control.

3.5. ELISA Assay for Secreted Adiponectin

The hSCFs were treated with various concentrations of each chemical (SG, KCED-1, and KCED-2) and differentiated for 14 days. The culture medium was collected and centrifuged at 13,000 rpm for 15 min to remove any debris. The secreted adiponectin was measured using adiponectin ELISA kit (Enzo Life Sciences, Farmingdale, NY, USA), following the manufacturer's instructions.

3.6. Oil Red O Staining

The differentiated hSCFs were washed twice with cold PBS and fixed with 3.7% formaldehyde (Sigma-Aldrich, St. Louis, MO, USA) for 1 h. The fixed cells were washed with 60% propylene glycol

(Sigma-Aldrich, St. Louis, MO, USA) in PBS and were stained with a working solution of Oil Red O (ORO; 0.3% ORO in 60% propylene glycol; Sigma-Aldrich, St. Louis, MO, USA) for 30 min. The cells were washed with 85% propylene glycol thrice and rinsed with tap water. Lipid droplets stained with ORO dye were visualized with an IX71 microscope (Olympus, Tokyo, Japan).

3.7. Statistical Analysis

All data are presented as the mean ± SD. Two-tailed Student's *t*-tests were used to analyze the differences between pairs of groups, and the threshold for statistical significance was set at 0.05 (* $p < 0.05$). Multiple groups were analyzed with one-way ANOVA.

4. Conclusions

We demonstrated that the kojyl cinnamate ester derivatives including SG, KCED-1, and KCED-2 induce APN production in vitro and stimulate adipogenesis in hSCFs. In addition, SG-, KCED-1-, or KCED-2-treated hSCF media increased the mRNA levels of hair growth-related growth factors in hDPCs. Based on our observations, we propose that SG, KCED-1, and KCED-2 are potent APN inducers and could be used in cosmetic and dermatological products for regulating adipogenesis in subcutaneous fat tissue and for promoting hair growth through stimulation of APN-associated hair growth signaling.

Author Contributions: P.J.P. conceived and designed the experiments. P.J.P. performed the experiments. P.J.P. and E.-G.C. analyzed the data. P.J.P. and E.-G.C. wrote the paper.

Funding: This research received no external funding.

Acknowledgments: None.

Conflicts of Interest: P.J.P. and E.-G.C. are employees of Amorepacific corporation.

Abbreviations

APN	Adiponectin
KCED	Kojyl cinnamate ester derivative
hSCFs	Human subcutaneous fat cells
AdioR	Adiponectin receptor
hDPCs	Human follicular dermal papilla cells
SG	Seletinoid G
ADSCs	Adipose tissue-derived stem cells
KA	Kojic acid
CA	Cinnamic acid
GC	Glibenclamide
IGF-1	Insulin-like growth factor 1
VEGF	Vascular endothelial growth factor
HGF	Hepatocyte growth factor
TGF-β1	Transforming growth factor β-1
HF	Hair follicle
dWAT	Dermal white adipose tissue
sWAT	Subcutaneous white adipose tissue

References

1. Kershaw, E.E.; Flier, J.S. Adipose tissue as an endocrine organ. *J. Clin. Endocrinol. Metab.* **2004**, *89*, 2548–2556. [CrossRef]
2. Avram, M.M.; Avram, A.S.; James, W.D. Subcutaneous fat in normal and diseased states: 1. Introduction. *J. Am. Acad. Dermatol.* **2005**, *53*, 663–670. [CrossRef]
3. Yosipovitch, G.; DeVore, A.; Dawn, A. Obesity and the skin: Skin physiology and skin manifestations of obesity. *J. Am. Acad. Dermatol.* **2007**, *56*, 901–916, quiz 917–920. [CrossRef] [PubMed]

4.   Ezure, T.; Amano, S. Influence of subcutaneous adipose tissue mass on dermal elasticity and sagging severity in lower cheek. *Skin Res. Technol.* **2010**, *16*, 332–338. [CrossRef] [PubMed]
5.   Kadowaki, T.; Yamauchi, T.; Kubota, N.; Hara, K.; Ueki, K.; Tobe, K. Adiponectin and adiponectin receptors in insulin resistance, diabetes, and the metabolic syndrome. *J. Clin. Invest.* **2006**, *116*, 1784–1792. [CrossRef]
6.   Lafontan, M.; Viguerie, N. Role of adipokines in the control of energy metabolism: Focus on adiponectin. *Curr. Opin. Pharmacol.* **2006**, *6*, 580–585. [CrossRef]
7.   Yamauchi, T.; Iwabu, M.; Okada-Iwabu, M.; Kadowaki, T. Adiponectin receptors: A review of their structure, function and how they work. *Best Pract. Res. Clin. Endocrinol. Metab.* **2014**, *28*, 15–23. [CrossRef] [PubMed]
8.   Holland, W.L.; Miller, R.A.; Wang, Z.V.; Sun, K.; Barth, B.M.; Bui, H.H.; Davis, K.E.; Bikman, B.T.; Halberg, N.; Rutkowski, J.M.; et al. Receptor-mediated activation of ceramidase activity initiates the pleiotropic actions of adiponectin. *Nat. Med.* **2011**, *17*, 55–63. [CrossRef] [PubMed]
9.   Won, C.H.; Yoo, H.G.; Park, K.Y.; Shin, S.H.; Park, W.S.; Park, P.J.; Chung, J.H.; Kwon, O.S.; Kim, K.H. Hair growth-promoting effects of adiponectin in vitro. *J. Invest. Dermatol.* **2012**, *132*, 2849–2851. [CrossRef] [PubMed]
10. Cho, J.C.; Rho, H.S.; Baek, H.S.; Ahn, S.M.; Woo, B.Y.; Hong, Y.D.; Cheon, J.W.; Heo, J.M.; Shin, S.S.; Park, Y.H.; et al. Depigmenting activity of new kojic acid derivative obtained as a side product in the synthesis of cinnamate of kojic acid. *Bioorg. Med. Chem. Lett.* **2012**, *22*, 2004–2007. [CrossRef]
11. Rho, H.S.; Hong, S.H.; Park, J.; Jung, H.I.; Park, Y.H.; Lee, J.H.; Shin, S.S.; Noh, M. Kojyl cinnamate ester derivatives promote adiponectin production during adipogenesis in human adipose tissue-derived mesenchymal stem cells. *Bioorg. Med. Chem. Lett.* **2014**, *24*, 2141–2145. [CrossRef] [PubMed]
12. Kim, M.S.; Lee, S.; Rho, H.S.; Kim, D.H.; Chang, I.S.; Chung, J.H. The effects of a novel synthetic retinoid, seletinoid G, on the expression of extracellular matrix proteins in aged human skin in vivo. *Clin. Chim. Acta* **2005**, *362*, 161–169. [CrossRef] [PubMed]
13. Ahmadi, A.; Khalili, M.; Khatami, K.; Farsadrooh, M.; Nahri-Niknafs, B. Synthesis and investigating hypoglycemic and hypolipidemic activities of some glibenclamide analogues in rats. *Mini Rev. Med. Chem.* **2014**, *14*, 208–213. [CrossRef] [PubMed]
14. Guerre-Millo, M. Adiponectin: An update. *Diabetes Metab.* **2008**, *34*, 12–18. [CrossRef] [PubMed]
15. Iwabu, M.; Yamauchi, T.; Okada-Iwabu, M.; Sato, K.; Nakagawa, T.; Funata, M.; Yamaguchi, M.; Namiki, S.; Nakayama, R.; Tabata, M.; et al. Adiponectin and AdipoR1 regulate PGC1α and mitochondria by Ca^{2+} and AMPK/SIRT1. *Nature* **2010**, *464*, 1313–1319. [CrossRef]
16. Kadowaki, T.; Yamauchi, T.; Waki, H.; Iwabu, M.; Okada-Iwabu, M.; Nakamura, M. Adiponectin, adiponectin receptors, and epigenetic regulation of adipogenesis. *Cold Spring Harb. Symp. Quant. Biol.* **2011**, *76*, 257–265. [CrossRef] [PubMed]
17. Tao, C.; Sifuentes, A.; Holland, W.L. Regulation of glucose and lipid homeostasis by adiponectin: Effects on hepatocytes, pancreatic β cells and adipocytes. *Best Pract. Res. Clin. Endocrinol. Metab.* **2014**, *28*, 43–58. [CrossRef]
18. Festa, E.; Fretz, J.; Berry, R.; Schmidt, B.; Rodeheffer, M.; Horowitz, M.; Horsley, V. Adipocyte lineage cells contribute to the skin stem cell niche to drive hair cycling. *Cell* **2011**, *146*, 761–771. [CrossRef]
19. Guerrero-Juarez, C.F.; Plikus, M.V. Emerging nonmetabolic functions of skin fat. *Nat. Rev. Endocrinol.* **2018**, *14*, 163–173. [CrossRef]
20. Kruglikov, I.L.; Scherer, P.E. Dermal adipocytes and hair cycling: Is spatial heterogeneity a characteristic feature of the dermal adipose tissue depot? *Exp. Dermatol.* **2016**, *25*, 258–262. [CrossRef]
21. Kruglikov, I.L.; Zhang, Z.; Scherer, P.E. The Role of Immature and Mature Adipocytes in Hair Cycling. *Trends Endocrinol. Metab.* **2019**, *30*, 93–105. [CrossRef] [PubMed]
22. Kruglikov, I.L.; Scherer, P.E. Skin aging: Are adipocytes the next target? *Aging (Albany NY)* **2016**, *8*, 1457–1469. [CrossRef] [PubMed]

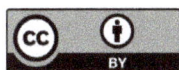

International Journal of
Molecular Sciences

MDPI

Article

Interaction of Nerve Growth Factor β with Adiponectin and SPARC Oppositely Modulates its Biological Activity

Yuu Okura [1], Takeshi Imao [1], Seisuke Murashima [1], Haruki Shibata [2], Akihiro Kamikavwa [1], Yuko Okamatsu-Ogura [1], Masayuki Saito [1] and Kazuhiro Kimura [1,*]

[1] Department of Biomedical Sciences, Graduate School of Veterinary Medicine, Hokkaido University, Sapporo 060-0818, Japan; okura.yuu@icloud.com (Y.O.); t-imao@mfour.med.kyoto-u.ac.jp (T.I.); murashima@daktari.info (S.M.); akami@obihiro.ac.jp (A.K.); y-okamatsu@vetmed.hokudai.ac.jp (Y.O.-O.); ms-consa@krf.biglobe.ne.jp (M.S.)

[2] Morinaga Institute of Biological Science, Yokohama 236-0003, Japan; h.shibata@miobs.com

* Correspondence: k-kimura@vetmed.hokudai.ac.jp; Tel./Fax: +81-11-757-0703

Received: 2 March 2019; Accepted: 25 March 2019; Published: 27 March 2019

Abstract: Both adiponectin and secreted protein, acidic and rich in cysteine (SPARC) inhibit platelet-derived growth factor-BB (PDGF-BB)-induced and basic fibroblast growth factor (FGF2)-induced angiogenic activities through direct and indirect interactions. Although SPARC enhances nerve growth factor (NGF)-dependent neurogenesis, the physical interaction of NGFβ with adiponectin and SPARC remains obscure. Therefore, we first examined their intermolecular interaction by surface plasmon resonance method. NGFβ bound to immobilized SPARC with the binding constant of 59.4 nM, comparable with that of PDGF-BB (24.5 nM) but far less than that of FGF2 (14.4 µM). NGFβ bound to immobilized full length adiponectin with the binding constant of 103 nM, slightly higher than those of PDGF-BB (24.3 nM) and FGF2 (80.2 nM), respectively. Treatment of PC12 cells with SPARC did not cause mitogen-activated protein kinase (MAPK) activation and neurite outgrowth. However, simultaneous addition of SPARC with NGFβ enhanced NGFβ-induced MAPK phosphorylation and neurite outgrowth. Treatment of the cells with adiponectin increased AMP-activated protein kinase (AMPK) phosphorylation but failed to induce neurite outgrowth. Simultaneous treatment with NGFβ and adiponectin significantly reduced cell size and the number of cells with neurite, even after silencing the adiponectin receptors by their siRNA. These results indicate that NGFβ directly interacts with adiponectin and SPARC, whereas these interactions oppositely regulate NGFβ functions.

Keywords: adiponectin; AMPK; BIAcore; extracellular signal-regulated kinase (ERK); matricellular proteins; neuritogenesis; NGFβ; PC12 cells; Secreted protein; acidic and rich in cysteine (SPARC)

1. Introduction

Adiponectin, a member of the C1q/tumor necrosis factor (TNF)-related proteins, is secreted exclusively by adipocytes. Circulating adiponectin exists in several homo-oligomeric forms consisting of elemental homo-trimeric subunit with a collagen-like triple-helical structure [1–4] and its levels are lower in obese subjects compared with lean subjects [5]. Subjects carrying a missense mutation in the adiponectin gene associated with hypo-adiponectinemia exhibit the phenotype of the metabolic syndrome, including insulin resistance and coronary artery disease [1–4,6]. Administration of adiponectin has been shown to be beneficial in animal models of diabetes, obesity and atherosclerosis [1–4,6].

The hallmark of atherosclerosis is the uncontrolled proliferation and migration of vascular smooth muscle cells, resulting in thickening of the vascular wall [7]. Physiological concentrations of adiponectin significantly suppress both the proliferation and migration of vascular smooth muscle cells induced by platelet-derived growth factor (PDGF)-BB, through direct interaction between adiponectin and PDGF-BB [8]. Moreover, it was also shown that adiponectin binds with basic fibroblast growth factor (FGF2), thereby precluding the biological activity [9].

Matricellular proteins are defined as extracellular matrix (ECM)-associated proteins that have no structural roles in ECM-like collagens and laminins. Secreted protein, acidic and rich in cysteine (SPARC), also known as osteonectin and BM-40, is a collagen-binding matricellular protein that regulates tissue remodeling and repair, morphogenesis and angiogenesis in vivo [10,11]. SPARC also plays pivotal roles in altering cancer cell activity and the microenvironment of tumors as well as in the pathologies of obesity and diabetes [12–14]. Some SPARC functions are mediated by its binding to target molecules and alterations in their biological functions. For example, like adiponectin, SPARC binds to PDGF-AB and PDGF-BB, resulting in inhibiting the ligand binding to their receptors [15]. However, SPARC influences biological activities of FGF2 not through their direct binding [10,16].

SPARC protein has been detected in the brain, mainly in glia and astrocytes [17]. Although no obvious neural defects were observed in SPARC null mice [18], recent findings suggest that SPARC is involved in synaptogenesis [19] and synapse elimination [20] as well as nerve growth factor (NGF)-dependent neurite outgrowth [21,22] and axon regeneration [23]. However, it remains unclear whether SPARC directly interacts with NGF.

NGF is a member of a family of neurotrophic factors, which is responsible for the survival, development and function of basal forebrain cholinergic neuron in the central nervous system and of peripheral sympathetic and embryonic sensory neurons [24]. NGF gene is also expressed in white adipose tissues [25]. NGF expression and secretion in 3T3-L1 adipocyte culture are markedly increased in response to inflammatory cytokine such as TNF [25]. Moreover, circulating NGF levels are upregulated in a group of women with obesity and metabolic syndrome, which are related to a low-grade systemic inflammation [26,27]. As NGF modulates various immune cell functions [28,29], it is likely that NGF plays roles as an inflammatory mediator in adipose tissues, in addition to roles as a neurotrophic factor.

It currently remains unclear whether adiponectin affect biological activity of NGF through physical interaction. Therefore, we examined the interactions of adiponectin and SPARC with NGF using a surface plasmon resonance (SPR) method and their effects on NGF-dependent morphological changes in PC12 rat pheochromocytoma.

2. Results

The interactions of PDGF-BB and FGF2 with SPRAC were examined using the SPR method. Infusion of different doses of two growth factors on the surface of immobilized SPARC increased RU, reflecting their binding to the ligand, while the cessation of this infusion decreased RU, reflecting their dissociation from the ligand (Figure S1). An analysis of binding kinetics revealed that K_D of PDGF-BB was 24.3 nM, while that of FGF2 was 14.4 µM, triple-digit difference from the former (Table 1). On the other hand, the infusion of increasing concentrations of NGFβ gave clear sensorgrams with a K_D of 59.4 nM, comparable with that of PDGF-BB.

Table 1. Summary of analyte binding to SPARC.

Analytes	Association Constant (ka)	Dissociation Constant (kd)	Binding Constant (K_D = kd/ka)
PDGF-BB	3.71×10^4	9.03×10^{-4}	2.43×10^{-8}
VEGF-165	7.58×10^4	4.13×10^{-3}	5.44×10^{-8}
FGF2	1.35×10^2	1.95×10^{-3}	1.44×10^{-5}
TGFβ1	7.90×10^2	1.92×10^{-2}	2.43×10^{-5}
NGFβ	1.86×10^5	1.10×10^{-2}	5.94×10^{-8}

Interactions of PDGF-BB and FGF2 with full length adiponectin were also examined and found the K_D of PDGF-BB and FGF2 were 24.5 nM and 80.2 nM, respectively (Figure S2, Table 2). Infusion of NGFβ but not the boiled protein, increased RU in a dose-dependent manner. The K_D of NGFβ to adiponectin was 103 nM, comparable to those of PDGF-BB and FGF2. To determine whether the interactions of growth factors with full length adiponectin occurred through its globular region, the SPR analyses with globular adiponectin-immobilized chip were performed. Both PDGF-BB and NGFβ bound selectively to the chip with K_D of 70.4 nM and 1260 nM, respectively (Figure S2, Table 2).

In order to investigate the effects of the NGFβ and SPARC interaction on NGFβ-induced neuronal differentiation of PC12 rat pheochromocytoma, we initially examined the NGFβ-dependent activation of p44/p42 MAPK (ERK1/2) as its phosphorylated state. In the cells, among the neurotrophin receptor genes, mRNAs of TrkA, TrkC and p75NTR but not TrkB were detected (Figure S3A). Addition of NGFβ to the PC12 culture for 10 min dose-dependently induced the phosphorylation of ERK1/2, whereas neurotrophin (NT)-3 and NT4 failed to stimulate its phosphorylation (Figure S3B), suggesting that NGFβ activates the ERK signal through a TrkA neurotrophin receptor. Addition of SPARC alone did not change the phosphorylated state of ERK1/2 (Figure 1A). However, simultaneous addition of SPARC with NGFβ enhanced NGFβ-induced ERK1/2 phosphorylation. Similar to this short-term synergistic effect of SPARC and NGF, simultaneous addition of both for 96 h enhanced NGF-induced neurite outgrowth; however, SPARC alone did not influence neuritogenesis (Figure 1B).

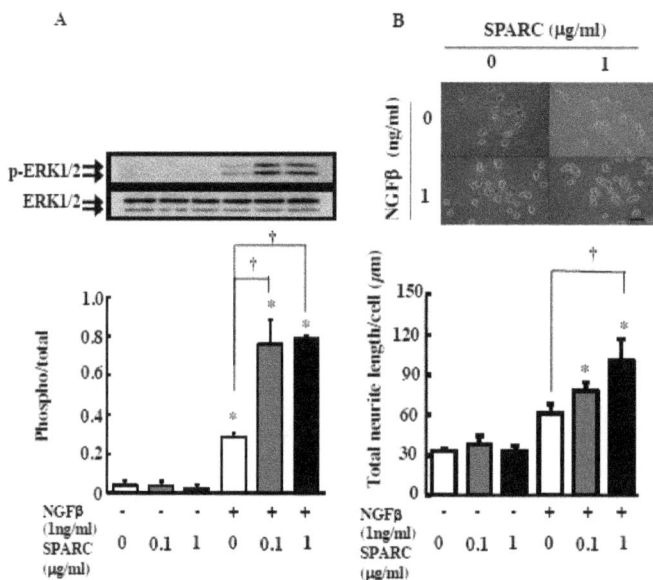

Figure 1. SPARC enhances NGFβ-dependent ERK activation and neurite outgrowth in PC12 cells. (**A**) PC12 cells were treated with NGFβ (1 ng/mL) in the presence or absence of SPARC (0.1 or 1 µg/mL) for 10 min. Representative results of Western blots for ERK and its phosphorylation are shown in the upper panel, Results from four independent experiments are summarized in the bottom panel. (**B**) PC12 cells were treated with or without NGFβ (0 or 1 ng/mL) either in the presence or absence of SPARC (0.1 or 1 µg/mL) for 96 h. Representative results of cells with neurites are shown in the upper panel and results (total neurite length per cell) from three independent experiments are summarized in the bottom. The length of the scale bar in the picture is 50 µm. * and † indicate significant differences ($p < 0.05$) between *no* NGFβ treatment (0 ng/mL) vs NGF treated and *no* SPARC treatment (0 µg/mL) vs SPARC treated, respectively.

Table 2. Summary of analyte binding to adiponectin.

Analytes	Association Constant (ka)	Dissociation Constant (kd)	Binding Constant (K_D = kd/ka)
	(ligand: full length adiponectin)		
PDGF-BB	1.15×10^3	2.82×10^{-5}	2.45×10^{-8}
FGF2	7.16×10^2	5.76×10^{-5}	8.02×10^{-8}
NGFβ	5.76×10^4	5.97×10^{-3}	1.03×10^{-7}
	(ligand: globular adiponectin)		
PDGF-BB	1.05×10^5	7.38×10^{-3}	7.04×10^{-8}
NGFβ	1.15×10^4	1.45×10^{-2}	1.26×10^{-6}

We next examined the interaction between NGFβ and adiponectin in the physiological condition. PC12 cells treated with NGFβ induced neurite outgrowth as well as enlargement of cell size, while the cells treated with full length adiponectin or globular adiponectin alone did not (Figure 2A). The cells treated simultaneously with NGFβ and full length adiponectin induced morphological changes of the cells but the degrees of neurite outgrowth (Figure 2B,C) and cell enlargement (Figure 2D) were significantly decreased, compared with those of low-dose NGFβ alone (e.g., 1ng/mL). It is interesting to note that full length adiponectin failed to suppress high-dose NGFβ (20 ng/mL)-induced number of cells with neurite (Figure 2A,B). Simultaneous addition of NGFβ and globular adiponectin also suppressed morphological changes of the cells in some cases but the magnitudes of suppression by globular adiponectin, if present, were less than those induced by full length adiponectin (Figure 2B–D).

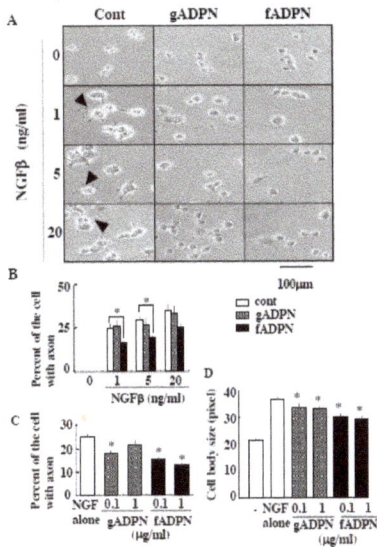

Figure 2. Adiponectin suppressed NGFβ-induced neurite outgrowth and cell swelling. (**A,B**) PC12 cells were treated with increasing concentration of NGFβ either in the presence or absence of full-length adiponectin (fADPN, 1 µg/mL) and globular adiponectin (gADPN, 1 µg/mL). Representative results of the cells (arrowhead: neurite) are shown in A and results (percentage of the cells with axon) from five independent experiments are summarized in B. (**C,D**) PC12 cells were treated with NGFβ (1 ng/mL) either in the presence or absence of full length adiponectin and globular adiponectin (0.1 and 1 g/mL). The ratio of the cell with axon (**C**) and the changes in cell body size (**D**) are determined and summarized from three independent experiments. * indicates the statistically significant difference ($p < 0.05$) from NGFβ treatment alone (Cont).

RT-PCR analysis was performed on adiponectin receptors in PC12 cells. As shown in Figure 3A, both AdipoR1 and AdipoR2 mRNA were detected. The cells treated with either full length or globular adiponectin alone did enhance the activity-related site-specific phosphorylation of AMP-activated protein kinase (AMPK) α (Figure 3B), indicating the PC12 cells expresses two types of functional adiponectin receptors. To examine whether these receptors' activation was necessary for the adiponectin inhibition of NGFβ functions, we tested the effect of adiponectin on NGFβ-induced neurite outgrowth in the AdipoR1- and/or AdipoR2-silenced PC12 cells. Transfection of siRNA for either AdipoR1, AdipoR2 or both successfully silenced the respective receptors in mRNA levels (Figure 3C) and AMPK activation (Figure 3D). Treatment of PC12 cells with NGFβ, irrespective of silencing of either AdipoR1 or AdipoR2, induced neurite outgrowth and the addition of full length adiponectin suppressed the effect of NGFβ (Figure 3E).

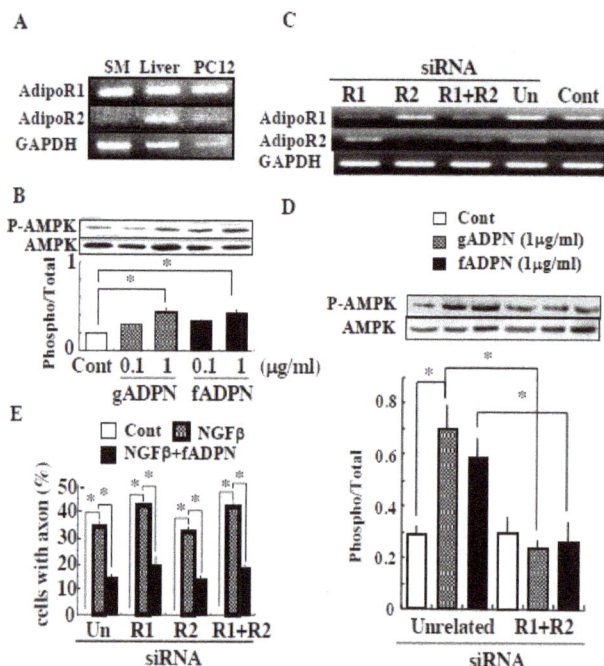

Figure 3. Adiponectin suppressed NGFβ-induced neurite outgrowth independently of its receptor activation. (**A**) Expression of AdipoR1 and AdipoR2 mRNA in the rat skeletal muscle (SM), liver and PC12 cells are shown. (**B**) PC12 cells were treated with full length adiponectin or globular adiponectin and the amounts of phosphorylated and total AMPK were determined. Representative results and the ratio of phosphorylated and total AMPK are shown ($n = 5$). (**C–E**) PC12 cells were treated with unrelated (un), AdipoR1, AdipoR2 and R1 plus R2 siRNA and (**C**) mRNA expression of AdipoR1 and AdipoR2 are shown. (**D**) The transfected cells were treated with vehicle (cont.), globular adiponectin (1 μg/mL) and full length adiponectin (1 μg/mL) and the state of AMPK activation are shown ($n = 3$). (**E**) The transfected cells were treated with vehicle (cont.), NGFβ (1 ng/mL) or NGFβ plus full length adiponectin (1 μg/mL) and the ratios of the cell with axon are shown ($n = 3$). The transfected cells treated with vehicle did not induce any neurite (axon) as shown in Figure 2A and the ratio calculated was 0 as in Figure 2B. Thus, bar for control value of each siRNA was not seen. * indicates the statistically significant difference ($p < 0.05$) from cont. or NGFβ treatment alone.

3. Discussion

In the present study, we showed the apparent interaction of SPARC with NGFβ, PDGF-BB and FGF2 with the K_D of 59.4 nM, 24.3 nM and 14.4 μM, respectively. As SPARC is reported to interfere with FGF2-induced functions not through direct binding [16], the interaction between SPARC and FGF2 on the sensor chip was unexpected although its K_D value was a triple-digit difference from those of two other growth factors tested. Since in vitro binding studies between SPARC and FGF2 were performed by using the RIPA buffer containing various detergents during the washing procedure, this weak interaction might be masked. Similarly, no apparent binding of SPARC to transforming growth factor (TGF) β1 is reported by in vitro binding assay [30]. However, we observed weak interaction between SPARC and TGFβ1 with the K_D of 24.3 μM. This weak interaction might also contribute to chimeric TGF-receptor II binding to SPARC, as the binding occurred only in the presence of TGFβ1 [30]. In contrast, it is reported that SPARC prevents PDGF-induced and vascular endothelial growth factor (VEGF)-induced biological activities through their direct interactions [31]. SPR analysis revealed that SPARC interacted selectively with VEGF-165 with the K_D of 54.4 nM. As the K_D between SPARC and NGFβ is almost the same as those of PDGF-BB and VEGF-165, direct binding of NGFβ to SPARC might be able to influence NGF activity.

Similarly, we demonstrated that NGFβ but not denatured NGFβ by boiling, bound to full length adiponectin with the K_D of 103 nM, while those of PDGF-BB and FGF2 were 24.5 nM and 80.2 nM, respectively. Different from SPARC, it is reported that adiponectin binds with FGF2 as well as PDGF-BB, thereby precluding their biological activity [8,9]. As the interaction between NGFβ and adiponectin shows comparative K_D value with those of PDGF-BB and FGF2, the interaction might also modulate NGF activity. We also showed that NGFβ bound to globular adiponectin with much greater reduction of K_D value (>10-fold), compared with its binding to full length adiponectin. As the K_D values between PDGF-BB and either adiponectin were relatively unchanged (<3-fold), it is likely that trimeric or a much higher dimensional structure of adiponectin might be necessary for NGFβ interaction. This lower ability to bind NGFβ may lead to weaker suppressive activity by globular adiponectin of NGFβ function.

NGFβ binds to two different receptors: the TrkA tyrosine kinase receptor with high affinity and the p75 NTR with low affinity [32]. In PC12 cells, NGFβ activates the ERK signal through the TrkA, that leading to neurite outgrowth [33]. In the present study, we confirmed the NGFβ activities, whereas SPARC alone did not change the phosphorylated state of ERK1/2 and subsequent neuritogenesis. However, simultaneous addition of SPARC with NGFβ enhanced NGFβ-induced ERK1/2 phosphorylation and NGFβ-induced neurite outgrowth. This synergistic effect of SPARC and NGF on neurite outgrowth was also found in superior cervical ganglion neurons and Schwann cells [21,22]. The basal forebrain cholinergic system is one of the target neuronal networks for NGF as a survival factor of cholinergic neurons [24]. NGF is also involved in nurturing the peripheral nervous system [34]. On the other hand, SPARC in the brain is suggested to facilitate cholinergic synapse formation [35], whereas other studies show that SPARC antagonizes the synaptogenesis by having, another matricellular protein [19] and triggers a cell-autonomous program of synapse elimination in cholinergic neurons [20]. Collectively, the present results suggest that a direct interaction between SPARC and NGFβ enhances the biological activity of this growth factor in the central and peripheral nervous systems. However, the mechanism by which the SPARC and NGFβ interaction enhanced NGF-signals remains obscure and further works are needed to clarify it.

PC12 cells treated with full length adiponectin alone did not induce any morphological changes, while it activated intracellular signal such as AMPK. The cells treated simultaneously with NGFβ and full length adiponectin induced neurite outgrowth and cell swelling but the degrees of the changes were significantly less than those of NGFβ alone. In addition, increasing the concentration of NGFβ prevented suppression by the constant amount of adiponectin, suggesting that at high concentrations of NGF, excess unbound NGFβ is able to induce neuritogenesis. Moreover, as this adiponectin suppression of NGFβ-dependent morphological changes were seen even after silencing adiponectin receptor signaling in PC12 cells, therefore our present results indicate that full length adiponectin interacts with NGFβ, thereby inhibits NGFβ functions, possibly through interfering its interaction with TrkA, in contrast to SPARC.

The physiological relevance of full length adiponectin and NGF interaction remains to be elucidated. However, it is interesting to note that NGF production in adipocytes is enhanced and adiponectin production is suppressed, by inflammatory stimuli like TNF [25]. In addition, proteases secreted from activated monocytes and/or neutrophils cleave full-length adiponectin to generate globular adiponectin [36]. Supportively, blood NGF levels are upregulated in a group of women with obesity and the metabolic syndrome [26,27], while circulating adiponectin levels are lower in obese subjects [27]. Therefore, in an adipose tissue from obese subjects where inflammation develops, it is likely to occur that the amounts of NGF and full length adiponectin are increased and decreased, respectively and as a consequence dominance of NGF over adiponectin becomes clear. Furthermore, the expression of SPARC is increased in the adipose tissue of obese animals [14]. In such conditions, NGF and SPARC interaction is expected to facilitate recruitment and activation of mast cells [37], that sustain chronic low-grade inflammation within adipose tissue [38] (see also Figure S4). In an adipose tissue from lean subjects, it is plausible that locally produced NGF is associated with full length adiponectin, resulting in the masking of NGF bioactivity (Figure S4).

In summary, we showed that NGFβ interacted substantially with both SPARC and full length adiponectin and that SPARC enhanced, but adiponectin suppressed, NGFβ-dependent function in PC12 cells. Other than a neurotrophic factor, NGF plays roles in obesity-related inflammation as described above, in the proliferation and survival of various cancers [39,40] and in pain control [41]. Further works should be undertaken to investigate the involvement of NGF interactions with adiponectin and/or SPARC in each NGF-mediated process in detail.

4. Materials and Methods

4.1. Materials

Recombinant murine full-length adiponectin was purchased from Biovender Laboratory Medicine, Inc. (Bmo, Czech Republic), while recombinant murine globular adiponectin and recombinant human PDGF-BB were purchased from Wako Pure Chemical (Osaka, Japan). NGFβ from mouse submaxillary glands was bought from Alomone Labs (Jerusalem, Israel). Recombinant human basic FGF was purchased from Acris Antibodies GmbH (Hiddenhausen, Germany), while recombinant human VEGF-165 was purchased from Becton Dickison (Bedford, MA, USA). Recombinant human TGFβ1 was purchased from R&D systems (Minneapolis, MN, USA).

4.2. Analysis of Protein-Protein Interaction with Surface Plasmon Resonance (SPR) Method

The interactions of a growth factor with either adiponectin or SPARC were examined using the BIAcore X instrument (GE healthcare, Tokyo, Japan) and the binding kinetics were analyzed with BIAevaluation software [42,43]. Briefly, full length adiponectin, globular adiponectin or SPARC (Sangi, Tokyo, Japan) as a ligand was immobilized onto the carboxymethylated dextran surface of the CM5 sensor chip, respectively. The relative responses for the immobilized full length and globular adiponectin and SPARC were 2025, 12707 and 3574 resonance units (RU), respectively, where 1000 RU is equivalent to 1ng of protein/mm^2. The surface of the adiponectin-chip or the SPARC-chip was perfused with HBS-EP buffer (10 mM HEPES, 150 mM NaCl and 0.005% Surfactant P20, pH 7.4) at 37 °C and then with increasing concentrations of a number of growth factors (as analytes) dissolved in buffer at a flow rate of 20 μL/min for 105 s. Following the addition of each analyte, dissociation was evaluated by passing the buffer alone over the chip for 120 s. If an analyte bound to a ligand, the surface showed a change in reflected light, which was directly proportional to the mass bound and measured in arbitrary RU. Based on the dissociation constant (kd) (s^{-1}) and association constant (Ka) (M^{-1}s^{-1})

obtained, the binding constant K_D (M) was calculated by dividing Kd by Ka. The regeneration of the surface of the sensor chip was performed by injecting 1 M NaCl at 20 µL/min for 90 s.

4.3. Assay of Biological Activity of NGF

Rat pheochromocytoma, PC12 cells were cultured in RPMI1640 medium (Wako) containing 10% fetal calf serum (FCS), 10% horse serum. To examine the effects of NGF on their morphological changes (neurite outgrowth and cell swelling), the cells (5×10^3 cells) were cultured on Type I-collagen-coated plates (Iwaki Techno Glass, Chiba, Japan) in RPMI1640 containing 1% FCS and 1% horse serum for 24 h and subsequently cultured with either NGFβ, adiponectin or both for 4 days. To quantify the morphological changes of PC12 cells, at least 100 randomly selected cells per experimental condition were photographed at the same scale under light transmission inverted photomicroscopy. The picture was analyzed using Adobe Photoshop and NIH Image J, a public-domain image processing and analysis program. Changes in cell body length were measured as a marker of cell swelling. Total neurite length measured and number of cells with neurite which length was longer than cell body length counted were used as an indicator of axonal elongation [44].

4.4. Expression of AdipoR1 and AdipoR2 in PC12 Cells and Their Silencing

Total RNA was isolated from PC12 cells and rat tissues by the guanidine-isothiocyanate method using ISOgen reagent (Takara, Tokyo, Japan) and RNA (2 µg) was used for reverse transcription. Rat AdipoR1 (GenBank accession number NM 207587), AdipoR2 (NM 001037979) and glyceraldehyde 3-phosphate dehydrogenase (GAPDH) (NM 017008) cDNA were amplified with the primer pairs as follow: AdipoR1 (201bp) Forward: 5′-TGC TTC AAG AGC ATC TTC CG-3′, Reverse: 5′-GAA TGA CAG TAG ACG GTG TG-3′ (annealing conditions 56 °C, 30 s, 29 cycles); AdipoR2 (206bp) Forward: 5′-TCT TCT TGG GAG CCA TTC TC-3′, Reverse: 5′-GCA CAC AGA TGA CAA TCA GG-3′ (56 °C, 30 s, 29 cycles); GAPDH (453 bp) Forward: 5′-ACC ACA GTC CAT GCC ATC AC-3′, Reverse: 5′-TCC ACC ACC CTG TTG CTG TA-3′ (62 °C, 30 s, 27 cycles).

Expression of AdipoR1 and AdipoR2 were suppressed by treating the cells with siRNA as essentially described by Fujioka et al [45]. In brief, siRNA specific for AdipoR1 and AdipoR2 and unrelated siRNA were transfected with Lipofectamine2000 (Invitrogen, Carlsbad, CA, USA) according to the instruction provided and cultured as described above.

4.5. MAP Kinase and AMP-Activated Protein Kinase Activation

PC12 cells were grown to 80% confluence in RPMI1640 containing 10% FCS and 10% horse serum and further cultured in RPMI1640 containing 1% FCS and 1% horse serum for 24 h. Subsequently the cells were treated with either vehicle, NGFβ, neurotrophin (NT)-3, NT-4 (Sigma-Aldrich, St. Louis, MO, USA), SPARC or adiponectin for 10 min. The cells were then lysed with the lysis buffer [50 mM Hepes (pH 7.5), 150 mM NaCl, 5 mM EDTA, 10 mM sodium pyrophosphate, 2 mM $NaVO_3$ containing protease inhibitor mixture (Complete; Boehringer Mannheim, GmbH, Germany) and 1% (*v/v*) Nonidet P40], centrifuged at 12,000× g for 15 min at 4 °C and the supernatant was saved at –70 °C.

Aliquot of the lysates (15 or 20 µg of protein) were separated by SDS-PAGE (10% gel) and transferred on PVDF membranes (Immobilon, Millipore, Bedford, MA, USA). The membranes were incubated first in a blocking buffer [20 mM Tris/HCl (pH 7.5), 150 mM NaCl] containing 0.1% Tween 20 and 5% (*v/v*) skimmed milk], then in the buffer containing anti-Erk1/2, anti-phosphorylated Erk1/2 (Thr202/Tyr204), anti-AMPKα or anti-phosphorylated AMPKα (Thr172) antibody (Cell Signaling Technology, Beverly, MA, USA) for 2 h. The bound antibody was detected with horseradish peroxidase-linked secondary antibodies (Zymed Laboratories, South San Francisco, CA, USA) and an enhanced chemiluminescence system (Millipore). The intensity of chemiluminescence for the corresponding proteins was analyzed by NIH Image J.

4.6. Statistical Analysis

Data were expressed as means ± standard errors of the mean (SEM) and analyzed by ANOVA followed by the Tukey-Kramer post-hoc test. A p value of less than 0.05 was considered statistically significant.

Supplementary Materials: Supplementary materials can be found at http://www.mdpi.com/1422-0067/20/7/1541/s1.

Author Contributions: Conceptualization, M.S. and K.K.; Methodology, A.K., Y.O.-O. and K.K.; Software, A.K. and Y.O.-O.; Validation, Y.O., T.I., H.S. and S.M.; Formal Analysis, Y.O., T.I., S.M. and K.K.; Investigation, Y.O., T.I., H.S. and S.M.; Resources, H.S., Y.O.-O. and K.K.; Data Curation, Y.O., T.I. and K.K.; Writing—Original Draft Preparation, Y.O., T.I.; Writing—Review & Editing, K.K.; Visualization, K.K.; Supervision, M.S. and K.K.; Project Administration, Y.O.-O. and K.K.; Funding Acquisition, K.K.

Funding: This work was supported by the Japan Society for the Promotion of Science (No. 16K08068).

Conflicts of Interest: The authors declare no conflict of interest.

Abbreviations

AMPK	AMP-activated protein kinase
ECM	extracellular matrix
ERK	extracellular signal regulated kinase
FCS	fetal calf serum
FGF	fibroblast growth factor
GAPDH	glyceraldehyde 3-phosphate dehydrogenase
MAPK	mitogen-activated protein kinase
NGF	nerve growth factor
NT	neurotrophin
PDGF	platelet-derived growth factor
RU	resonance unit
SPARC	secreted protein, acidic and rich in cysteine
SPR	surface plasmon resonance
TGF	transforming growth factor
TNF	tumor necrosis factor
VEGF	vascular endothelial growth factor

References

1. Matsuzawa, Y.; Funahashi, T.; Kihara, S.; Shimomura, I. Adiponectin and metabolic syndrome. *Arterioscler. Thromb. Vasc. Biol.* **2004**, *24*, 29–33. [CrossRef]
2. Oh, D.K.; Ciaraldi, T.; Henry, R.R. Adiponectin in health and disease. *Diabetes Obes. Metab.* **2007**, *9*, 282–289. [CrossRef] [PubMed]
3. Schäffler, A.; Buechler, C. CTRP family: Linking immunity to metabolism. *Trends Endocrinol. Metab.* **2012**, *23*, 194–204. [CrossRef]
4. Liu, M.; Liu, F. Regulation of adiponectin multimerization, signaling and function. *Best Pract. Res. Clin. Endocrinol. Metab.* **2014**, *28*, 25–31. [CrossRef]
5. Arita, Y.; Kihara, S.; Ouchi, N.; Takahashi, M.; Maeda, K.; Miyagawa, J.; Hotta, K.; Shimomura, I.; Nakamura, T.; Miyaoka, K.; et al. Paradoxical decrease of an adipose- specific protein, adiponectin, in obesity. *Biochem. Biophys. Res. Commun.* **1999**, *257*, 79–83. [CrossRef]
6. Kondo, H.; Shimomura, I.; Matsukawa, Y.; Kumada, M.; Takahashi, M.; Matsuda, M.; Ouchi, N.; Kihara, S.; Kawamoto, T.; Sumitsuji, S.; et al. Association of adiponectin mutation with type 2 diabetes: A candidate gene for the insulin resistance syndrome. *Diabetes* **2002**, *51*, 2325–2328. [CrossRef] [PubMed]
7. Orlandi, A.; Bochaton-Piallat, M.L.; Gabbiani, G.; Spagnoli, L.G. Aging, smooth muscle cells and vascular pathobiology: Implications for atherosclerosis. *Atherosclerosis* **2006**, *188*, 221–230. [CrossRef] [PubMed]

8. Arita, Y.; Kihara, S.; Ouchi, N.; Maeda, K.; Kuriyama, H.; Okamoto, Y.; Kumada, M.; Hotta, K.; Nishida, M.; Takahashi, M.; et al. Adipocyte-derived plasma protein adiponectin acts as a platelet-derived growth factor-BB–binding protein and regulates growth factor–induced common postreceptor signal in vascular smooth muscle cell. *Circulation* **2002**, *105*, 2893–2898. [CrossRef] [PubMed]

9. Wang, Y.; Lam, K.S.L.; Xu, J.U.; Lu, G.; Xu, L.Y.; Cooper, G.J.S.; Xu, A. Adiponectin inhibits cell proliferation by interacting with several growth factors in an oligomerization-dependent manner. *J. Biol. Chem.* **2005**, *280*, 18341–18347. [CrossRef]

10. Rivera, L.B.; Bradshaw, A.D.; Brekken, R.A. The regulatory function of SPARC in vascular biology. *Cell Mol. Life Sci.* **2011**, *68*, 3165–3173. [CrossRef]

11. Bradshaw, A.D. Diverse biological functions of the SPARC family of proteins. *Int. J. Biochem. Cell Biol.* **2012**, *44*, 480–488. [CrossRef] [PubMed]

12. Bradshaw, A.D.; Sage, E.H. SPARC, a matricellular protein that functions in cellular differentiation and tissue response to injury. *J. Clin. Invest.* **2001**, *107*, 1049–1054. [CrossRef] [PubMed]

13. Nagaraju, G.P.; Dontula, R.; El-Rayes, B.F.; Lakka, S.S. Molecular mechanisms underlying the divergent roles of SPARC in human carcinogenesis. *Carcinogenesis* **2014**, *35*, 967–973. [CrossRef] [PubMed]

14. Kos, K.; Wilding, J.P.H. SPRAC: A key player in the pathologies associated with obesity and diabetes. *Nat. Rev. Endocrinol.* **2010**, *6*, 225–235. [CrossRef] [PubMed]

15. Raines, E.W.; Lane, T.F.; Iruela-Arispe, M.L.; Ross, R.; Sage, E.H. The extracellular glycoprotein SPARC interacts with platelet-derived growth factor (PDGF)-AB and -BB and inhibits the binding of PDGF to its receptors. *Proc. Natl. Acad. Sci. USA* **1992**, *89*, 1281–1285. [CrossRef] [PubMed]

16. Motamed, K.; Blake, D.J.; Angello, J.C.; Allen, B.L.; Rapraeger, A.C.; Hauschka, S.D.; Sage, E.H. Fibroblast growth factor receptor-1 mediates the inhibition of endothelial cell proliferation and the promotion of skeletal myoblast differentiation by SPARC: A role for protein kinase A. *J. Cell. Biochem.* **2003**, *90*, 408–423. [CrossRef] [PubMed]

17. Jayakumar, A.R.; Apeksha, A.; Norenberg, M.D. Role of matricellular proteins in disorders of the central nervous system. *Neurochem. Res.* **2017**, *42*, 858–875. [CrossRef]

18. Gilmour, D.T.; Lyon, G.J.; Carlton, M.B.; Sanes, J.R.; Cunningham, J.M.; Anderson, J.R.; Hogan, B.L.; Evans, M.J.; Colledge, W.H. Mice deficient for the secreted glycoprotein SPARC/osteonectin/BM40 develop normally but show severe age-onset cataract formation and disruption of the lens. *EMBO J.* **1998**, *17*, 1860–1870. [CrossRef]

19. Kucukdereli, H.; Allen, N.J.; Lee, A.T.; Feng, A.; Ozlu, M.I.; Conatser, L.M.; Chakraborty, C.; Workman, G.; Weaver, M.; Sage, E.H.; et al. Control of excitatory CNS synaptogenesis by astrocyte-secreted proteins Hevin and SPARC. *Proc. Natl. Acad. Sci. USA* **2011**, *108*, E440–E449. [CrossRef] [PubMed]

20. López-Murcia, F.J.; Terni, B.; Llobet, A. SPARC triggers a cell-autonomous program of synapse elimination. *Proc. Natl. Acad. Sci. USA* **2015**, *112*, 13366–13371. [CrossRef]

21. Au, E.; Richter, M.W.; Vincent, A.J.; Tetzlaff, W.; Aebersold, R.; Sage, E.H.; Roskams, A.J. SPARC from olfactory ensheathing cells stimulates Schwann cells to promote neurite outgrowth and enhances spinal cord repair. *J. Neurosci.* **2007**, *27*, 7208–7221. [CrossRef]

22. Ma, C.H.; Palmer, A.; Taylor, J.S. Synergistic effects of osteonectin and NGF in promoting survival and neurite outgrowth of superior cervical ganglion neurons. *Brain Res.* **2009**, *1289*, 1–13. [PubMed]

23. Lorber, B.; Chew, D.J.; Hauck, S.M.; Chong, R.S.; Fawcett, J.W.; Martin, K.R. Retinal glia promote dorsal root ganglion axon regeneration. *PLoS ONE* **2015**, *10*, e0115996. [CrossRef]

24. Pepeu, G.; Grazia Giovannini, M. The fate of the brain cholinergic neurons in neurodegenerative diseases. *Brain Res.* **2017**, *1670*, 173–184. [CrossRef] [PubMed]

25. Peeraully, M.R.; Jenkins, J.R.; Trayhurn, P. NGF gene expression and secretion in white adipose tissue: Regulation in 3T3-L1 adipocytes by hormones and inflammatory cytokines. *Am. J. Physiol. Endocrinol. Metab.* **2004**, *287*, E331–E339. [CrossRef]

26. Bulló, M.; Peeraully, M.R.; Trayhurn, P.; Folch, J.; Salas-Salvadó, J. Circulating nerve growth factor levels in relation to obesity and the metabolic syndrome in women. *Eur. J. Endocrinol.* **2007**, *157*, 303–310. [CrossRef] [PubMed]

27. Atanassova, P.; Hrischev, P.; Orbetzova, M.; Nikolov, P.; Nikolova, J.; Georgieva, E. Expression of leptin, NGF and adiponectin in metabolic syndrome. *Folia Biol.* **2014**, *62*, 301–306. [CrossRef]

28. Skaper, S.D. Nerve growth factor: A neuroimmune crosstalk mediator for all seasons. *Immunology* **2017**, *151*, 1–15. [CrossRef]

29. Minnone, G.; De Benedetti, F.; Bracci-Laudiero, L. NGF and its receptors in the regulation of inflammatory response. *Int. J. Mol. Sci.* **2017**, *18*, 1028. [CrossRef]

30. Francki, A.; McClure, T.D.; Brekken, R.A.; Motamed, K.; Murri, C.; Wang, T.; Sage, E.H. SPARC regulates TGF-beta1-dependent signaling in primary glomerular mesangial cells. *J. Cell. Biochem.* **2004**, *91*, 915–925. [CrossRef] [PubMed]

31. Kupprion, C.; Motamed, K.; Sage, E.H. SPARC (BM-40, osteonectin) inhibits the mitogenic effect of vascular endothelial growth factor on microvascular endothelial cells. *J. Biol. Chem.* **1998**, *273*, 29635–29640. [CrossRef] [PubMed]

32. Meldolesi, J. Neurotrophin receptors in the pathogenesis, diagnosis and therapy of neurodegenerative diseases. *Pharmacol. Res.* **2017**, *121*, 129–137. [CrossRef] [PubMed]

33. Ravichandran, A.; Low, B.C. SmgGDS antagonizes BPGAP1-induced Ras/ERK activation and neuritogenesis in PC12 cell differentiation. *Mol. Biol. Cell.* **2013**, *24*, 145–156. [CrossRef] [PubMed]

34. Lombardi, L.; Persiconi, I.; Gallo, A.; Hoogenraad, C.C.; De Stefano, M.E. NGF-dependent axon growth and regeneration are altered in sympathetic neurons of dystrophic mdx mice. *Mol. Cell. Neurosci.* **2017**, *80*, 1–17. [CrossRef]

35. Albrecht, D.; López-Murcia, F.J.; Pérez-González, A.P.; Lichtner, G.; Solsona, C.; Llobet, A. SPARC prevents maturation of cholinergic presynaptic terminals. *Mol. Cell. Neurosci.* **2012**, *49*, 364–374. [CrossRef] [PubMed]

36. Waki, H.; Yamauchi, T.; Kamon, J.; Kita, S.; Ito, Y.; Hada, Y.; Uchida, S.; Tsuchida, A.; Takekawa, S.; Kadowaki, T. Generation of globular fragment of adiponectin by leukocyte elastase secreted by monocytic cell line THP-1. *Endocrinology* **2005**, *146*, 790–796. [CrossRef]

37. Kritas, S.K.; Saggini, A.; Cerulli, G.; Caraffa, A.; Antinolfi, P.; Pantalone, A.; Frydas, S.; Rosatt, M.; Tei, M.; Speziali, A.; et al. Neuropeptide NGF mediates neuro-immune response and inflammation through mast cell activation. *J. Biol. Regulators Homeostatic agents* **2014**, *28*, 177–181.

38. Żelechowska, P.; Agier, J.; Kozłowska, E.; Brzezińska-Błaszczyk, E. Mast cells participate in chronic low-grade inflammation within adipose tissue. *Obes. Rev.* **2018**, *19*, 686–697.

39. Demir, I.E.; Tieftrunk, E.; Schrn, S.; FriEss, H.; Ceyhan, G.O. Nerve growth factor & TrkA as novel therapeutic targets in cancer. *Biochim. Biophys. Acta* **2016**, *1866*, 37–50.

40. Aloe, L.; Rocco, M.L.; Balzamino, B.O.; Micera, A. Nerve growth factor: Role in growth, differentiation and controlling cancer cell development. *J. Exp. Clin. Cancer Res.* **2016**, *35*, 116. [CrossRef]

41. Denk, F.; Bennett, D.L.; McMahon, S.B. Nerve growth factor and pain mechanisms. *Annu. Rev. Neurosci.* **2017**, *40*, 307–325. [CrossRef] [PubMed]

42. O'Shannessy, D.J.; Brigham-Burke, M.; Soneson, K.K.; Hensley, P.; Brooks, I. Determination of rate and equilibrium binding constants for macromolecular interactions by surface plasmon resonance. *Methods Enzymol.* **1994**, *240*, 323–349.

43. Schuster, S.C.; Swanson, R.V.; Alex, L.A.; Bourret, R.B.; Simon, M.I. Assembly and function of a quaternary signal transduction complex monitored by surface plasmon resonance. *Nature* **1993**, *365*, 343–347. [CrossRef]

44. Komagome, R.; Shuto, B.; Moriishi, K.; Kimura, K.; Saito, M. Neuronal and glial differentiation of neuroblastoma and glioma cell lines by Rho inhibitory exoenzyme C3. *Neuropathology* **1999**, *19*, 288–293. [CrossRef]

45. Fujioka, D.; Kawabata, K.; Saito, Y.; Kobayashi, T.; Nakamura, T.; Kodama, Y.; Takano, H.; Obata, J.E.; Kitta, Y.; Umetani, K.; et al. Role of adiponectin receptors in endothelin-induced cellular hypertrophy in cultured cardiomyocytes and their expression in infarcted heart. *Am. J. Physiol. Heart Circul. Physiol.* **2006**, *290*, H2409–H2416. [CrossRef] [PubMed]

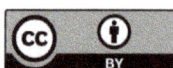

MDPI

St. Alban-Anlage 66

4052 Basel

Switzerland

Tel. +41 61 683 77 34

Fax +41 61 302 89 18

www.mdpi.com

International Journal of Molecular Sciences Editorial Office

E-mail: ijms@mdpi.com

www.mdpi.com/journal/ijms